Capsule Endoscopy by Case Study, 2nd Edition

Edited by Daniel L. Raines, MD

11333 Woodglen Drive, Suite 100
North Bethesda, MD 20852-3071
www.gi.org

2nd Edition

Edited by Daniel Raines, MD, FACG
Editorial Project Management by Claire Neumann, MA, CMPP
Editorial Staff: Neen LeMaster, MLIS and Angélica Bermúdez, MA
Design is updated from the 1st Edition based on template by Kristen Cherry, Cherry-Tree Designs, and Kristen Leotti, American College of Gastroenterology.
Cover design by Emily Garel

Educational Access
Video capsule studies can be accessed at www.gi.org/CECaseStudy_Videos
Password: Raines2025

Published by The American College of Gastroenterology

CAPSULE ENDOSCOPY BY CASE STUDY

Table of Contents

CASE-BASED CHAPTERS

Preface

Daniel L. Raines, MD, FACG

Project Background

Video capsule endoscopy (VCE) has captivated my attention since the beginning of my gastroenterology fellowship training. My early adoption of VCE technology in 2004 led me to integrate device-assisted enteroscopy (DAE) into my clinical practice. Through the advice and mentorship of established small bowel endoscopists, including Drs. Jonathan Leighton, Daniel Mishkin, and Oleh Haluszka, I became proficient in examination of the small bowel using DAE. These interests and skills have afforded me the privilege of providing subspecialty care to thousands of patients while contributing to the education of hundreds of physicians.

The First Edition of Capsule Endoscopy by Case Study was created through collaboration among leading small bowel experts in response to recognized variability in video capsule image interpretation, and new requirements for VCE training during gastroenterology fellowship. This body of work was developed as an educational resource supported and published by the American College of Gastroenterology in 2012. It has since become widely adopted as an educational resource for gastroenterology fellowship programs as well as practicing gastroenterologists.

This Second Edition presents a new collection of capsule endoscopy studies which reflect technological advancements, new indications, and current presentations for capsule endoscopy. By completing this course, readers will develop proficiency in interpreting video capsule studies and in recognizing the broad spectrum of small bowel pathology.

The preparation of this edition has created new opportunities to collaborate and learn with a distinguished group of small bowel experts, including senior colleagues, emerging leaders,

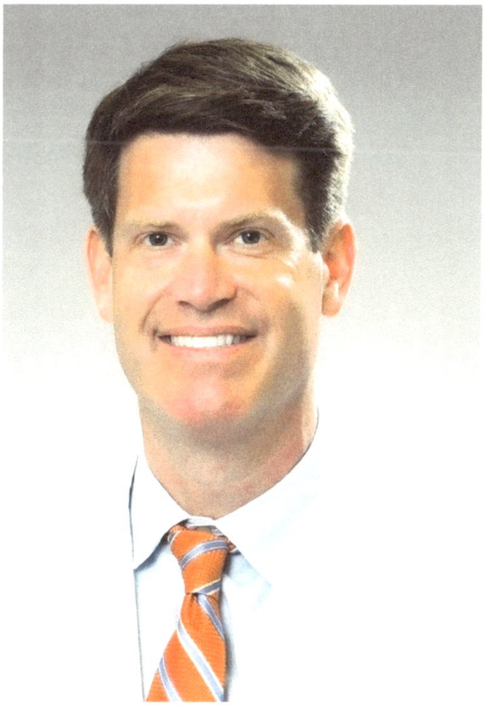

Editor, Daniel L. Raines, MD, FACG

and international contributors. Their collective expertise and commitment have greatly enriched this publication. It is with great satisfaction that we present the ACG's Second Edition of Capsule Endoscopy by Case Study as a resource for training in video capsule endoscopy and small bowel disease.

Instructions for Users

For trainees: Instruction in capsule endoscopy should start with review of the introductory chapters pertaining to indications, performance, and interpretation of VCE. Interpretation of the case study set should then be performed under the supervision of a faculty mentor. Each case is associated with a history combined with pertinent objective findings which should be read prior to interpretation of the capsule video. Read the complete capsule video with recording of first gastric image, first duodenal image, first cecal image, and any abnormalities. For early users, it is best to mark all frames which appear abnormal so that each of these can be reviewed with the supervising faculty. Your interpretation of the capsule video should be accompanied by a plan for management as future practice will require you to use your study observations, combined with patient information, to make recommendations for additional testing or treatment. It may be appropriate to request additional history, lab studies or imaging to make a final diagnosis. Your management may also include plans for device-assisted enteroscopy for additional evaluation or therapy. Once you have discussed your observations and management plan with a faculty supervisor, read the expert interpretation of the capsule video, subsequent post-capsule findings, and chapter which corresponds with each case. This process will provide exposure to a broad spectrum of small bowel pathologies which would require many years to encounter in routine practice.

For practicing clinicians: Use of the information included in this publication should be adapted to your specific needs and level of experience. Clinicians will little or no capsule experience, should consider following the above listed recommendations for trainees while using the expert interpretation in the post-capsule findings to oversee your reading. Gastroenterologists who have already received training in capsule endoscopy may elect to read only the remarkable images or segments noted in the post-capsule findings then review the associated small bowel disease chapters. Even experienced capsule readers will find value in this resource through review of case study examples and current medical knowledge relevant to each condition.

The ACG website maintains a password protected website to allow readers to download the video capsule study case set. The link is: www.gi.org/CECaseStudy_Videos and the password is Raines2025.

In order to read the capsule videos included in this publication, please download and install the Rapid Reader version 9.7 or higher from the Medtronic Website.

Pillcam Software V9.7 or higher
https://www.medtronic.com/covidien/en-gb/products/capsule-endoscopy/pillcam-software.html#

Contributors

Oscar Alvarez, MD
Honorary Professor, CES University (Medellin, Colombia), Texas Digestive Specialists, Harlingen, Texas

Jose Aponte-Pieras, MD
Assistant Professor, Department of Internal Medicine, University of Las Vegas, Las Vegas, Nevada

Nikki Arceneaux, MD
Department of Internal Medicine, LSU Health Sciences Center, New Orleans, Louisiana

Jodie A. Barkin, MD, FACG
Associate Professor of Clinical Medicine, University of Miami, Miller School of Medicine, Miami, Florida

Matthew G. Bell, MD
Mayo Clinic in Rochester, Minnesota

Pegah Carroll, MD
Associate Professor, Section of Gastroenterology, Department of Medicine, University of Mississippi Medical Center, Jackson, Mississippi

David R. Cave, MD, PhD, FACG
Brigham and Women's Hospital, Division of Gastroenterology, Hepatology and Endoscopy, Boston, Massachusetts

Abraham Z. Cheloff, MD, MS
NYU Langone Health, New York, New York

Autumn Collins, MD
Department of Internal Medicine, LSU Health Sciences Center, New Orleans, Louisiana

Yichun Fu, MD
Assistant Professor of Medicine, University of Chicago Medicine, Chicago, Illinois

Peter H.R. Green, MD, FACG
Department of Medicine, Celiac Disease Center, Columbia University, New York, New York

Seth A. Gross, MD, FACG
Division of Gastroenterology and Hepatology, New York University Langone Health System, New York, New York

Oleh Haluzska, MD
Clinical Professor of Medicine, Division of Gastroenterology and Hepatology, University of Arizona, Tucson, Arizona

David Hass, MD, FACG
Clinical Professor of Medicine, Yale University School of Medicine, Hamden, Connecticut

Erika Haviland, DO
Department of Internal Medicine, LSU Health Sciences Center, New Orleans, Louisiana

Catherine Hudson, MD
Assistant Professor of Clinical Medicine, Section of Gastroenterology, LSU Health Sciences Center, New Orleans, Louisiana

John J. Hutchings, MD, FACG
Professor of Clinical Medicine, Section of Gastroenterology, LSU Health Sciences Center, New Orleans, Louisiana

Michelle Kang Kim MD, PhD
Chair, Department of Gastroenterology, Hepatology, and Nutrition, Cleveland Clinic, Cleveland, Ohio

Martin Keuchel, MD
Agaplesion Bethesda Krankenhaus Bergedorf, Hamburg, Germany

Stephen Landreneau, MD, FACG
Professor of Clinical Medicine, Section of Gastroenterology, LSU Health Sciences Center, New Orleans, Louisiana

Suzanne K. Lewis, MD
Department of Medicine, Celiac Disease Center, Columbia University, New York, New York

Contributors

Nisha Loganantharaj, MD
Assistant Professor of Clinical Medicine, Section of Gastroenterology, LSU Health Sciences Center, New Orleans, Louisiana

Pablo Machado, MD
Uruguayan Association of Gastroenterology and Endoscopy (AUGE); Director of Small Bowel Committee, Interamerican Endoscopy Society (SIED); Montevideo, Uruguay

Brooke F. Mishkin
Division of Gastroenterology, Beth Israel Deaconess Medical Center, Harvard Medical School, Boston, Massachusetts

Daniel S. Mishkin, MD, CM, FRCP(C), FACG
Division of Gastroenterology, Beth Israel Deaconess Medical Center, Harvard Medical School, Boston, Massachusetts

Claire Neumann, MA, CMPP
Director, Scholarly Publications & Managing Editor, American College of Gastroenterology, North Bethesda, Maryland

Stephany Nguyen, MD
Department of Internal Medicine, LSU Health Sciences Center, New Orleans, Louisiana

Muna Okafor, MD
Case Western Reserve/UH Cleveland Medical Center, Cleveland, Ohio

Shirley Paski, MD
Department of Gastroenterology, Hepatology, and Human Nutrition, Cleveland Clinic, Cleveland, Ohio

Shabana F. Pasha, MD, FACG
Professor of Medicine, Medical Director, Division of Gastroenterology and Hepatology, Mayo Clinic, Phoenix, Arizona

Essam Quraishi, MD
Gastrointestinal and Liver Consultants, Santa Ana, California

Ryne Ramaker, MD
Department of Medicine, Duke University School of Medicine, Durham, North Carolina

Michael D. Rice, MD
Clinical Associate Professor of Internal Medicine, Division of Gastroenterology, University of Michigan Medical School, Ann Arbor, Michigan

Barry Rubin, MD
Assistant Professor of Clinical Medicine, Section of Gastroenterology, LSU Health Sciences Center, New Orleans, Louisiana

Felice Schnoll-Sussman, MD, FACG
Professor of Clinical Medicine, Division of Gastroenterology, Weill Cornell Medical College, New York

Carol E. Semrad, MD, FACG
Professor of Medicine, Division of Gastroenterology, University of Chicago, Chicago, Illinois

Reena Sidhu, MD
Honorary Professor, University of Sheffield; Consultant Gastroenterologist, Sheffield Teaching Hospitals NHS Trust, United Kingdom

Ryan Stidham, MD
Associate Professor, Department of Internal Medicine, University of Michigan Medical School, Ann Arbor, Michigan

F. Otis Stephen, MD, FACG
Director, Small Bowel Diseases and Nutrition Program, Cedars-Sinai Medical Center, Los Angeles, California

Jason Stibbe, MD
Fellowship Program Director, Section of Gastroenterology, LSU Health Sciences Center, New Orleans, Louisiana

Daniel Wild, MD, FACG
Professor of Medicine, Division of Gastroenterology, Duke University Medical Center, Durham, North Carolina

Charles Woodall, DO
Department of Internal Medicine, LSU Health Sciences Center, New Orleans, Louisiana

DEDICATION

To my remarkable wife, Heidi, who has given me more than I could have imagined and everything I truly need. And to our daughters, Marie, Cecilia, and Camille, the three most precious gifts in my life.

Special Thanks To

Dave Hass

and

The American College of Gastroenterology Editorial Staff

Project support provided by

American College of Gastroenterology

Chapter A: Small Bowel Video Capsule Endoscopy — Clinical Use, Applications, and Performance Protocols

Jodie A. Barkin, MD, FACG

Introduction

Video capsule endoscopy (VCE) is a cornerstone of the diagnostic toolbox for evaluation of small bowel diseases. This chapter will review the clinical use of small bowel VCE with focus on indications for VCE, use of VCE in special patient populations, bowel preparation in VCE, and key points to improve quality of VCE procedures.

Indications for VCE

Small bowel VCE is most commonly utilized in the evaluation of suspected small bowel bleeding (SSBB) and Crohn's disease. The American College of Gastroenterology (ACG) and American Society for Gastrointestinal Endoscopy (ASGE) jointly issued the first American guidelines on quality metrics in small bowel VCE in 2022.[1,2] Per the guidelines, high-yield indications for VCE include suspected SBB, iron deficiency anemia, known or suspected Crohn's disease, inherited polyposis syndromes, abnormal small bowel imaging, and complicated/refractory Celiac disease (**Table 1**). Non-standard indications such as abdominal pain, diarrhea, malabsorption, and iron-deficiency anemia without evidence of gastrointestinal (GI) bleeding typically have lower diagnostic yield.

Suspected Small Bowel Bleeding

SSBB is defined as gastrointestinal bleeding of undefined source after upper endoscopy and colonoscopy and was previously referred to as obscure gastrointestinal bleeding prior to 2015.[3] SSBB accounts for 5%-10% of cases of gastrointestinal bleeding.[4,5] The diagnostic yield of VCE in SSBB is affected by patient and procedural factors including hemoglobin < 10 g/dl, longer bleeding duration of over 6 months, multiple bleeding episodes, overt bleeding (60% vs 46% in occult bleeding), and timing of VCE within 2 weeks of a bleed.[6-9] VCE has the highest diagnostic yield in SSBB in those who undergo VCE within 48-72 hours of a bleeding episode.[10-12] Data from a subsequent meta-analysis confirmed that earlier VCE after SSBB episode is associated with increased odds of finding active bleeding, positive diagnosis, and enable therapeutic intervention.[13] In contrast, patients with negative VCE after a SSBB episode are significantly less likely to rebleed compared to those with positive VCE.[14]

VCE has been compared with other diagnostic modalities for evaluation of SSBB in multiple studies. A large meta-analysis of 14 studies demonstrated that VCE had higher diagnostic yield than push enteroscopy for clinically significant findings in SBB (56% vs 26%), with complete outperformance of VCE over small bowel series (diagnostic yield 42% vs 6%).[15] VCE was then compared to double balloon enteroscopy in a large meta-analysis of 17 studies of 1,477 bleeding lesions. Of these lesions, 58.5% were discovered by VCE, whereas only 41.5% were found by double balloon enteroscopy (DBE), with a 7% increased diagnostic yield if DBE was performed sequentially after VCE, which models real-world clinical practice where VCE may guide enteroscopy.[16] Based on this data, VCE is positioned as the primary study for evaluation of the small bowel in SSBB after negative upper endoscopy and colonoscopy, except in patients with ongoing unstable gastrointestinal bleeding with SSBB where an approach that is

High-Yield Indications for VCE	Non-Standard Indications for VCE
Suspected Small Bowel Bleeding (Previously obscure gastrointestinal bleeding)	Abdominal Pain
Iron Deficiency Anemia	Diarrhea
Crohn's Disease (Known or Suspected)	Malabsorption
Intestinal Polyposis Syndromes	Iron deficiency anemia without evidence of GI bleeding
Abnormal Small Bowel Imaging	
Complicated/Refractory Celiac Disease	

Table 1. Indications for VCE. Adapted from Leighton et al.[1]

both diagnostic and therapeutic such as DBE or angiography is preferred.[3,17]

Small Bowel Crohn's Disease

VCE has 3 key functions in patients with known or suspected small bowel Crohn's disease: diagnosis, staging, and surveillance — including assessing disease activity, response to therapy, or recurrence postoperatively. In those with a suspected diagnosis of Crohn's disease, a meta-analysis by Choi et al found that VCE had comparable diagnostic yield to CT enterography (CTE) and magnetic resonance enterography (MRE), with superior yield compared to small bowel follow-through and enteroclysis.[18] A prior meta-analysis showed VCE was superior to small bowel radiography, CTE and ileocolonoscopy in diagnosis of patients with suspected Crohn's disease.[19] VCE may be considered as complementary to MRE in Crohn's disease diagnosis with VCE identifying small bowel mucosal lesions that may not be visible on MRE, whereas MRE may detect transmural inflammation and potential extraluminal complications.[20] These subtleties and small mucosal lesions may be missed on MRE in the absence of significant or transmural inflammation and may also be missed on ileocolonoscopy secondary to distribution of disease.[21] In contrast, for those with VCE with no evidence of Crohn's disease, there is high negative predictive value to VCE, with less than 3% of patients being diagnosed with Crohn's disease on long-term prospective follow up data.[22]

In patients with established Crohn's disease, VCE demonstrates comparable or superior performance to other modalities in assessing disease activity. One meta-analysis noted that VCE discovered significantly more terminal ileal lesions than ileocolonoscopy, while another meta-analysis demonstrated that VCE was similar to MRE and superior to small bowel radiography, push enteroscopy and CTE.[18,19] A prospective multi-center study of 74 patients with Crohn's disease compared VCE to ileocolonoscopy for disease activity surveillance, with high correlation of VCE and ileocolonoscopy disease activity scoring indices over time, proving feasibility of VCE as a valid Crohn's disease monitoring tool.[23] Unfortunately, endoscopic scores from neither VCE nor ileocolonoscopy correlated with clinical parameters. In addition to monitoring disease activity, VCE may have a role in predicting Crohn's disease flares with better short and long-term predictive values than even stool markers such as fecal calprotectin that only predicted short-term flares.[24] Importantly, in those with known or suspected small bowel Crohn's disease and especially in those with any potential obstructive symptoms, there is a substantially increased risk of VCE retention that merits careful preprocedural conversation and evaluation with the patient, which will be further discussed in a subsequent section.

Celiac Disease

VCE in celiac disease (CeD) may serve both diagnostic and monitoring functions for disease surveillance. VCE has been studied for use as a diagnostic modality for celiac disease. A large meta-analysis of 22 studies and 46 abstracts of 1,585 patients demonstrated an approximately 60% effect size using VCE to identify pathology consistent with CeD diagnosis.[25] In terms of specific performance characteristics of VCE for CeD diagnosis, VCE has a sensitivity of 70%-100%, specificity of 60%-100%, positive predictive value of 96%-100%, and negative predictive value of 71%-93%, but these studies are limited in that there is high pre-test probability secondary to positive serologies.[26-30] This led the European Society of Gastrointestinal Endoscopy in 2015 to recommend against VCE use for initial first-line CeD diagnosis, except in patients unable or unwilling to undergo esophagogastroduodenoscopy or in those whom the diagnosis is equivocal.[31] VCE also has a role in assessing celiac disease activity, refractory celiac disease, and complications such as lymphoma. A comprehensive review of 20 studies of 1,337 patients with VCE performed for a variety of indications including positive CeD serologies, suspected or known refractory CeD, or persistent symptoms, found 243 of the 1,337 patients had refractory CeD, 32 had ulcerative jejunoileitis, 18 had T-cell lymphoma, and 1 had a small bowel tumor.[32] Moreover, the application of machine learning algorithms to better assess VCE images for CeD activity is a continually emerging field of substantial interest with promising data to date.[33] While the absolute yield may be variable, patients with suspected CeD unable to undergo an endoscopy and patients with known CeD with concern for refractory CeD or associated complications are very reasonable candidates for VCE.

Intestinal Polyposis Syndromes

VCE has a screening and surveillance role to detect

small bowel polyps in those with inherited intestinal polyposis syndromes, such as those with familial adenomatous polyposis (FAP) or Peutz-Jeghers syndrome (PJS), and is recommended by the ASGE 2020 guidelines.[34] VCE is the preferred imaging modality for detection of small bowel polyps over prior contrast studies such as small bowel follow through or enteroclysis, primarily due to high false-negative rates of up to 42% for lesions of >10 mm in size in small bowel follow through or enteroclysis.[35,36] Further, VCE has a higher sensitivity than MRE for detecting smaller polyps and similar test performance in detection of lesions > 15 mm in size, but MRE has the benefit of improved lesion localization given its cross-sectional nature.[37] Given limitations in ampullary visualization, VCE should not be substituted for side-viewing duodenoscopy or forward-viewing endoscopy with a clear cap for ampullary surveillance in FAP.[34]

Abnormal Small Bowel Imaging

VCE is a reasonable modality to assess abnormal findings discovered on other types of small bowel imaging. This practice dates back to even the initial studies of the efficacy of VCE. For example, VCE was initially evaluated in patients with small bowel follow through with barium-based studies with improved diagnostic abilities.[38] While there is limited additional or newer data after the initial decade of VCE's entry into the diagnostic algorithm of small bowel disorders, abnormal small bowel imaging remains considered as a high-yield indication for VCE.[1,2] Of importance, one must take caution if there is concern for a small bowel obstructing tumor prior to performance of VCE, with appropriate pre-procedure surgical evaluation and discussion with the patient.

Contraindications and Special Situations

There are both absolute and relative contraindications to VCE. The absolute contraindications include a known small bowel stenosis without surgery planned, known perforation, either known or suspected intestinal obstruction in a patient who refuses surgical intervention or is not a surgical candidate.[1,2] The goal of evaluation in these patients is to prevent VCE retention, which remains the most significant potential complication and will be further discussed in the section below. There are multiple special scenarios and potential relative contraindications to VCE.

Implanted cardiac devices (pacemakers, defibrillators, left-ventricular assist devices)

Presence of implantable cardiac devices was initially thought to be an absolute contraindication to VCE due to potential for interference between VCE signaling and the cardiac device. Now after over 2 decades of clinical practice, this contraindication is indeed theoretical only. There is no interference with the functioning of the cardiac device from the VCE, and there are only a small number of cases of interference due to left-ventricular assist devices with VCE image acquisition. It is thought to be safe to perform VCE in these populations per multiple society guidelines from the United States and Europe, albeit that there is not clear U.S. Food and Drug Administration (FDA) approval for the manufacturers in these populations due to lack of extensive in vivo studies for the devices in these populations, which would not be feasible.[1,2,39,40]

Dysphagia

Oral VCE ingestion is relatively contraindicated in the presence of swallowing difficulties or gastric motility disorders. Patients with oropharyngeal dysphagia may have aspiration, and there may be capsule retention in patients with esophageal dysphagia, Zenker's diverticulum, or impaired gastric emptying. This also applies in patients with swallowing difficulties due to altered mental status. In these situations, endoscopic deployment may be considered (**Figure 1**).

Pregnancy

VCE use in pregnancy is contraindicated due to theoretical harm to the fetus, which has not been confirmed nor established in vivo. However, given

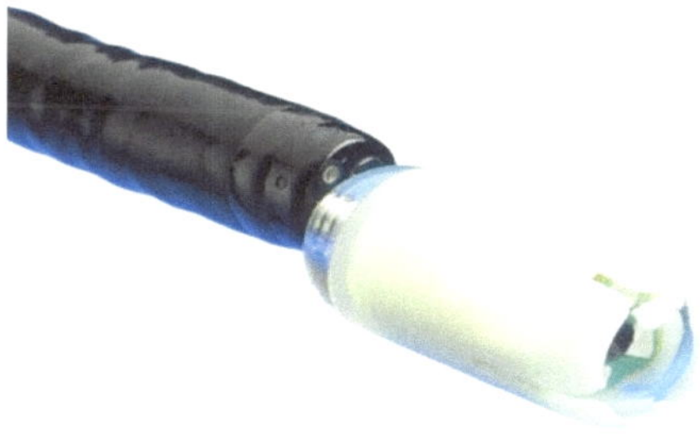

Figure 1. The endoscopic delivery system uses a catheter passed through the working channel of the endoscope with a holster connected at the tip protruding through the end of the endoscope. The capsule device is placed in the holster and then can be advanced and deployed into the stomach or small bowel.

lack of safety data, it is recommended to delay VCE until after delivery if possible. Further, if endoscopic or surgical interventions are required primarily for VCE device retrieval, this may increase fetal risk. The use of VCE in pregnancy should therefore be considered on an individualized basis.

Magnetic Resonance Imaging (MRI)

Due to metallic VCE components, if there is concern for potential VCE retention, passage of the VCE device should be confirmed either visually or via x-ray prior to undergoing MRI, though limited data suggests this may be more of a theoretical than actual concern.[1,2,41,42]

Capsule Endoscopy Equipment

Video capsule endoscopy requires minimal resource allocation from a systems perspective and can be performed in an office/clinic-based setting, outpatient endoscopy unit, or for inpatients. There are multiple different commercially available VCE systems.[40,42] Most VCE studies are primarily performed with administration of a swallowed or endoscopically deployed capsule device that wirelessly transmits images to an external receiver worn by the patient, which captures the images (**Figure 2**). These capsule devices primarily have a forward-facing camera that captures images, similar to a standard endoscopic view. The receiver is then returned and connected to a local computer workstation for image download and video creation to be able to be interpreted by the provider. In the case of inpatient VCE studies, one may be able to view a small image in real-time on the receiver or on a paired tablet device depending on the device manufacturer. One specific VCE device (CapsoCam Plus® SV-3; CapsoVision, Inc, Saratoga, CA) has lateral-facing cameras and no external receiver. The images are stored internally, and the device is passed in the stool and then collected and mailed to a central processing site for image download and video creation for interpretation via the cloud. Other capsule systems also provide cloud-based reading as an option. One of the most recent VCE device technology advancements introduced a single-use disposable receiver belt which allows patients to extend their recording time at home and then either return physically to the provider or return via mail, with additional cloud-based options (**Figure 3**).

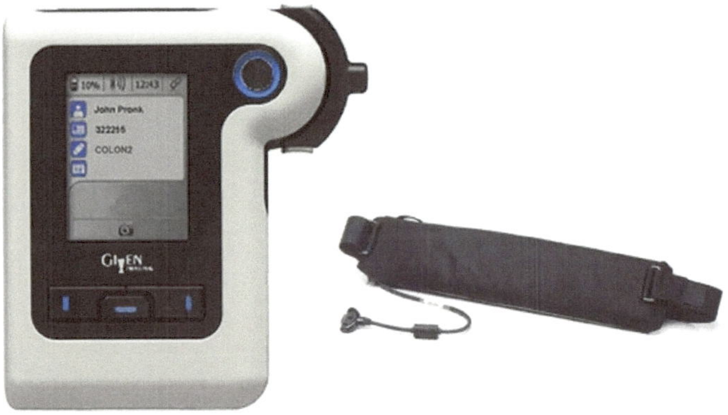

Figure 2. VCE sensor belt and video recorder. The belt sits across the abdomen and does not use adhesive pads. The recorder is connected to the belt via a cable.

Procedure Standards and Recommendations

Informed consent should be obtained as part of the VCE procedure as would be the case in any other endoscopic procedure.[1,2,40] This includes discussion of risks, benefits, and alternatives with the patient, including but not limited to capsule retention, and any specific situations or conditions unique to the patient. Patients are recommended to fast for 8 to 12 hours prior to VCE to allow for gastric and small bowel emptying to facilitate small bowel mucosal visualization. After ingestion or deployment, patients are generally allowed to have clear liquids at 2 hours post, a light snack at 4 hours post, and resume full oral intake at 8 hours post, provided there are otherwise no contraindications. Additional medication adjustments may be needed in patients undergoing VCE with endoscopic deployment due to restrictions and requirements of endoscopy with sedation. Periprocedural anticoagulation and antiplatelet agent management is unique in VCE. In swallowed VCE, especially in those with concern for bleed,

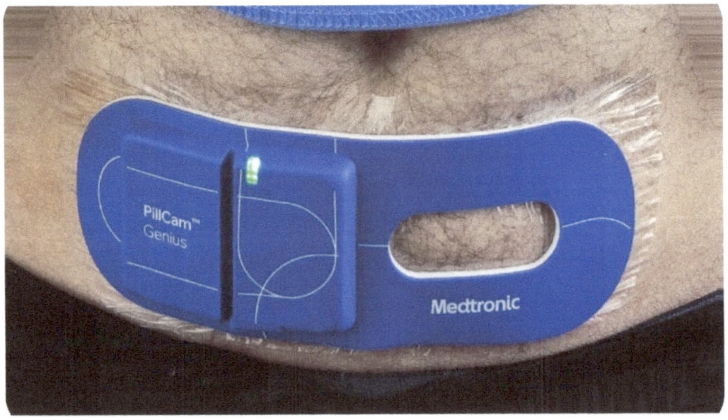

Figure 3. PillCam™ Genius SB link device is applied directly to the lower abdomen with adhesive pads as a single use VCE receiver device.

provided there is not a contraindication to continued anticoagulant/antiplatelet therapy, it may be of benefit to continue these medications to closely reflect daily conditions for the patient during VCE evaluation and potentially improve VCE yield. In the setting of endoscopic deployment, these medications may need to be held depending on endoscopy periprocedural requirements.

Improving Mucosal Visualization

The overall adequacy of a VCE study is defined by adequate bowel preparation to enable mucosal visualization, a complete study with VCE device traversing the entirety of the small bowel during the video period, and a small bowel transit time of at least 2 hours. The overall quality of the bowel preparation affects mucosal visualization, which theoretically impacts diagnostic yield. If the bowel is filled with food debris, bubbles, or viscous fluid, then mucosal visualization may be impacted. There are 2 general categories of agents that have been studied to affect mucosal visualization including purgative bowel preparation agents and agents to decrease bubbles, such as simethicone.

Bowel preparation for VCE has been evaluated with a variety of different purgative agents, but polyethylene glycol (PEG) solution has been studied most extensively. In a meta-analysis of 12 randomized controlled trials of 2,072 patients, 2 or 4 liters of PEG solution had improved mucosal visualization compared to 1 liter of PEG or no preparation; however, there were no differences found in diagnostic yield or completion rate.[43] In a separate meta-analysis of 40 studies of 4,380 patients with laxatives agents and 2,185 patients without laxatives, those with laxative bowel preparation had improved mucosal visualization, with a number needed to treat of 14, but again had no change in overall diagnostic yield with use of laxative agents.[44] This theoretical disconnect of improved mucosal visualization without change in overall diagnostic yield has led to guideline statements that have been equivocal even dating back to the 2009 European Society of Gastrointestinal Endoscopy guidelines.[45] Similarly, despite over 10 years of additional data, in the more recent joint American guidelines, this level of ambiguity led to bowel preparation remaining a research question needing further study, with some institutions using simply an overnight fast and other considering use of a 2-liter PEG purgative regimen.[1,2] There may be a benefit to the use of simethicone to improve mucosal visualization by decreasing intraluminal bubbles. The largest and most recent meta-analysis of 10 studies (8 randomized controlled trials, 1 prospective trial, and 1 retrospective trial) of 843 total patients evaluating use of simethicone, found that simethicone decreased bubbles and improved small bowel mucosal visualization, but similarly to laxative agents did not affect diagnostic yield or completion rate.[46] Use of simethicone as with purgative laxative agents remained a research question in the 2022 ACG/ASGE guidelines, though many institutions may use this benign and low-risk medication prior to VCE ingestion in practice.[1,2]

Maximizing Completion Rate

There are 3 general categories of factors that have been investigated to attempt to affect study completeness: prokinetic agents, endoscopic deployment, and increased battery length of the VCE device itself. It is estimated that approximately 16%-20% of VCE studies will be incomplete with capsule remaining in small bowel at end of video recording, despite only an average of 1%-2% of patients with eventual true capsule retention.[47-49] The use of prokinetic agents to promote gastric emptying of the VCE device and improve small bowel motility with the goal of increasing study completeness is theoretically attractive. Trials of metoclopramide and erythromycin have yielded heterogeneous results at best regarding perhaps improved completion rates.[50-52] Given lack of substantial data to support their use, prokinetic agents were not recommended to be routinely administered in patients undergoing VCE.[1,2]

Endoscopic deployment should be considered in those at increased risk of incomplete studies including bedbound patients, inpatients with limited mobility, those with delayed gastric emptying, and those with concern for or history of prior incomplete VCE study.[1,2,42] Increased battery life of the VCE device has also been explored with original VCE devices having 8 hours of battery life and newer versions having 12 or more hours of battery life. Two large studies compared the traditional 8-hour to the longer 12-hour VCE device. The first study with 200 patients in each group demonstrated a significantly increased completion rate in the 12-hour battery device (88% vs 79.5%; $P = 0.03$). A similar study of

408 total patients found a higher completion again with the 12-hour device (93.2% vs 88.2%, odds ratio 1.78; $P = 0.111$). Interestingly, neither study found difference in diagnostic yield despite increased rates of completion.[53,54] In the newest updated VCE device on the market (PillCam™ Genius SB Capsule Endoscopy Kit; Medtronic Inc, Minneapolis, MN; Given Imaging, Yoqneam, Israel), the 12-hour battery life has been integrated as a standard feature, whereas prior iterations had the option for an 8-hour or a 12-hour version.

Video Capsule Retention

Capsule retention is the primary complication of VCE, with an overall prevalence for all VCE indications of 1.4%-2.5%, and higher in known Crohn's disease (4.6%).[48,55,56] It is defined as the capsule remaining in the small bowel for 14 days or more. Patients planned for VCE should undergo screening for risks for VCE retention. These risks include Crohn's disease specifically if history of small bowel stricturing disease, chronic high-dose use of nonsteroidal anti-inflammatory medications (NSAIDs), known small bowel stricture or mass, history of small bowel obstruction or resection, symptoms of small bowel obstruction, or prior abdominal/pelvic radiation therapy.[40,48,55] A prior history of radiation therapy is particularly important as symptoms of chronic radiation enteritis, such as small bowel bleeding or chronic diarrhea, may be considered as indications for VCE. However, the risk of capsule retention in this population is high while capsule retrieval from irradiated bowel may be challenging.

In patients at risk for VCE retention, evaluation prior to VCE should be performed with a dissolvable patency capsule or CTE/MRE to reduce risk of capsule retention.[1,2] Small bowel follow through exams and traditional CT with oral and IV contrast are not sufficient to assess risk of retention.[57] Retention is still possible, even with a negative patency capsule or CTE/MRE, albeit at a minimal rate. A meta-analysis of 5 studies involving 203 patients estimated a 97% sensitivity and 83% specificity for the patency capsule, with other studies showing similar performance between patency capsule and CTE/MRE.[58,59] In the presence of positive patency capsule or CTE/MRE, one should not perform VCE unless it is to guide surgical removal or surgery is on standby if obstruction occurs.

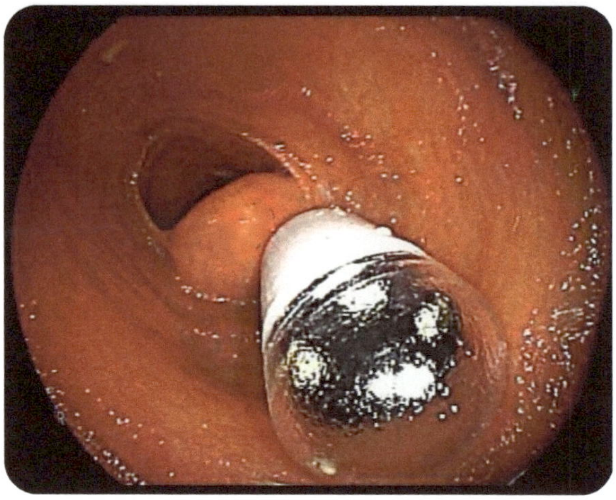

Figure 4. Video capsule retention aids in localization of a malignant tumor.

Recommendations for management of capsule retention are based on the presence (or absence) of symptoms.[40,47] Video capsule retention should not be considered as an indication for emergency surgery unless there is evidence of small bowel obstruction. Although retention is technically a complication of VCE, it can be useful in certain cases to localize malignant tumors or other pathology requiring surgery (**Figure 4**). In cases of symptomatic retention or a high suspicion for malignancy, endoscopic retrieval via enteroscopy or surgical intervention is recommended. In patients with asymptomatic retention, a watch and wait approach with repeat abdominal x-ray is reasonable along with any indicated disease specific medical therapies, as approximately 50% of retained VCE will eventually pass spontaneously in these situations.[40,47,60] Endoscopic or surgical interventions should be contemplated only after careful consideration of the likely etiology of retention and the risks of retrieval.

Conclusion

Video capsule endoscopy is an essential tool for visualization of the small bowel lumen and plays a key role in the diagnosis and management of small bowel diseases. Use of VCE for high-yield indications, with appropriate timing, pre-procedural evaluation and preparation, is key to the overall diagnostic yield. The utility and performance of VCE will continue to improve over time through a combination of technological advancements, procedure optimization, and applications which support study interpretation.

References

1. Leighton JA, Brock AS, Semrad CE, et al. Quality Indicators for Capsule Endoscopy and Deep Enteroscopy. Am J Gastroenterol. 2022;117(11):1780-1796.
2. Leighton JA, Brock AS, Semrad CE, et al. Quality Indicators for Capsule Endoscopy and Deep Enteroscopy. Gastrointest Endosc. 2022;96(5):693-711.
3. Gerson LB, Fidler JL, Cave DR, et al. ACG Clinical Guideline: diagnosis and management of small bowel bleeding. Am J Gastroenterol. 2015;110(9):1265-1287.
4. Lau WY, Fan ST, Wong SH, et al. Preoperative and intraoperative localisation of gastrointestinal bleeding of obscure origin. Gut. 1987;28:869–877.
5. Longstreth GF. Epidemiology and outcome of patients hospitalized with acute lower gastrointestinal hemorrhage: a population-based study. Am J Gastroenterol. 1997;92:419–424.
6. Bresci G, Parisi G, Bertoni M, et al. The role of video capsule endoscopy for evaluating obscure gastrointestinal bleeding: usefulness of early use. J Gastroenterol. 2005;40:256–259.
7. Carey EJ, Leighton JA, Heigh RI, et al. A single-center experience of 260 consecutive patients undergoing capsule endoscopy for obscure gastrointestinal bleeding. Am J Gastroenterol 2007;102:89–95.
8. May A, Nachbar L, Ell C. Double-balloon enteroscopy (push-and-pull enteroscopy) of the small bowel: feasibility and diagnostic and therapeutic yield in patients with suspected small bowel disease. Gastrointest Endosc. 2005;62:62–70.
9. Mishkin DS, Chuttani R, Croffie J, et al. ASGE Technology Status Evaluation Report: wireless capsule endoscopy. Gastrointest Endosc. 2006;63:539–545.
10. Goenka MK, Majumder S, Kumar S et al. Single center experience of capsule endoscopy in patients with obscure gastrointestinal bleeding. World J Gastroenterol. 2011;17:774–778.
11. Singh A, Marshall C, Chaudhuri B, et al. Timing of video capsule endoscopy relative to overt obscure GI bleeding: implications from a retrospective study. Gastrointest Endosc. 2013;77:761–766.
12. Yamada A, Watabe H, Kobayashi Y, et al. Timing of capsule endoscopy influences the diagnosis and outcome in obscure-overt gastrointestinal bleeding. Hepatogastroenterology. 2012;59(115):676–679.
13. Estevinho MM, Pinho R, Fernandes C, et al. Diagnostic and therapeutic yields of early capsule endoscopy and device-assisted enteroscopy in the setting of overt GI bleeding: a systematic review with meta-analysis. Gastrointest Endosc. 2022;95(4):610-625.
14. Ribeiro I, Pinho R, Rodrigues A, et al. What is the long-term outcome of a negative capsule endoscopy in patients with obscure gastrointestinal bleeding? Rev Esp Enferm Dig. 2015;107(12):753-8.
15. Triester SL, Leighton JA, Leontiadis GI, et al. A meta-analysis of the yield of capsule endoscopy compared to other diagnostic modalities in patients with obscure gastrointestinal bleeding. Am J Gastroenterol 2005;100:2407–2418.
16. Brito HP, Ribeiro IB, de Moura DTH, et al. Video capsule endoscopy vs double-balloon enteroscopy in the diagnosis of small bowel bleeding: A systematic review and meta-analysis. World J Gastrointest Endosc. 2018;10(12):400-421.
17. ASGE Standards of Practice Committee; Gurudu SR, Bruining DH, et al. The role of endoscopy in the management of suspected small-bowel bleeding. Gastrointest Endosc. 2017;85(1):22-31.
18. Choi M, Lim S, Choi MG, et al. Effectiveness of Capsule Endoscopy Compared with Other Diagnostic Modalities in Patients with Small Bowel Crohn's Disease: A Meta-Analysis. Gut Liver. 2017;11:62–72.
19. Dionisio PM, Gurudu SR, Leighton JA, et al. Capsule endoscopy has a significantly higher diagnostic yield in patients with suspected and established small-bowel Crohn's disease: a meta-analysis. Am J Gastroenterol. 2010;105:1240–1248.
20. Albert JG, Martiny F, Krummenerl A, et al. Diagnosis of small bowel Crohn's disease: a prospective comparison of capsule endoscopy with magnetic resonance imaging and fluoroscopic enteroclysis. Gut. 2005;54:1721–1727.
21. McCurdy JD, Weng R, Parlow S, et al. Video Capsule Endoscopy can Identify Occult Luminal Crohn's Disease in Patients with Isolated Perianal Fistulas. J Crohns Colitis. 2023;17(10):1624-1630.
22. Hall B, Holleran G, Costigan D, et al. Capsule endoscopy: High negative predictive value in the long term despite a low diagnostic yield in patients with suspected Crohn's disease. United European Gastroenterol J. 2013;1(6):461-466.
23. Melmed GY, Dubinsky MC, Rubin DT, et al. Utility of video capsule endoscopy for longitudinal monitoring of Crohn's disease activity in the small bowel: a prospective study. Gastrointest Endosc. 2018 Dec;88(6):947-955.e2.
24. Ben-Horin S, Lahat A, Amitai MM, et al. Assessment of small bowel mucosal healing by video capsule endoscopy for the prediction of short-term and long-term risk of Crohn's disease flare: a prospective cohort study. Lancet Gastroenterol Hepatol. 2019;4(7):519-528.
25. Shapiro M, Niv Y. Diagnostic yield of video capsule endoscopy (VCE) in Celiac Disease (CD): A systematic review and meta-analysis. J Clin Gastroenterol. 2025;59(7):598-606.
26. Murray JA, Rubio-Tapia A, van Dyke CT et al. Mucosal atrophy in celiac disease: extent of involvement,

correlation with clinical presentation, and response to treatment. Clin Gastroenterol Hepatol. 2008;6:186-193.
27. Petroniene R, Dubcenco E, Baker JP, et al. Given capsule endoscopy in celiac disease: evaluation of diagnostic accuracy and interobserver agreement. Am J Gastroenterol. 2005;100:685-694.
28. Hopper AD, Sidhu R, Hurlstone DP, et al. Capsule endoscopy: an alternative to duodenal biopsy for the recognition of villous atrophy in coeliac disease? Dig Liver Dis. 2007;39:140-145.
29. Lidums I, Cummins AG, Teo E. The role of capsule endoscopy in suspected celiac disease patients with positive celiac serology. Dig Dis Sci. 2011;56:499-505.
30. Rondonotti E, Spada C, Cave D, et al. Video capsule enteroscopy in the diagnosis of celiac disease: a multicenter study. Am J Gastroenterol. 2007;102:1624-1631.
31. Pennazio M, Spada C, Eliakim R, et al. Small-bowel capsule endoscopy and device-assisted enteroscopy for diagnosis and treatment of small-bowel disorders: European Society of Gastrointestinal Endoscopy (ESGE) Clinical Guideline. Endoscopy. 2015;47(4):352-376.
32. Rossi RE, Poletti V, Masoni B, et al. The role of videocapsule endoscopy in the diagnosis and follow-up of celiac disease: a scoping review. Expert Rev Gastroenterol Hepatol. 2024;18(10):673-679.
33. Chetcuti Zammit S, McAlindon ME, Greenblatt E, et al. Quantification of Celiac disease severity using video capsule endoscopy: A comparison of human experts and machine learning algorithms. Curr Med Imaging. 2023;19(12):1455-1662.
34. Yang J, Gurudu SR, Koptiuch C, et al. American Society for gastrointestinal endoscopy guideline on the role of endoscopy in familial adenomatous polyposis syndromes. Gastrointest Endosc. 2020;91:963–82.
35. Plum N, May A, Manner H, et al. Small bowel diagnosis in patients with familial adenomatous polyposis: comparison of push enteroscopy, capsule endoscopy, ileoscopy, and enteroclysis. Z Gastroenterol. 2009;47:339-346.
36. Mata A, Llach J, Castells A, et al. A prospective trial comparing wireless capsule endoscopy and barium contrast series for small-bowel surveillance in hereditary GI polyposis syndromes. Gastrointest Endosc. 2005;61:721-725.
37. Caspari R, von Falkenhausen M, Krautmacher C, et al. Comparison of capsule endoscopy and magnetic resonance imaging for the detection of polyps of the small intestine in patients with familial adenomatous polyposis or with Peutz-Jeghers' syndrome. Endoscopy. 2004; 36:1054-1059.
38. Costamanga C, Shah SK, Riccioni ME, et al. A prospective trial comparing small bowel radiographs and video capsule endoscopy for suspected small bowel disease. Gastroenterology. 2002;123(4):999-1005.
39. Enns RA, Hookey L, Armstrong D, et al. Clinical practice guidelines for the use of video capsule endoscopy. Gastroenterology. 2017;152:497-514.
40. Rondonotti E, Spada C, Adler S, et al. Small-bowel capsule endoscopy and device-assisted enteroscopy for diagnosis and treatment of small bowel disorders: European society of gastrointestinal endoscopy (ESGE) technical review. Endoscopy. 2018;50:423-46.
41. Bandorski D, Kurniawan N, Baltes P, et al. Contraindications for video capsule endoscopy. World J Gastroenterol. 2016;22:9898–908.
42. Barkin JA, Barkin JS. Video capsule endoscopy: Technology, reading, and troubleshooting. Gastrointest Endosc Clin N Am. 2017;27:15–27.
43. Yang L, Wang X, Gan T, et al. Polyethylene Glycol for Small Bowel Capsule Endoscopy. Gastroenterol Res Pract. 2017;2017:7468728.
44. Yung DE, Rondonotti E, Sykes C, et al. Systematic review and meta-analysis: is bowel preparation still necessary in small bowel capsule endoscopy? Expert Rev Gastroenterol Hepatol. 2017;11(10):979-993.
45. Ladas SD, Triantafyllou K, Spada C, et al. European Society of Gastrointestinal Endoscopy (ESGE): Recommendations (2009) on clinical use of video capsule endoscopy to investigate small bowel esophageal and colonic diseases. Endoscopy. 2010;42(3):220-227.
46. Chen S, Guo L, Zhong L, et al. Preparation of small bowel capsule endoscopy (SBCE) with simethicone: A meta-analysis. Clin Res Hepatol Gastroenterol. 2022;46(10):102029.
47. Spada C, McNamara D, Despott EJ, et al. Performance measures for small-bowel endoscopy: a European Society of Gastrointestinal Endoscopy (ESGE) Quality Improvement Initiative. Endoscopy. 2019;51(6):574-598.
48. Liao Z, Gao R, Xu C, et al. Indications and detection, completion, and retention rates of small-bowel capsule endoscopy: a systematic review. Gastrointest Endosc. 2010;71:280-286.
49. Hoog CM, Bark LA, Arkani J, et al. Capsule retentions and incomplete capsule endoscopy examinations: an analysis of 2300 examinations. Gastroenterol Res Pract. 2012;2012:518718.
50. Selby W. Complete small bowel transit in patients undergoing capsule endoscopy: determining factors and improvement with metoclopramide. Gastrointest Endosc. 2005. 61(1):80-85.
51. Almeida N, Figueiredo P, Freire P, et al. The effect of metoclopramide in capsule enteroscopy. Dig Dis Sci. 2010;55(1):153-157.
52. Caddy GR, Moran L, Chong AKH, et al. The effect of

erythromycin on video capsule endoscopy intestinal transit time. Gastrointest Endosc. 2006;63(2):262-266.
53. Rahman M, Akerman S, DeVito B, et al. Comparison of the diagnostic yield and outcomes between standard 8 h capsule endoscopy and the new 12 h capsule endoscopy for investigating small bowel pathology. World J Gastroenterol. 2015;21(18):5542-7.
54. Ou G, Shahidi N, Galorport C, et al. Effect of longer battery life on small bowel capsule endoscopy. World J Gastroenterol. 2015;21(9):2677-82.
55. Rezapour M, Amadi C, Gerson LB. Retention associated with video capsule endoscopy: Systematic review and meta-analysis. Gastrointest Endosc 2017;85(6):1157-1168.
56. Pasha SF, Pennazio M, Rondonotti E, et al. Capsule retention in Crohn's disease: A meta-analysis. Inflamm Bowel Dis. 2020;26(1):33-42.
57. Hosoe N, Takabayashi K, Ogata H, et al. Capsule endoscopy for small-intestinal disorders: current status. Dig Endosc. 2019;31(5):498-507.
58. Yadav A, Heigh RI, Hara AK, et al. Performance of the patency capsule compared with nonenteroclysis radiologic examinations in patients with known or suspected intestinal strictures. Gastrointest Endosc. 2011;74(4):834-9.
59. Zhang W, Han ZL, Cheng Y, et al. Value of the patency capsule in pre-evaluation for capsule endoscopy in cases of intestinal obstruction. J Dig Dis. 2014;15(7):345-51.
60. Rondonotti E, Soncini M, Girelli C, et al. Small bowel capsule endoscopy in clinical practice: a multicenter 7-year survey. Eur J Gastroenterol Hepatol. 2010;22(11):1380-6.

Chapter B: Interpretation of Video Capsule Endoscopy

Blair Lewis, MD, FACG and Daniel Raines, MD FACG

Introduction

Video capsule endoscopy (VCE) was introduced to physicians across the world at the turn of the millennium as an aid to visualize the small bowel. Over 2 decades of experience has demonstrated that proficiency in standard endoscopy does not equate to competency in capsule endoscopy. Effective video capsule interpretation requires both efficiency and familiarity with small bowel pathology. Yet a skilled endoscopist must do more than simply distinguish normal from abnormal findings: the interpreter must synthesize thousands of images to formulate a diagnostic impression then provide management recommendations appropriate for the individual case. Capsule endoscopy can do this only with the best of reading which requires skills not easily acquired.

Video Capsule Review

The original PillCam™ SB (Given Imaging, Yoqneam, Israel) recorded images at a fixed rate of 2 frames per second, producing 57,600 images over 8 hours. Early studies reported mean review times of 50–120 minutes per case.[1,2] A multicenter trial later confirmed an average review time of 50 minutes, with considerable variability depending on study complexity.[3] Evolution of PillCam™ technology has since led to both improved image capture and a reduction in total frames presented for interpretation. The current PillCam™ SB3 system incorporates adaptive frame rate technology to capture 6 images per second during rapid transit, while integrated software reduces image volume by eliminating duplicate frames. Together, these advancements enable more detailed evaluation of the proximal small bowel while reducing the total number of images by 40%.

Interpretation of only small bowel images typically requires ~10 minutes per hour of small bowel transit. Considering that small bowel transit averages between 2 and 4 hours, reading times for small bowel images alone range from 17 to 42 minutes.[3,4] Considerably longer interpretation times (45–120 minutes) are commonly cited in discussions contrasting manual interpretation with artificial intelligence (AI)-assisted review. It is important to recognize that the perception of time required for study interpretation may vary with circumstance. Studies read during off-duty hours or at the end of the workday may feel disproportionately burdensome, contributing to the impression that interpretation requires an excessive amount of time.

VCE study interpretation time is strongly influenced by indication and findings. Studies performed for suspected small bowel bleeding are more time-consuming, as the reader is often searching for angioectasias that may appear on only 1 or 2 frames. Studies indicated for Crohn's disease are typically faster as the main objective is to determine the presence or absence of gross ulceration. Exams with grossly abnormal findings, such as obvious intraluminal blood, can be read quickly. Normal studies usually take the longest, as the reader must carefully confirm that every frame is free of pathology.

Because VCE study review involves prolonged interpretation of tens of thousands of images, reader vigilance directly affects accuracy and reading time. Human performance studies demonstrate that attention declines after about 50 minutes of continuous visual tasks.[5] For this reason, capsule reading is best performed in sessions of less than an hour, with

Strategy	Rationale
Schedule a 30-minute appointment for each capsule study interpretation	A protected time block ensures unhurried interpretation, similar to a scheduled colonoscopy or new patient visit.
Read in a comfortable, quiet room	Dim lighting and minimal interruptions promote concentration and reduce fatigue.
Prioritize the small bowel segment, allocating ~10 minutes of reading time per hour in the small bowel	The small bowel segment is the most clinically relevant portion of the study.
Modify focus and attention based on indication and likely abnormalities	Example: Studies indicated for Crohn's disease typically require identification or exclusion of gross ulceration.
Avoid extended continuous reading (>50 minutes)	Prolonged sessions increase fatigue and risk of error.
Use mild stimulants (ex: caffeine or carbohydrate drinks)	May improve sustained attention during interpretation.

Table 1. Strategies for success in reading video capsule studies.

breaks between segments. Reading efficiency and accuracy are optimized when the environment is comfortable, with dim lighting, ergonomic seating, and minimal distractions. Mild stimulants such as caffeine or carbohydrate intake may also improve sustained attention.[6,7] A summary of strategies for reading capsule endoscopy review can be found in **Table 1.**

Reading Software

Studies stored locally are accessed via Rapid Reader Study Manager. For centralized databases, studies are accessed through PillCam™ Cloud Reader procedures menu (**Figure 1**). Once a study has been selected, evaluation of images begins with navigating the colored segments of the Progress Bar. First, confirm that the capsule reached the colon, then locate the ileocecal valve and thumb-nail the first cecal image. After returning to the first image, gastric and small bowel emptying times are determined. Using single view mode at 25 frames/sec, the esophagogastric junction and first gastric image are marked, and the first duodenal image is identified. If the capsule refluxes back into the stomach, the final entry into the duodenum should be used as the first duodenal image landmark.

Designation of anatomic landmarks enables the Top 100 feature, which highlight images most likely to show pathology (**Figure 2**). Manual review then

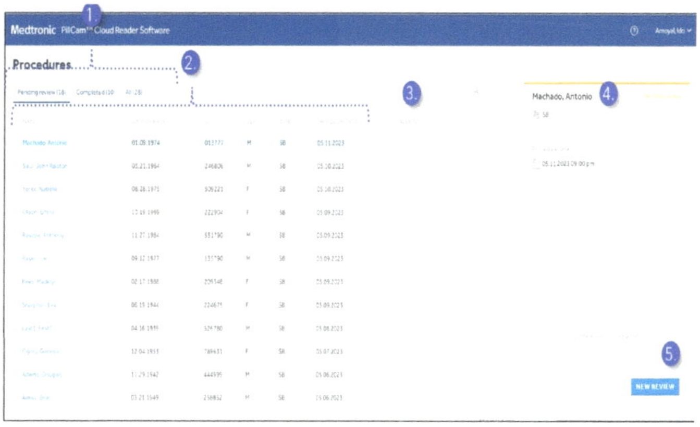

Figure 1. Pillcam™ Cloud Reader procedures menu including numbers of studies completed vs pending review (1), listing of studies uploaded (2), alerts (3), current study selected (4) and prompt for study interpretation (5).

proceeds at 7–8 frames/sec in full-screen mode, ideally with a mouse to aid navigation. If selected, the Dynamic Player Control can be found to the right of the viewing frame and used to advance or backtrack through images. Reading frame rate should be reduced in the proximal small bowel where transit may be swift and angioectasias are prevalent. Frame rate can be increased to up to 10-20 fps when viewing segments of distal small bowel where capsule transit slows. Basic steps for VCE study interpretation are listed in **Table 2**.

Rapid Reader™ includes accessory modes to single view (Dual View, Quad View, Mosaic View) that can

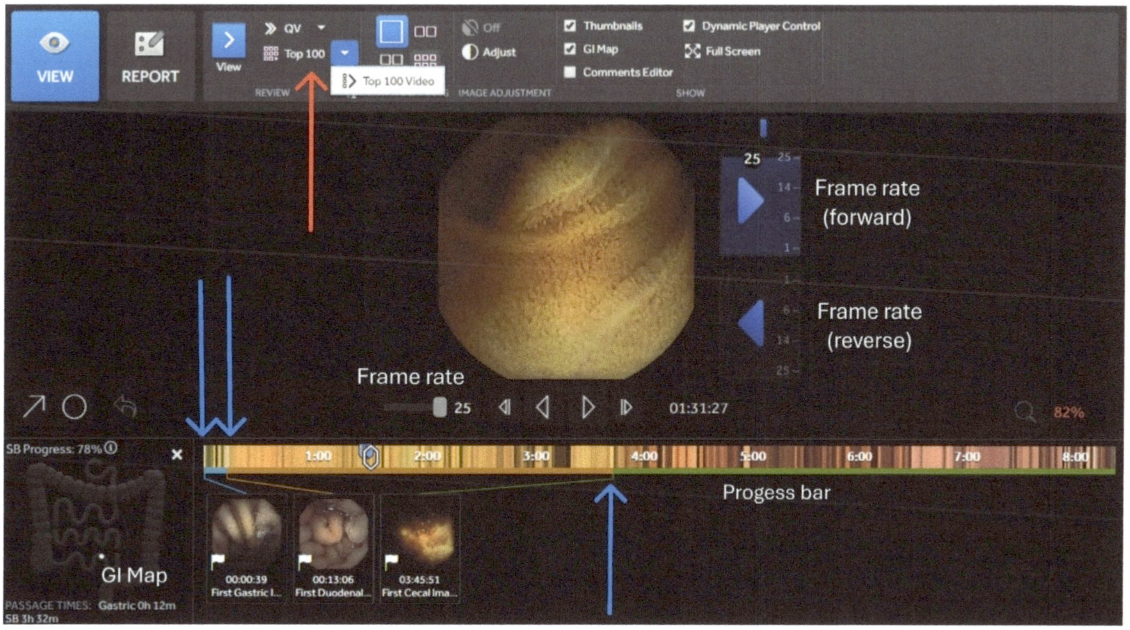

Figure 2. Rapid Reader™ (v9.7) single view mode with anatomic landmarks identified along the progress bar (blue arrows). The Top 100 feature is enabled after designation of a first duodenal and first cecal image (red arrow). Reading frame rate may be adjusted using the controls below the reading frame or the Dynamic Player Control located on the right. The GI Map sits in the bottom left corner, if selected, to provide estimation of capsule transit.

accelerate overview without flooding the reader with frame changes.QuickView can provide computer-aided triage of abnormal frames, while image adjustment tools (brightness/contrast, Blue Mode, and FICE) may improve lesion conspicuity in select cases.[8,9,10]

Table 2. Steps for Video Capsule Endoscopy Interpretation.

1	Review the clinical history relevant to the study
2	Confirm that the capsule reaches the colon, then mark the first cecal image
3	Identify and mark the first gastric image and the first duodenal image
4	Use the Top 100 feature to preview the small bowel segment for potential pathology
5	Apply the QuickView feature to screen the gastric and colonic images
6	For manual review of small bowel images, expand to Full Screen and read in single view mode at an initial frame rate of 7–8 frames/sec
7	Increase the frame rate to 10–20 frames/sec as capsule transit slows in the distal bowel
8	Create thumbnails for any abnormal or indeterminate images for later reinspection

Normal Variants & Non-pathologic Lesions

Readers of VCE studies must exclude or diagnose pathology based upon visual features. This requires experience in recognizing normal findings, including normal variants. Readers must also accurately characterize non-pathologic lesions. Examples of non-pathologic findings commonly encountered by VCE include lymphangiectasias, phlebectasias, lymphoid hyperplasia, and normal structures which mimic pathology.

Lymphangiectasias are dilated lymphatic vessels found in the lamina propria and submucosa. On VCE, lymphatic structures which accumulate chylomicrons stand out as bright white/yellow lesions which reflect light. Although their terminology has not been standardized, lymphangiectasias may be classified as microcystic or macrocystic.[11,12] Microcystic lymphangiectasias appear as focal clusters of tiny, superficial white dots. Macrocystic lymphangiectasias, also called chylous cysts or xanthomas, are larger, submucosal lesions which typically appear flat and well-circumscribed (**Figure 3a, b**).[13,14]

In the duodenum, lymphatic vessels involved in

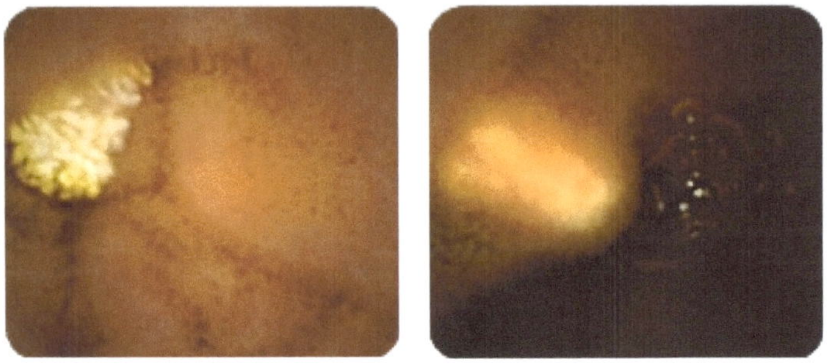

Figure 3. Microcystic lymphangiectasia (a) and macrocystic lymphangiectasia (b).

physiologic absorption of fat appear as white-tipped villi in "snow-dotted" mucosal pattern (**Figure 4**). This common VCE finding is considered as a normal variant. However, isolated, white-tipped villi in deep small bowel may indicate localized impairment of lymphatic drainage and should be considered as a feature suggestive of pathology.

Phlebectasias, or venous lakes, are dilated submucosal veins of the small bowel that appear on VCE as round or oval lesion with a bluish hue (**Figure 5**). Unlike angioectasias, which are fragile and prone to bleeding, phlebectasias are stable and rarely cause clinical symptoms. Lack of recognition of these lesions may lead to mischaracterization as possible small bowel varices or other vascular pathology.[11,14]
Lymphoid hyperplasia, particularly when prominent in the terminal ileum, may create the impression of premalignant polyps or even follicular lymphoma (**Figure 6**). Capsule retention in the proximal duodenum can also lead to misinterpretation of normal structures as if they were located deeper in the small bowel. The capsule may remain for minutes to hours at the junction of the duodenal bulb and descending duodenum, where repeated visualization of the ampulla confused for a polyp while Brunner gland hyperplasia may be misread as malignancy.

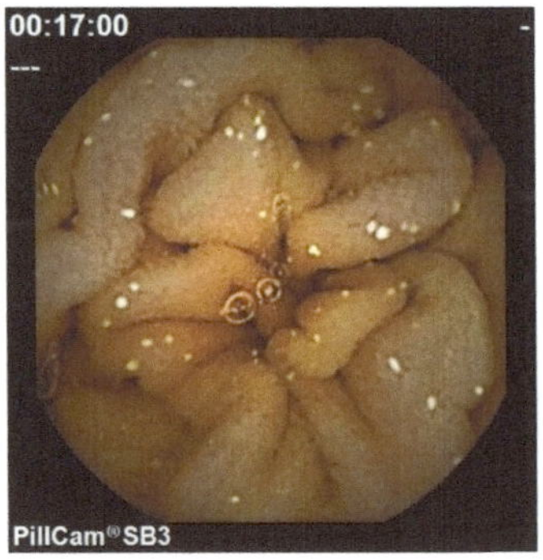

Figure 4. White tipped villi in the duodenum.

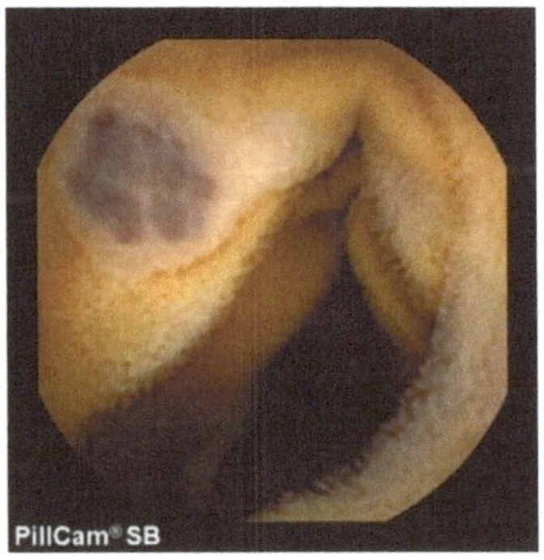

Figure 5. Venous lake (phlebectasia).

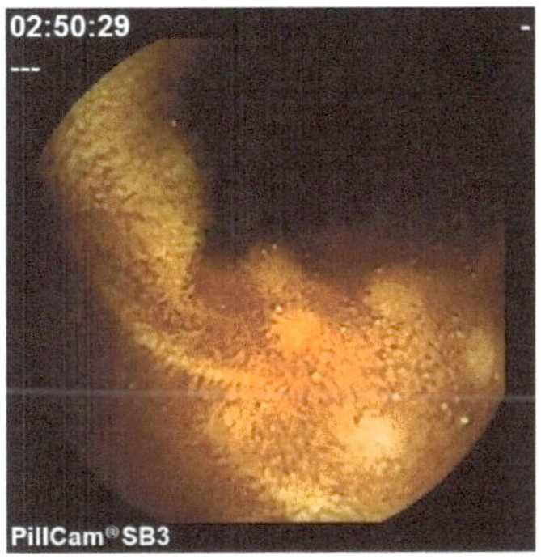

Figure 6. Lymphoid hyperplasia in the terminal ileum.

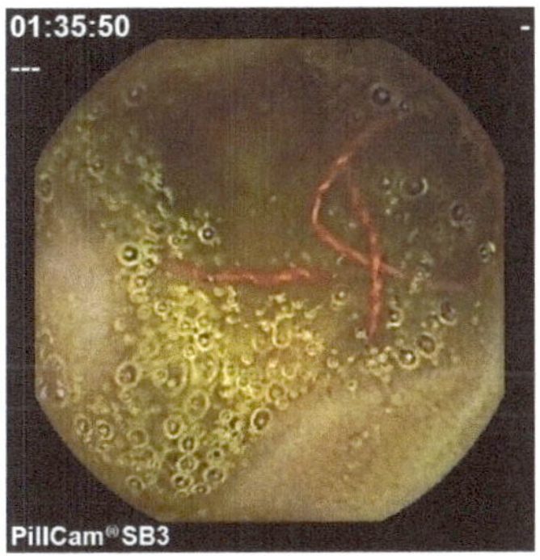

Figure 7. Synthetic textile fiber in the lumen which may appear as a segmented worm.

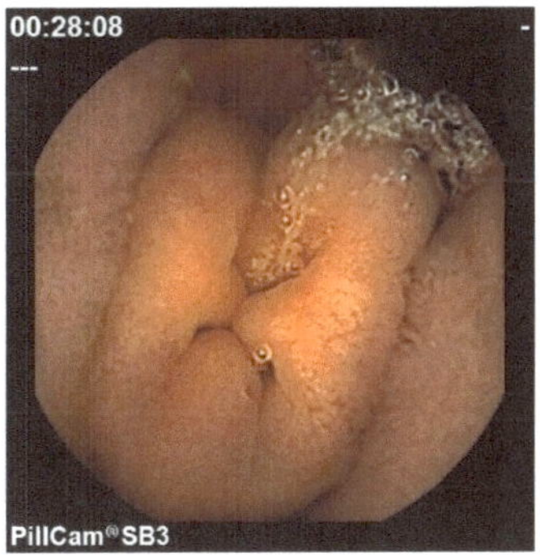

Figure 8. Retrograde view of the pylorus.

Retrograde views of the pylorus may give an impression of stenosis within the deep small bowel. Finally, food residue or other luminal contents can create pseudopathology that mimics true pathology such as tumors, blood, or parasites (**Figure 7**).

Capsule retention in the proximal duodenum can result in misinterpretation of normal structures as if they were located deeper in the small bowel (**Figure 8**).

Identifying Pathology

To identify pathology, evaluate any suspected abnormality in the context of the surrounding mucosa as well as images both proximal and distal to the finding. Ideally, pathologic findings will appear on more than one frame. If there is uncertainty about a particular frame, mark it for later review with fresh eyes. Rapid Reader contains an atlas of small bowel

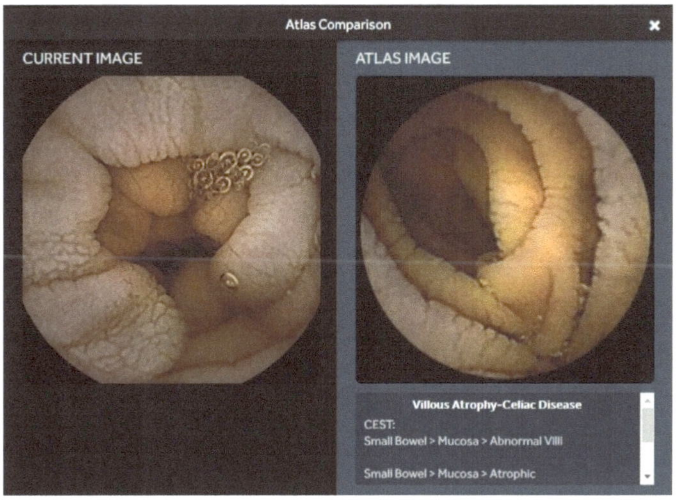

Figure 9. Rapid Atlas allows readers to compare individual study frames with a collection of frames demonstrating small bowel pathology and non-pathologic findings.

findings which can be used as a reference as well as for comparison with individual thumbnails saved during capsule study review (**Figure 9**).

Angioectasias are flat or slightly raised red lesions with irregular borders and radiating capillaries. They are often seen in only 1 or 2 frames and are most prevalent in the duodenum, proximal jejunum, and distal ileum. Since readers are often focused on identifying angioectasias, there is a tendency to overcall these lesions during capsule review. Common findings that may be misinterpreted as angioectasias include tiny red spots that are too small to characterize and prominent submucosal vessels (**Figure 10**).

Submucosal tumors must be differentiated from benign budges created by compression of the small bowel lumen by an adjacent segment of bowel. The easiest way to identify a benign bulge is to review the frames before and after the bulge to determine if it appears and disappears with peristalsis. Features indicative of submucosal small bowel tumors include bleeding, ulceration, abnormal mucosal architecture, central umbilication or cleft, and/or interruption of folds (**Figure 11**). The presence of white-tipped villi overlying a bulge is also indicative of underlying pathology.

Small bowel ulceration is observed in a variety of settings and requires clinical context to determine its etiology and significance. Idiopathic aphthous ulcers are encountered in the deep small bowel in approximately 10% of normal controls (**Figure 12**).

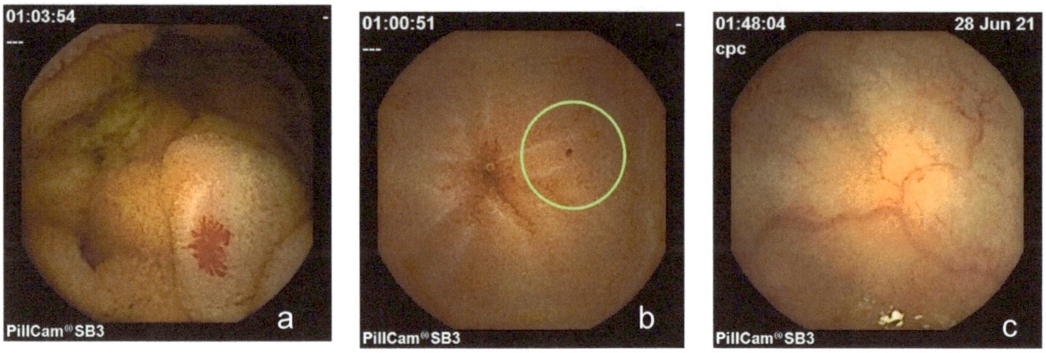

Figure 10. Angioectasias and their imposters: True angioectasias are bright red in appearance with a "fern-like" appearance (a). Tiny (1mm) red mucosal spots (b) and prominent submucosal vessels (c) are not sufficient for a diagnosis of angioectasia.

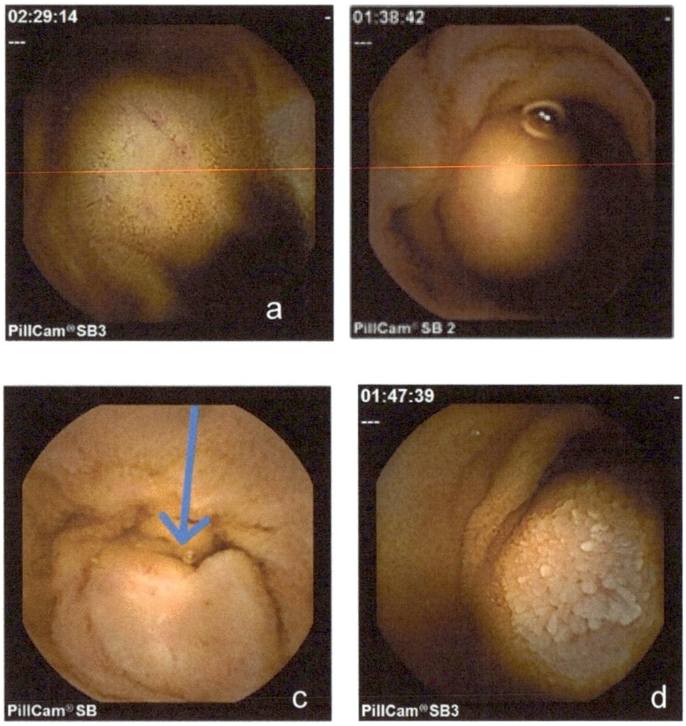

Figure 11. Identifying small bowel tumors: Benign mucosal bulges (a) may be differentiated from small bowel tumors by specific findings such as flat or "stretched' mucosa (b), central cleft (c), or overlying mucosa which differs in appearance relative to adjacent mucosa (d).

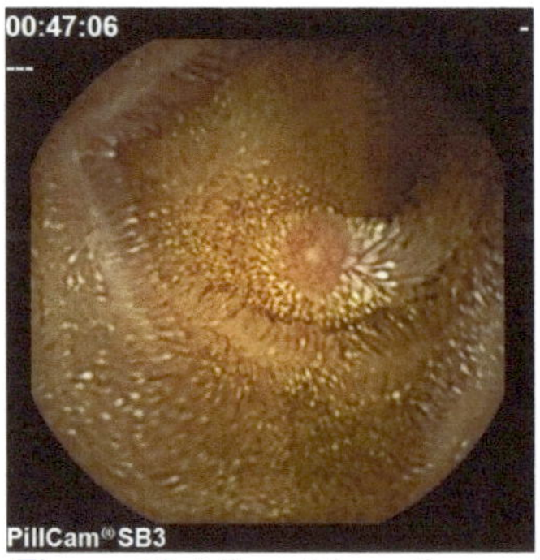

Figure 12. Idiopathic apthous ulcer.

One or a few small aphthae are typically incidental and should not be presumed to explain presentations with iron deficiency anemia or chronic diarrhea. Solitary ulcers are observed with multiple focal pathologies such as malignant tumors (primary or metastatic), ischemic injury, anastomotic ulceration, and opportunistic infection.

When multifocal or larger ulcers are present, the leading causes are Crohn's disease (CD) and Nonsteroidal anti-inflammatory drug (NSAID) enteropathy. Small bowel involvement occurs in 40%–70% of CD cases, with isolated small bowel disease present in up to 30%,[15,16] NSAID enteropathy can appear similarly and is prevalent in NSAID users. Ulcers and erosions have been shown to develop in 55% of patients after 14 days of naproxen and in up to 71% of chronic NSAID users.[17] Severe diaphragm disease is characterized by circumferential, rim-shaped ulcers with associated stenosis[18] **(Figure 13)**.

The Lewis score helps differentiate CD from NSAID injury by quantifying ulcer number, size, distribution, and villous edema across 3 time-based tertiles; stenoses are scored separately. The final score is the worst tertile plus the stenosis score: <135 normal/ clinically insignificant; 135–790 mild inflammation; >790 moderate–severe inflammation consistent with CD[19,20] (**Table 2; Figure 14**).

Prostaglandin-associated enteropathy is a very rare cause of multifocal small bowel ulceration with stricture formation. This spectrum of disorders includes chronic stenosing enteritis (CSE), cryptogenic multifocal ulcerative stenosing enteritis, and chronic nonspecific stenosing ulcers. The diaphragm-like lesions in CSE are broader than those typically seen with NSAID-related diaphragms. Multifocal ulceration may also be encountered in small bowel lymphoma and in multifocal neuroendocrine tumors.[21]

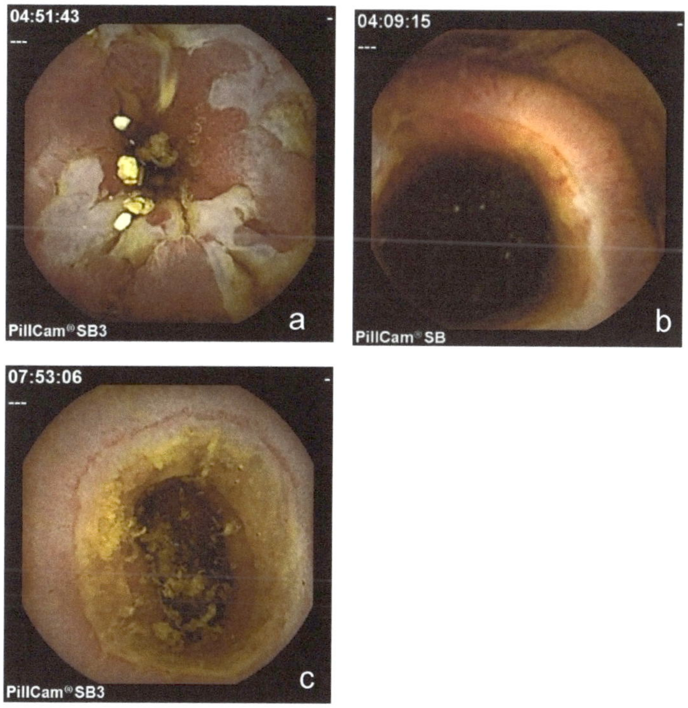

Figure 13. Ulcerated small bowel strictures: Crohn's disease of the small bowel is often complicated by stenotic lesions with deep, irregular ulceration (a). NSAID injury may result in either scattered ulcers in the proximal SB or thin, diaphragm stenoses of the ileum associated with superficial ulceration (b). Diaphragm-like stenoses with thick (>3mm) bands of ulceration are also observed in rare cases of prostaglandin deficiency, such as CSE (c).

Reporting

Interpretation is incomplete without effective reporting. RAPID™ software enables the generation of structured reports documenting study indications, preparation quality, transit times, and findings (**Figure 15**). Reports should include a clinical impression and recommendations for management.[22,23,24] Thumbnails can be attached to highlight key lesions, and the use of standardized terminology ensures clarity and facilitates comparison across institutions.[25]

Images saved in reporting mode can be exported as single JPEG files or as AVI clips containing sequential frames before and after the saved image. For backup or sharing, complete studies can be saved in a separate folder and stored on an external drive or transferred over the internet. PillCam™ Cloud provides secure, HIPAA-compliant upload and remote reading of capsule studies, supporting regional networks, second-reader review, and multidisciplinary case sharing. Cloud-based workflows improve efficiency and ensure that capsule expertise can be delivered even in settings without on-site readers.[26,27]

Ulcer	Number	Size	Distribution in Tertile
	None = 0	≤10% (small) = 8	<25% = 9
	Single = 3	11%-50% (moderate) = 12	25%-50% = 12
	2-7 = 5	>50% (large) = 15	>50% = 18
	≥8 = 10		
Villi	**Presence of Edema**	**Extent of Edema**	**Distribution of Edema**
	None = 0	<10% = 8	Single = 1
	Edema = 1	11-50% = 12	Patchy = 14
		>50% = 20	Diffuse = 17
Stenosis	**Number**	**Presence of Ulcer in the Stenosis**	**Did Capsule Traverse Stenosis?**
	None = 0	None = 2	Yes = 7
	Single = 14	Present = 24	No = 10
	Multiple = 20		

Table 2. Lewis Score - Incorporated into Pillcam™ Rapid Reader.

Step 1: Small bowel divided into three equal parts based on capsule transit time from first image in duodenum to first cecal image. ***Step 2***: Calculate each tertiles sub-score based on sum of ulcers (size, number, and distribution) and edema of villi (extent and distribution). ***Step 3***: Assess stenosis in the entire small bowel, irrespective of tertile. ***Step 4***: Lewis score = the highest or worst single tertile score plus the stenosis score.

Summary and Conclusions

Interpretation of video capsule endoscopy requires vigilance, systematic training, and accumulated experience. Readers must orient the capsule within the bowel using anatomic landmarks and reliably distinguish normal variants from clinically significant pathology. Proficiency in interpretation enables detection of subtle angioectasias, differentiation between tumors and benign bulges, and accurate diagnosis of ulcerative pathologies within the proper clinical context. Clear, structured reporting is essential to convey findings and provide actionable recommendations. In this way, capsule endoscopy is transformed from thousands of raw images into an effective diagnostic tool that meaningfully improves patient care.

References

1. Ell C, Remke S, May A, et al. The first prospective controlled trial comparing wireless capsule endoscopy with push enteroscopy in chronic gastrointestinal

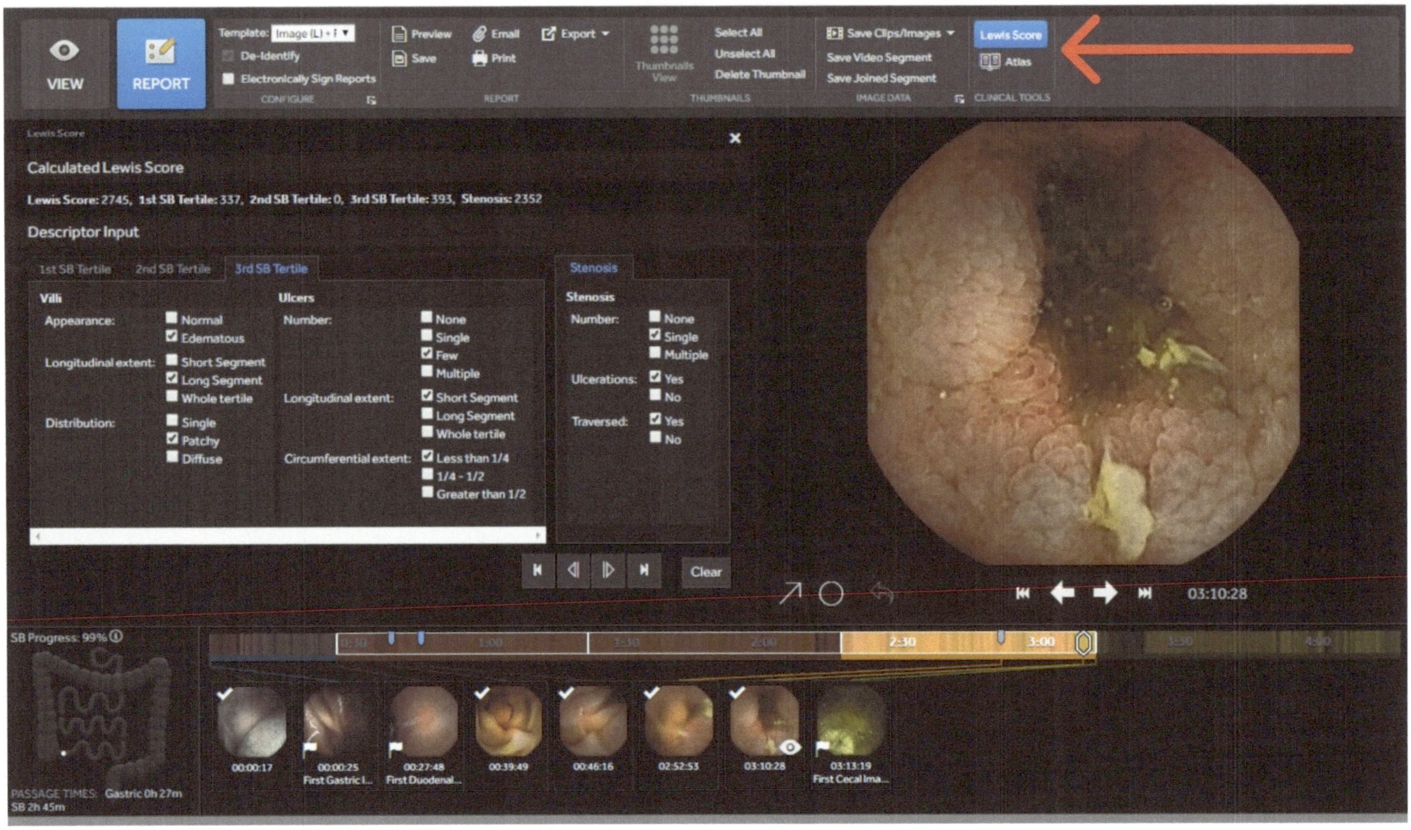

Figure 14. Lewis Score Calculation Tool

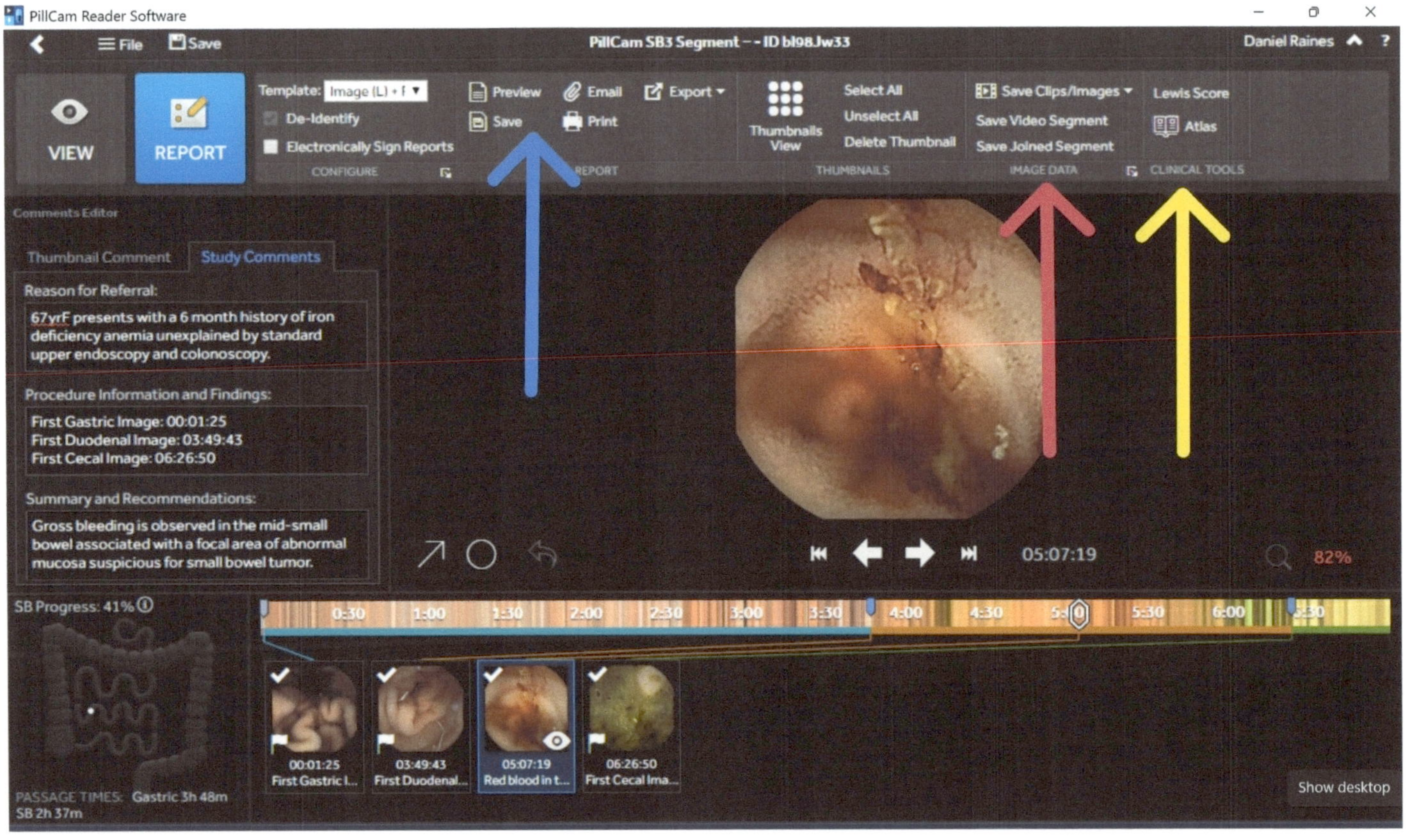

Figure 15. The Report tab (blue arrow) is used to preview, save, print, and transmit reports. The Image Data tab (red arrow) accesses tools to save individual VCE images and image series. Lewis Score and Rapid Atlas can be accessed through the Clinical Tools Tab (yellow arrow).

bleeding. Endoscopy. 2002;34:685–689.
2. Costamagna G, Shah S, Riccioni M, et al. A prospective trial comparing small bowel radiographs and video capsule endoscopy for suspected small bowel disease. Gastroenterology. 2002;123:999–1005.
3. Cave DR, Fleischer DE, Leighton JA, et al. A multicenter randomized comparison of the endocapsule and the Pillcam SB. Gastrointestinal Endoscopy. 2008;68(3):487-94.
4. Westerhof J, Koornstra JJ, Weersma RK. Can we reduce capsule endoscopy reading times? Gastrointestinal Endoscopy. 2009;69(3 Pt 1):497-502.
5. Galinsky TL, Rosa RR, Warm JS, Dember WN. Psychophysical determinants of sustained attention. Hum Factors. 1993;35:603–614.
6. Lieberman HR, Falco CM, Slade SS. Carbohydrate administration during a day of sustained activity improves vigilance. Am J Clin Nutr. 2002;76:120–127.
7. Lane JD, Phillips-Bute BG. Caffeine deprivation affects vigilance performance and mood. Physiol Behav. 1998;65(1):171-5.
8. Pohl J, May A, Rabenstein T, et al. Comparison of virtual chromoendoscopy with conventional white-light endoscopy in small-bowel capsule endoscopy. Endoscopy. 2012;44:236–241.
9. Imagawa H, Oka S, Tanaka S, et al. Improved detectability of small-bowel lesions with flexible spectral imaging color enhancement. Endoscopy. 2011;43:1099–1105.
10. Triantafyllou K, Viazis N, Tsibouris P, et al. FICE enhances small-bowel vascular lesion detection in capsule endoscopy. World J Gastroenterol. 2014;20:5317–5325.
11. Mergener K, Faigel DO, Cave DR. Normal small bowel and normal variants of the small bowel. In Faigel DO, Cave DR, eds, Capsule Endoscopy. Philadelphia, PA: Saunders Elsevier; 2008:61-68.
12. Shilkin KB, Zerman BJ, Blackwell JB. Lymphangiectatic cysts of the small bowel. J Pathol Bacteriol. 1968;96(2):353-8.
13. Bellutti M, Mönkemüller K, Fry LC, Dombrowski F, Malfertheiner P. Characterization of yellow plaques found in the small bowel during double-balloon enteroscopy. Endoscopy. 2007;39(12):1059-63.
14. Mishkin D. Normal variants. In Franchis R, Lews B, Mishkin D, eds, Capsule Endoscopy Simplified.Slack Inc.;2010:43-59.
15. Niu M, Chen ZH, Li M, Zhang X, Chen CX. Differentiation of isolated small bowel crohn's disease from other small bowel ulcerative diseases: clinical features and double-balloon enteroscopy characteristics. Gastroenterol Res Pract. 2022; 5374780.
16. Hall B, Holleran G, McNamara D. Small bowel Crohn's disease: an emerging disease phenotype? Dig Dis. 2015;33:42–51
17. Graham DY, Opekun AR, Willingham FF, Qureshi WA. Visible small-intestinal mucosal injury in chronic NSAID users. Clin Gastroenterol Hepatol. 2005;3(1):55-9.
18. Lang J, Price AB, Levi AJ et al. Diaphragm disease: pathology of disease of the small intestine induced by non-steroidal drugs. J Clin Pathol. 1988; 41;516-526.
19. Gralnek IM, Defranchis R, Seidman E, Leighton JA, Legnani P, Lewis BS. Development of a capsule endoscopy scoring index for small bowel mucosal inflammatory change. Aliment Pharmacol Ther. 2008; 27(2):146-54.
20. Omori T, Matsumoto T, Hara T, et al. A novel capsule endoscopic score for Crohn's disease. Crohns Colitis 360. 2020;2(2):otaa040.
21. Cave DR, Hanscom M, Bledsoe J, et al. Chronic stenosing enteritis: a variant of chronic non-specific stenosing ulceration (CNSU) that is distinct from Crohn's disease. Dig Dis Sci. 2025;70(4):1449-1456.
22. Cave D, Legnani P, de Franchis R, Lewis BS; ICCE. ICCE consensus for capsule retention. Endoscopy. 2005;37(10):1065-7.
23. Pennazio M, Rondonotti E, Despott EJ, et al. Small-bowel capsule endoscopy and device-assisted enteroscopy for diagnosis and treatment of small-bowel disorders: European Society of Gastrointestinal Endoscopy (ESGE) Guideline - Update 2022. Endoscopy. 2023 Jan;55(1):58-95.
24. Rondonotti E, Spada C, Adler S, et al. Small-bowel capsule endoscopy and device-assisted enteroscopy for diagnosis and treatment of small-bowel disorders: European Society of Gastrointestinal Endoscopy (ESGE) Technical Review. Endoscopy. 2018 Apr;50(4):423-446.
25. Gerson LB, Fidler JL, Cave DR, Leighton JA. ACG clinical guideline: Diagnosis and management of small-bowel bleeding. Am J Gastroenterol. 2015;110:1265–1287.
26. Leighton JA, Brock AS, Semrad CE, et al. Quality indicators for capsule endoscopy and deep enteroscopy. Am J Gastroenterol. 2022; 117(11):1780-1796
27. Adler SN, Metzger YC. Pillcam COLON capsule endoscopy: Recent advances and new insights. Ther Adv Gastroenterol. 2011 Jul;4(4):265-8.

Chapter C: Artificial Intelligence for Video Capsule Interpretation

Ryan Stidham, MD and Michael Rice, MD

Introduction

The introduction of VCE in 2001 dramatically improved our ability to examine the small bowel.[1,2] This non-invasive technology created access into regions of the bowel that were once difficult or impossible to examine. As adoption of VCE increased, so did the recognition of practical limitations related to the time and expertise required to review the tens of thousands of images included in each study.[3] Manual interpretation can be tedious, variable, and vulnerable to fatigue-related oversight. For the clinician faced with increasing procedural workloads and growing expectations for diagnostic accuracy, the development of artificial intelligence (AI) models to assist in study interpretation are highly anticipated as transformative improvements in VCE. In this chapter, we review AI development for VCE study interpretation, including basic principles, advancements, and current status.

VCE Interpretation with AI: Basic Principles

Artificial intelligence (AI) is an umbrella term for all systems designed to perform a task which traditionally requires human intelligence. Within AI, machine learning (ML) refers to algorithms that learn from data input without explicit programming. Deep learning (DL), a subset of ML, uses multi-layered artificial neural networks to process complex data. A key deep learning architecture used in VCE is the convolutional neural network (CNN) **(Figure 1)**. CNNs are specifically designed for image recognition tasks, making them ideal for classifying and interpreting capsule endoscopy images. CNNs can identify the presence of abnormalities such as bleeding, ulcers, or masses and can also distinguish normal from abnormal tissue.

Computer vision (CV) is a field of AI which focuses on image analysis. CV tools interpret digital images to allow for automated detection, characterization, and localization of specific findings. Key CV tools employed for VCE interpretation include image classifiers, image segmenters, and spatial localization tools.[4] Image classification identifies the presence or absence of features within an individual image. Image classifiers powered by CNN's are ideal for classification of VCE images.[5] CNN image classifiers are trained for VCE interpretation using large data sets of images containing a wide range of clinically relevant findings. Images in these data sets have been labeled or "classified" by experts as containing data pertaining to important features (e.g., blood, ulcer, healthy tissue), image quality, and even clinical information. A trained CNN image classifier mimics the structure of interconnected neurons to find visual patterns associated with specific labels **(Figure 2)**.

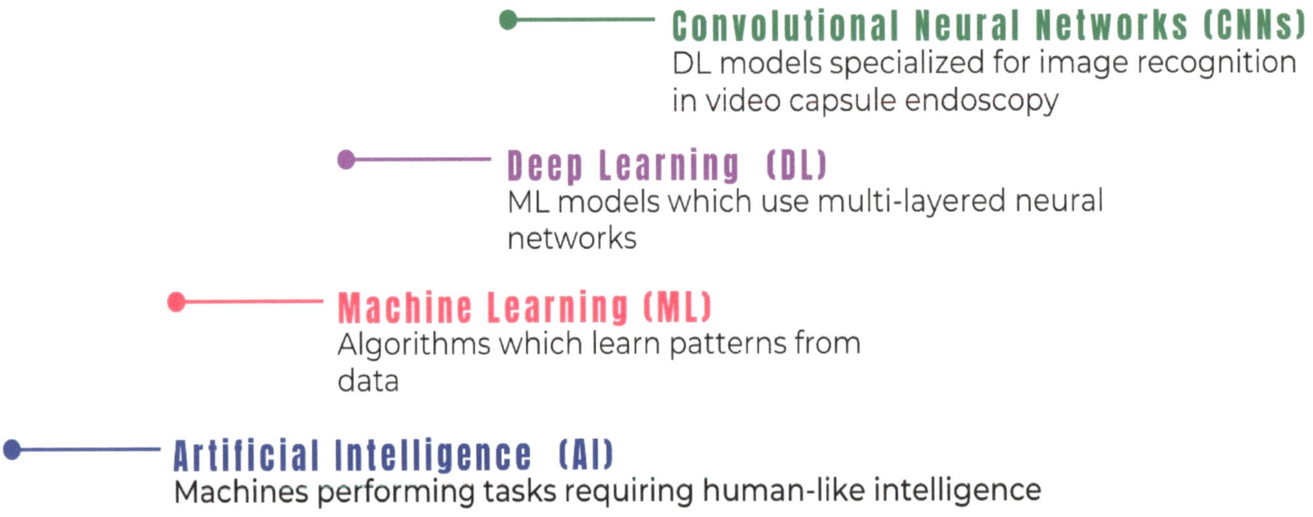

Figure 1. Hierarchy of terms in the field of artificial intelligence (AI): Convolutional neural networks (CNN's) are the primary models used for interpretation of VCE studies. DL, deep learning.

Once optimized, CNN model performance is evaluated using a testing image set and often compared to human performance.

Image segmentation identifies the precise boundaries of a finding within an image, Segmentation enables quantification of lesion size, surface area and morphology, offering more nuanced descriptions of disease **(Figure 3).** Developing image segmentation models requires more extensive image annotation but catalogues the presence, location, and characteristics of disease findings more comprehensively than image classifiers alone. Image segmentation models can be used to highlight the exact location of a finding (e.g., angioectasia) on an image, aiding human review of automated findings.[6]

Spatial localization tools estimate the capsule's position within the small bowel. Monocular visual odometry assists with anatomic localization by analyzing sequential frames to gauge the relative distance traveled by the capsule.[7] Depth estimation tools determine lesion distance from the VCE camera, helping distinguish a large lesion at a distance from a small lesion close to the camera. Finally, integrative methods such as simultaneous localization and mapping (SLAM) combine visual odometry with depth perception to generate 3-dimensional context from 2-dimensional images, improving both localization and spatial description of lesions. Used in combination, spatial localization tools have successfully reconstructed capsule trajectories with high accuracy allowing for precise localization of findings in the gut.[8]

Evolution of AI Tools for VCE

Following the advent of VCE, software applications were

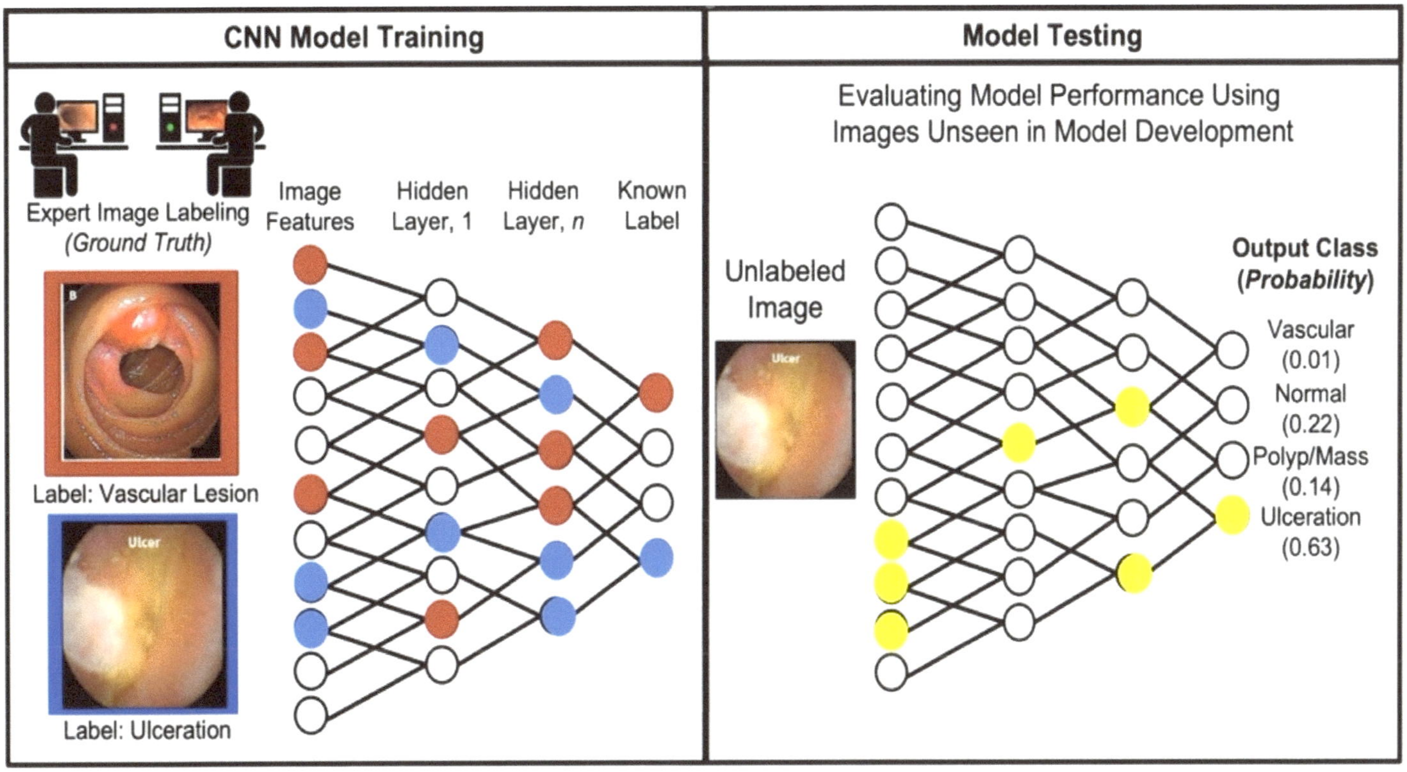

Figure 2. Video capsule endoscopy image classification.
(Left) During training, a convolutional neural network (CNN) evaluates the common relationships of values among groups of pixels within individual image classifications (e.g. the presence of bleeding vs. not containing bleeding), learning hierarchical features from edges and color gradients in early layers to more complex patterns in deeper layers. The CNN model type has initial preset values of both the strength of signal needed to "activate" each neuron/node and the strength of the weights of connections between neurons. As thousands of images that are positive or negative for a class pass through the network, the neuronal activation patterns are associated with the positive or negative classification label. Using a process called backpropagation, the CNNs repeated adjusts the magnitude of network neurons and weighting between neuron connections to optimize a CNN model that best matches the patterns for each visual feature. (Right) Once the model has been developed, it is tested on expert labeled images that were not used in model training. Based on the network activation pattern output probabilities for each possible image classification are generated with the output having the highest value being selected as the predicted image class.

developed to support readers in identifying pathology and reducing reading time. Suspected blood indicator (SBI) was introduced as a feature that highlighted individual frames based on pixel intensity suggestive of blood. Although the utility of SBI was limited as stand-alone feature, it may be considered as the first AI tool for VCE interpretation.[9] Frame-reduction tools such as QuickView® were subsequently introduced to prioritize key frames and eliminate redundant images. These applications resulted in meaningful reductions in capsule reading time, particularly for experienced users.[10]

AI-assisted VCE interpretation improved dramatically with the introduction of CNN-powered VCE image classifiers.[11] In 2019, Ding et al published a study comparing VCE interpretation using a CNN image classifier model. The results of this study were sensational with a reported 99.9% sensitivity of AI for lesion detection compared to 76.9% for human readers accompanied by a reduction in reading time of 6 minutes using AI compared to 97 minutes with standard reading.[12] The details of this study demonstrate that "inflammation" accounted for the majority of VCE abnormalities while the superior performance AI was primarily driven by labeling normal variants.Although these details limit the external validity of the study results, the performance of CNN models in VCE interpretation was reinforced by subsequent research published by Otani et al[13] and Aoki et al.[14]

Studies using CNN image classifiers to identifying vascular lesions have demonstrated promising results. These models have demonstrated sensitivities from 88%-100% and specificities of 96%-97%[15,16] The reported negative predictive value of these models for vascular lesions is high (95%-99%).[17,18] CNN images classifiers can also subclassify lesions based upon Saurin's classification of bleeding propensity (P0, P1,P2) with sensitivity and specificity ranges of 88%-100% and 94%-100%, respectively.[19]

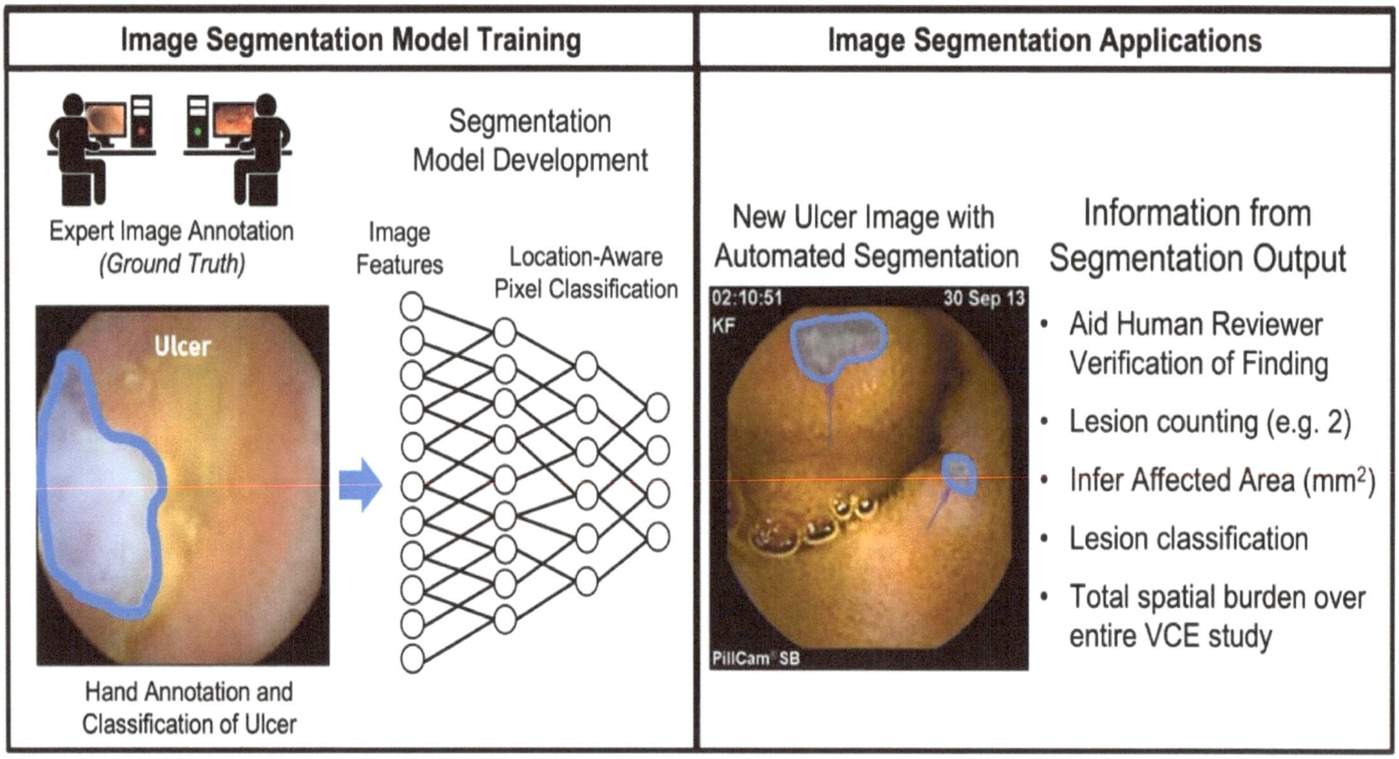

Figure 3. Video capsule endoscopy image segmentation.
(Left) The training image set undergoes manual hand annotation to define the boundary of findings of interest, here shown is an example of an ulcer annotation but any finding could be substituted. Thousands of annotated images are then used to train specialized neural networks (e.g. U-Net) to replicate identification and segmentation of key mucosal findings. (Right) New images can then be introduced in the testing phase to assess both the classification and localization performance of the image segmentation model. Segmentation enables new disease quantification capabilities including quantification of discrete lesions such as ulcers or vascular lesions by count, size, area of involvement in 3 dimensions, and also improved spatial localization.

CNN model performance is excellent in differentiating normal tissue from strictures (AUC 0.99) and ulcerated mucosa (AUC 0.94).[20] This capability makes CNN models useful in the diagnosis, staging, and surveillance of Crohn's disease (CD). Majtner and colleagues demonstrated excellent diagnostic accuracy of CNN detection for both small bowel (98.5%) and colonic ulcerations (98.1%).[21] Another group automatically graded CD ulceration severity in 49 patients compared to 3 expert reviewers, with overall agreement on severity classifier was 67%, increasing to 91% when distinguishing between mild and severe ulcerations, similar to the agreement between human reviewers.[22]

Current Commercial Landscape

Clinicians as well as societies have advocated for the development of AI tools for use in VCE study interpretation to improve lesion detection and reduce read time.[23, 24] Currently available tools which highlight specific frames for inspection, such as Top100 for Pillcam™, provide time savings and improve reader confidence, especially in high-volume clinical settings[25] **(Figure 4)**.

Current research describes CNN models with lesion detection performance equal or superior to standard reading. A recent multicenter study reported an 88% sensitivity CNN model detection of angioectasias, ulcer, venous angioma, suspected tumor, or blood, compared to sensitivity of 80% with standard reading. This difference in sensitivity was primarily related to the angioectasia miss rate for standard readers (18/80) compared to AI (9/80).[26] The capabilities of AI-assisted reading in the setting of IBD have also been described. In one study of localization of inflammatory lesions, the sensitivity and specificity of AI-assisted reading ranged from 92%-95% and 90%-93%, respectively.[27] Further, overall agreement on CD vs ulcerative colitis diagnosis was excellent (k=0.84) and comparable to paired human reviewers (k=0.91). Reading time is dramatically reduced using models which present only images classified as abnormal, reducing the number of frames by 87%-91%. This reduction in images can reduce average standard reading time from 33.7 min to 3.8 min using AI-assisted review of only abnormal images.[26]

Despite these advancements, regulatory hurdles remain. As of this writing, no AI-driven capsule platform has received FDA clearance for autonomous diagnosis. Major investments in VCE technology are currently being made to develop and validate AI models which perform at a level equal or superior to human readers, reliably identify all abnormalities, and classify abnormalities with a high degree of accuracy.

Conclusion

VCE study interpretation can be time consuming and tedious. It is also imperfect, with miss rates of ~5% for bleeding sources and up to 15% for dysplastic lesions.[28] Advances in AI technology for use in VCE study interpretation provide tangible benefits in regard to detection of as well as reduction in reading time. AI-assisted grading of mucosal inflammation, especially in CD, offers potential for objective monitoring of disease activity. Automated lesion labeling and feedback loops also have the potential to improve training as new users learn to identify abnormalities and calibrate their diagnostic thresholds. Commercial platforms for AI-assisted capsule interpretation technology will soon become comprehensive, providing detailed lesion detection, classification, and precise anatomic localization.[29,30]

References

1. Lewis B, Goldfarb N. The advent of capsule endoscopy--a not-so-futuristic approach to obscure gastrointestinal bleeding. Aliment Pharmacol Ther. 2003;17(9):1085-96.
2. Akpunonu B, Hummell J, Akpunonu JD, Ud Din S. Capsule endoscopy in gastrointestinal disease: Evaluation, diagnosis, and treatment. Cleve Clin J Med. 2022;89(4):200-211.
3. Mohan BP, Khan SR, Kassab LL, et al. High pooled performance of convolutional neural networks in computer-aided diagnosis of GI ulcers and/or hemorrhage on wireless capsule endoscopy images: a systematic review and meta-analysis. Gastrointest Endosc. 2021;93(2):356-364.e4.
4. Esteva A, Chou K, Yeung S, Naik N, Madani A, Mottaghi A, Liu Y, Topol E, Dean J, Socher R. Deep learning-enabled medical computer vision. NPJ Digit Med. 2021;4(1):5.
5. Chen C, Mat Isa NA, Liu X. A review of convolutional neural network based methods for medical image classification. Comput Biol Med. 2025;185:109507.
6. Azad R, Aghdam EK, Rauland A, Jia Y, Avval AH, Bozorgpour A, Karimijafarbigloo S, Cohen JP, Adeli E, Merhof D. Medical Image Segmentation Review: The Success of U-Net. IEEE Trans Pattern Anal Mach Intell. 2024;46(12):10076-10095.

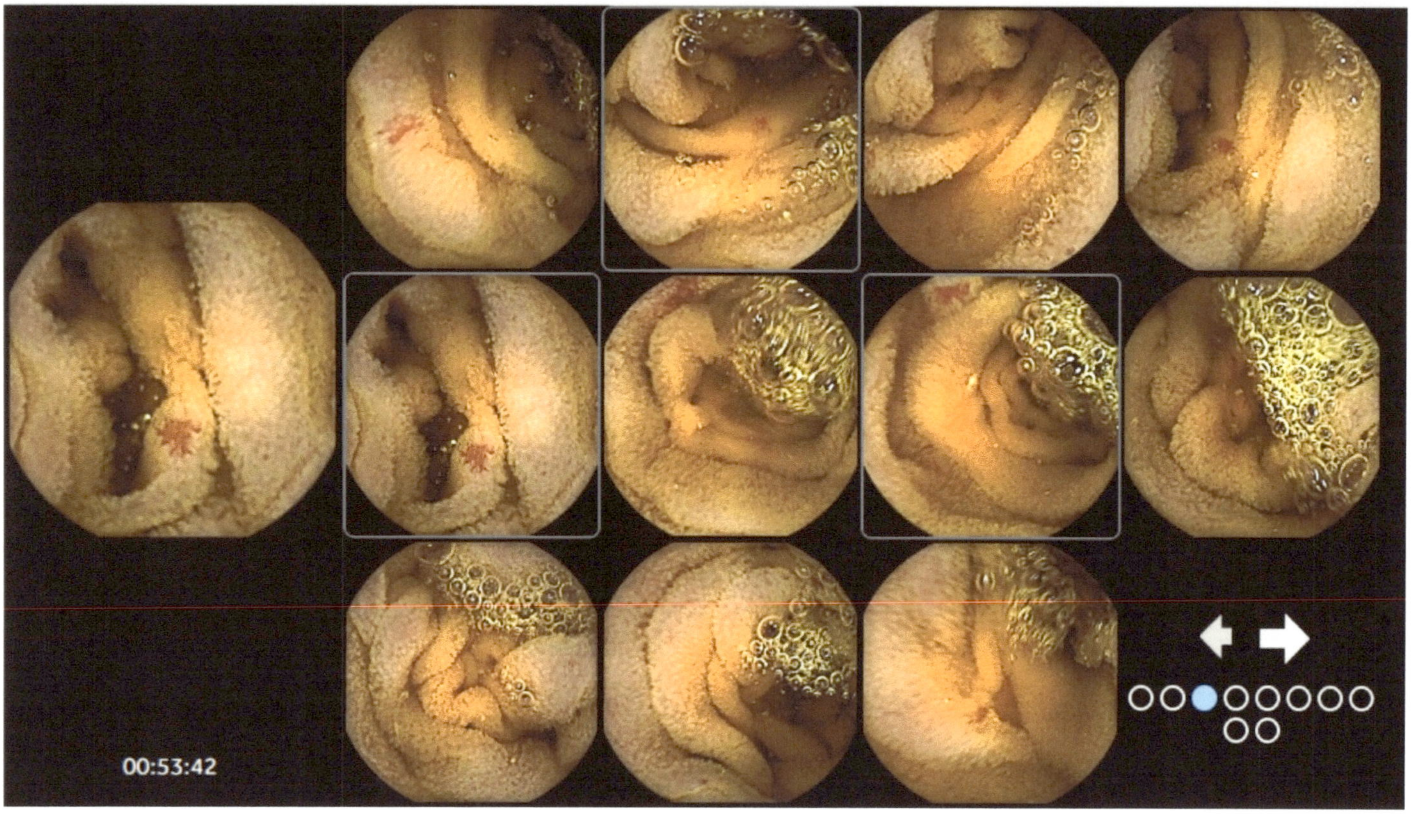

Figure 4. Example of Top100 (Pillcam™). This tool presents the reader with a series of 100 frames identified as most likely to be abnormal. In this example, multiple frames containing angioectasias are highlighted for review. Top100 is available with PillCam™ SB3 version 9 and is enabled after the first duodenal image and first cecal image are identified.

7. Turan M, Almalioglu Y, Araujo H, Konukoglu E, Sitti M. Deep EndoVO: A recurrent convolutional neural network (RCNN) based visual odometry approach for endoscopic capsule robots. Neurocomputing, 2018;275:1861–1870.
8. Ozyoruk KB, Gokceler GI, Bobrow TL, et al. EndoSLAM dataset and an unsupervised monocular visual odometry and depth estimation approach for endoscopic videos. Med Image Anal. 2021;71:102058.
9. Han S, Fahed J, Cave DR. Suspected Blood Indicator to Identify Active Gastrointestinal Bleeding: A Prospective Validation. Gastroenterology Res. 2018;11(2):106-111.
10. Shiotani A, Honda K, Kawakami M, et al. Analysis of small-bowel capsule endoscopy reading by using Quickview mode: training assistants for reading may produce a high diagnostic yield and save time for physicians. J Clin Gastroenterol. 2012;46(10):e92-5.
11. Ghosh T, Fattah SA, Shahnaz C, Wahid KA. An automatic bleeding detection scheme in wireless capsule endoscopy based on histogram of an RGB-indexed image. Annu Int Conf IEEE Eng Med Biol Soc. 2014;2014:4683-6.
12. Ding Z, Shi H, Zhang H, et al. Gastroenterologist-level identification of small-bowel diseases and normal variants by capsule endoscopy using a deep-learning model. Gastroenterology. 2019;157(4):1044-1054.e5.
13. Otani K, Nakada A, Kurose Y, et al. Automatic detection of different types of small-bowel lesions on capsule endoscopy images using a newly developed deep convolutional neural network. Endoscopy. 2020;52(9):786-791.
14. Aoki T, Yamada A, Kato Y, et al. Automatic detection of various abnormalities in capsule endoscopy videos by a deep learning-based system: a multicenter study. Gastrointest Endosc. 2021;93(1):165-173.e1.
15. Mascarenhas Saraiva M, Ribeiro T, Afonso J, Andrade P, Cardoso P, Ferreira J, Cardoso H, Macedo G. Deep learning and device-assisted enteroscopy: Automatic detection of gastrointestinal angioectasia. Medicina (Kaunas). 2021;57(12):1378.I
16. Leenhardt R, Vasseur P, Li C, et al; CAD-CAP Database Working Group. A neural network algorithm for detection of GI angiectasia during small-bowel capsule endoscopy. Gastrointest Endosc. 2019 ;89(1):189-194.
17. Chu Y, Huang F, Gao M, Zou DW, Zhong J, Wu W, Wang Q, Shen XN, Gong TT, Li YY, Wang LF. Convolutional neural network-based segmentation network applied to image recognition of angiodysplasias lesion under capsule endoscopy. World J Gastroenterol. 2023;29(5):879-889.
18. Mascarenhas M, Martins M, Afonso J, et al. Deep learning and capsule endoscopy: Automatic multi-brand

and multi-device panendoscopic detection of vascular lesions. Endosc Int Open. 2024;12(4):E570-E578.
19. Mascarenhas Saraiva MJ, Afonso J, Ribeiro T, et al. Deep learning and capsule endoscopy: Automatic identification and differentiation of small bowel lesions with distinct haemorrhagic potential using a convolutional neural network. BMJ Open Gastroenterol. 2021;8(1):e000753.
20. Klang E, Kopylov U, Mortensen B, et al. A convolutional neural network deep learning model trained on CD ulcers images accurately identifies NSAID ulcers. Front Med (Lausanne). 2021;8:656493.
21. Majtner T, Brodersen JB, Herp J, Kjeldsen J, Halling ML, Jensen MD. A deep learning framework for autonomous detection and classification of Crohn's disease lesions in the small bowel and colon with capsule endoscopy. Endosc Int Open. 2021;9(9):E1361-E1370.
22. Barash Y, Azaria L, Soffer S, et al. Ulcer severity grading in video capsule images of patients with Crohn's disease: an ordinal neural network solution. Gastrointest Endosc. 2021;93(1):187-192.
23. Rondonotti E, Pennazio M, Toth E, Koulaouzidis A. How to read small bowel capsule endoscopy: A practical guide for everyday use. Endosc Int Open. 2020;8(10):E1220-E1224.
24. Messmann H, Bisschops R, Antonelli G, et al. Expected value of artificial intelligence in gastrointestinal endoscopy: European Society of Gastrointestinal Endoscopy (ESGE) position statement. Endoscopy. 2022;54(12):1211-1231.
25. Arieira C, Monteiro S, Dias de Castro F, et al Capsule endoscopy: Is the software TOP 100 a reliable tool in suspected small bowel bleeding? Dig Liver Dis. 2019;51(12):1661-1664.
26. Spada C, Piccirelli S, Hassan C, et al. AI-assisted capsule endoscopy reading in suspected small bowel bleeding: A multicentre prospective study. Lancet Digit Health. 2024;6(5):e345-e353.
27. Brodersen JB, Jensen MD, Leenhardt R, et al. Artificial intelligence-assisted analysis of pan-enteric capsule endoscopy in patients with suspected Crohn's disease: A study on diagnostic performance. J Crohns Colitis. 2024;18(1):75-81.
28. Trasolini R, Byrne MF. Artificial intelligence and deep learning for small bowel capsule endoscopy. Dig Endosc. 2021;33(2):290-297.
29. Cao Q, Deng R, Pan Y, etal. Robotic wireless capsule endoscopy: recent advances and upcoming technologies. Nat Commun. 2024;15(1):4597.
30. Huang YH, Lin Q, Jin XY, et al. Classification of pediatric video capsule endoscopy images for small bowel abnormalities using deep learning models. World J Gastroenterol. 2025;31(21):107601.

Case Study Number 1

Presented by Nikki Arceneaux, MD, Daniel Raines, MD, FACG

Pre-capsule Findings (included in capsule study)

A 63-year-old man with a history of hypertension, dyslipidemia, type 2 diabetes mellitus, and cirrhosis due to metabolic dysfunction-associated steatohepatitis (MASH) presents to the emergency room due to shortness of breath. He reports progressive dyspnea on exertion of the past few days without associated cough, wheezing, or chest pain. Physical exam is notable for a mild tachycardia with regular rhythm, lungs clear to auscultation/ percussion, and a non-distended abdomen. Initial lab draw is revealing for a hemoglobin of 6.6 gm/dl, much lower than his baseline hemoglobin of 11 gm/dl. Following initiation of medical therapy and transfusion of 2 units packed red blood cells, endoscopic evaluation of the upper GI tract is negative for luminal blood or bleeding sources. A colonoscopy is performed the following day after a full bowel prep. This exam identifies dark red blood in the right colon and within the terminal ileum.

An inpatient capsule endoscopy study is performed to evaluate for small bowel bleeding. Review the capsule endoscopy study and report your findings, including: gastric passage time, small bowel passage time, and observed abnormalities. Be prepared to discuss your findings and management plan with your staff prior to reviewing the diagnosis and case discussion.

Capsule Endoscopy Findings
First Gastric Image = 0h 0min 32sec
First Duodenal Image = 0h 10min 31sec
Gastric passage time = 0h 10min
First Cecal Image = 4h 43min 43sec
Small bowel passage time = 4h 33min

Figure 1

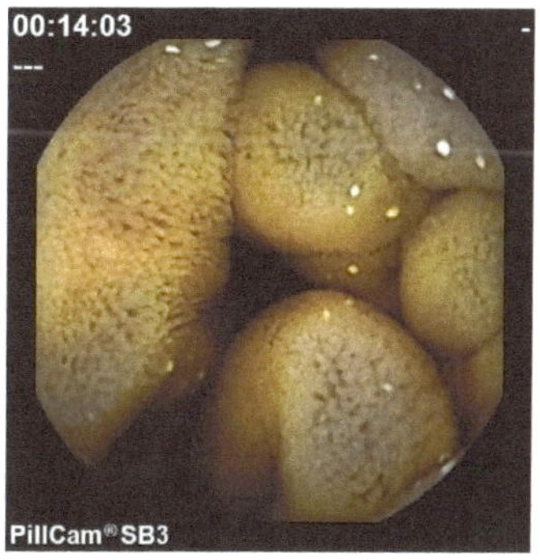

Figure 2

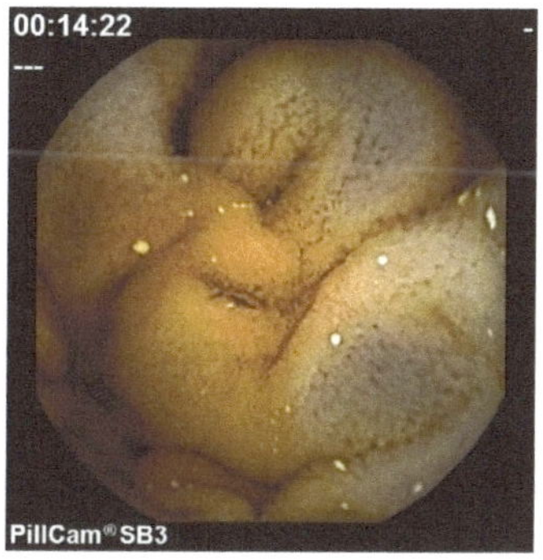

Figure 3

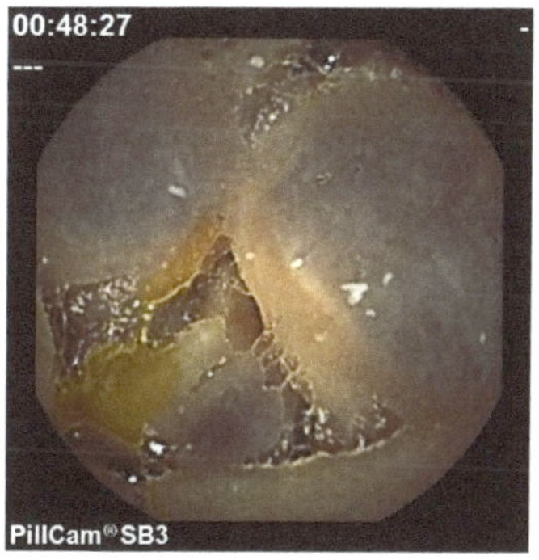

Figure 4

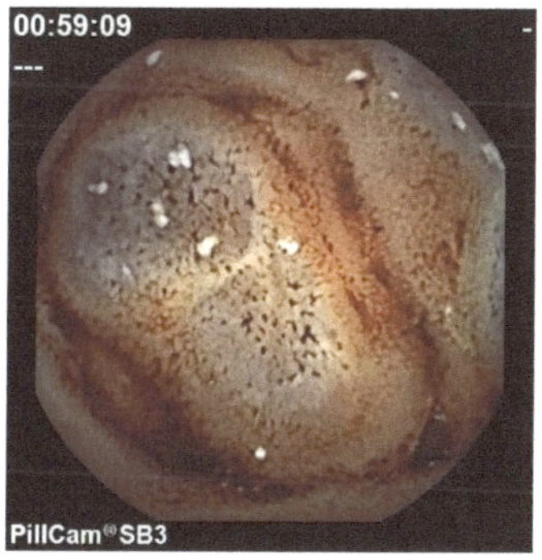

Examination of the esophagus and stomach are unremarkable. Within the duodenum, submucosal venous structures consistent with non-bleeding duodenal varices are observed (**Figure 1:** 0hr 14min 3sec**; Figure 2:** 0hr 14min 2sec). A second cluster of small bowel varices is encountered with a segment of jejunum (likely mid-jejunum) and associated with active bleeding (**Figure 3:** 0hr 48min 27sec; **Figure 4:** 0hr 59min 9sec). Visualization of the remaining small bowel is generally obscured by gross blood within the lumen.

Follow-up

An anterograde single balloon enteroscopy was performed to access the site of hemorrhage. Small bowel varices were observed in the third portion of the duodenum prior to discovery of a bleeding varix with fibrin plug in the mid-jejunum. Multiple hemoclips were placed across the varix on both sides of the fibrin plug for interruption of blood flow (**Figure 5a, 5b**). The following day, a multidisciplinary discussion was organized, including gastroenterology, hepatology, surgery, and interventional radiology. The consensus

A

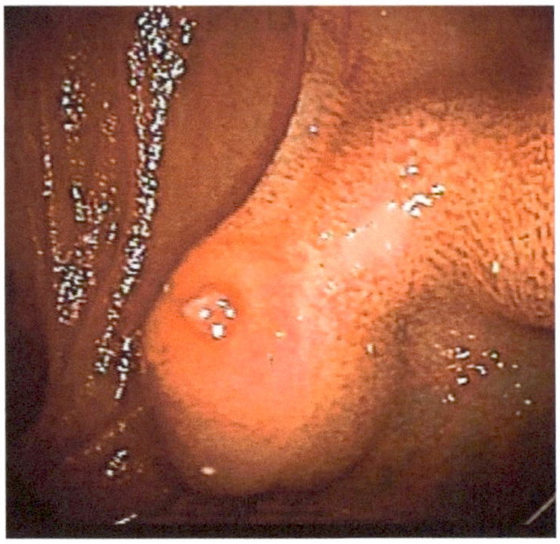

Figure 5a. Jejunal varix localized by anterograde DAE. A fibrin plug is identified as the site of hemorrhage.

B

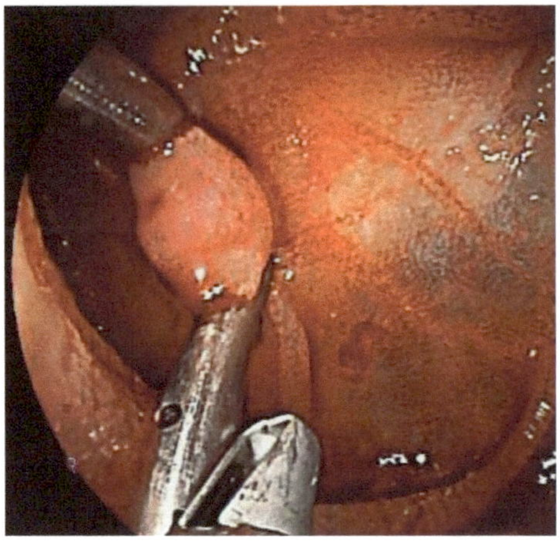

Figure 5b. Jejunal varix ligated with hemoclips placed across the vessel on each side of the fibrin plug.

recommendation for management was to perform a transhepatic anterograde embolization of the mid-jejunal varices in combination with a transjugular intrahepatic portosystemic shunt (TIPS) for decompression of duodenal varices.

Chapter 1: Small Bowel Varices

Nikki Arceneaux, MD and Daniel Raines, MD, FACG

Introduction

Small bowel varices (SBVs) including duodenal, jejunal, and ileal varices, are a rare but clinically significant source of gastrointestinal bleeding. Small bowel varices represent a subset of ectopic varices, defined as portosystemic collaterals occurring outside the gastroesophageal region.[1] While SBVs can occur throughout the small intestine, the duodenum is the most commonly affected site, followed by the jejunum and ileum. Ectopic varices may also develop within sites of small bowel anastomosis or stomas. In one study of 169 patients with variceal bleeding due to ectopic varices, 26% occurred at sites of previous abdominal surgery followed by the duodenum (17%), jejunum/ileum (17%), colon (14%), rectum (8%), and peritoneum (9%).[2]

Small bowel varices typically arise in the setting of elevated portal venous pressure, most commonly due to decompensated cirrhosis. They may also develop in cases of non-cirrhotic portal hypertension, such as chronic thrombosis of the portal or mesenteric veins. Surgical interventions involving bowel resection and anastomosis can predispose patients to the formation of small bowel varices, especially when normal venous return is disrupted or when segmental areas of venous congestion develop. In such postoperative settings, varices may form near anastomotic sites as localized collateral circulation compensates for altered venous flow[1] (**Figure 1**).

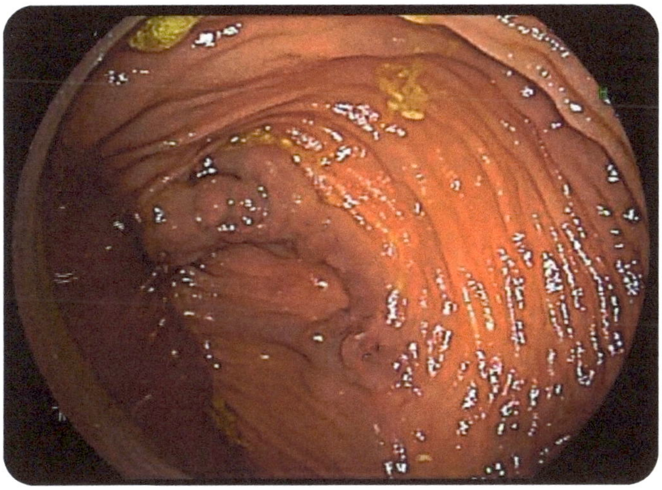

Figure 1. Endoscopic view of varices within a small bowel anastomosis.

Pathophysiology

Portal hypertension is the most common driver of varices development within the gastrointestinal tract. Portal hypertension results from increased resistance to portal flow and increased portal venous inflow secondary to a systemic hyperdynamic state and increased splanchnic circulation. As a result, collaterals between the portal and systemic circulation form. The most common location of collateral formation includes the gastroesophageal varices.[3,4] Esophageal varices can be classified by size (small, medium, large), location and endoscopic appearance. Gastric varices can be categorized by Sarin classification as gastroesophageal varices type 1 (GOV1), which are located along the lesser curvature and continuous with esophageal varices. Type 2 (GOV2) are found along the greater curvature and fundus. Isolated gastric varices are divided into type 1 (IGV1), limited to the fundus, and type 2 (IGV2) which are located elsewhere in the stomach other than the gastric fundus.[5]

Small bowel varices form in the setting of portal hypertension as well as in cases in which blood flow is diverted through the submucosal veins of the duodenum, jejunum, or ileum due to surgery or thrombosis.[2,3] Duodenal varices have also developed after band ligation of esophageal varices, presumably as alternate sites of spontaneous portosystemic shunting.[6] These varices are formed by the collateral veins originating from the portal vein trunk or superior mesenteric vein draining into the inferior vena cava through retroperitoneal veins of Retzius.[7,8]

Clinical Features

The clinical presentation of small bowel variceal bleeding varies by location. Duodenal varices typically present with melena, hematochezia, or hematemesis and can often mimic bleeding from gastric varices.[7] Bleeding from jejunal or ileal varices tends to manifest as melena or hematochezia and is frequently classified as obscure following negative evaluation by standard upper endoscopy and colonoscopy. Patients who experience slow or intermittent bleeding from small bowel varices may present with iron deficiency anemia. A potential diagnosis of SBV should be considered in any patient with unexplained gastrointestinal bleeding and a history of either portal hypertension or abdominal surgery with intestinal anastomosis.

Diagnosis

Small bowel varices often remain undetected by esophagogastroduodenoscopy (EGD) and/or colonoscopy. Duodenal varices may be diagnosed by EGD if located in the duodenal bulb or second portion (**Figure 2**). Video capsule endoscopy is a valuable non-invasive tool for the evaluation of patients with suspected small bowel bleeding. SBV may appear as dilated or saccular submucosal veins on VCE.[9] They are particularly conspicuous if associated with adherent blood or active bleeding. Device-assisted enteroscopy (DAE) allows for direct visualization of the small bowel via anterograde and/or retrograde approach. Although more invasive than VCE, DAE allows for therapeutic interventions for bleeding SBV, such as ligation with hemoclips, injection with sclerosant, or treatment with cyanoacrylate glue.[10,11] CT enterography (CTE) can identify vascular abnormalities, including varices, by demonstrating dilated, enhancing venous structures within the small bowel wall or mesentery. CTE is particularly useful for mapping the extent and location of varices and for procedural planning.

Management

Management of small bowel varices is highly individualized. Primary factors which influence management include anatomic location of the varices, severity of bleeding, underlying liver dysfunction, and the feasibility of available therapeutic modalities. Established treatment algorithms for the management of esophagogastric varices, including non-selective beta-blockers, band ligation, and TIPS, may not be applicable in cases of SBV. As there are no standardized guidelines for the treatment of SBV, clinical decision-making often relies on case reports, small series, and multidisciplinary expertise.

Duodenal varices, due to their proximity to the stomach, are sometimes accessible with standard upper endoscopy. If within reach of the gastroscope, they may be treated with band ligation. Other endoscopic options include injection of sclerosants, cyanoacrylate glue, or application of hemoclips.[2,12]

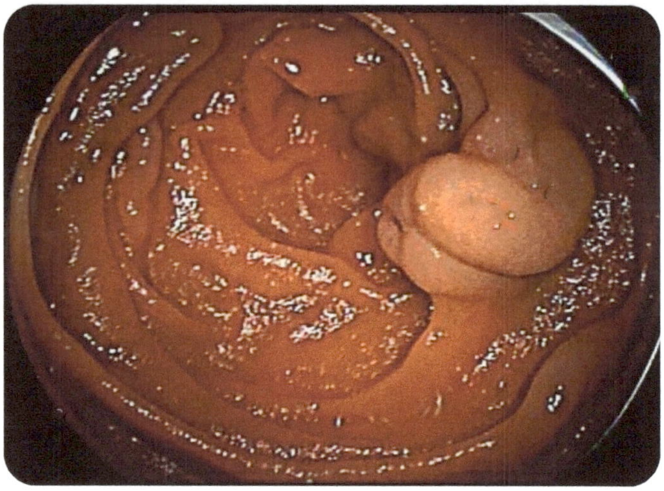

Figure 2. Duodenal varix diagnosed by standard EGD.

In cases where endoscopic therapy is not feasible or fails to achieve hemostasis, TIPS may be effective, particularly for duodenal varices that are part of the main portosystemic circuit.[13]

Jejunal and ileal varices pose greater diagnostic and therapeutic challenges. These lesions frequently arise in ectopic or surgically altered anatomy and often lie beyond the reach of conventional endoscopy, necessitating DAE for direct visualization and potential intervention. As jejunal and ileal varices typically drain into peripheral mesenteric venous branches, they are not reliably decompressed by TIPS. Multiple reports describe continued or recurrent hemorrhage from jejunal or ileal varices despite technically successful TIPS placement, likely due to insufficient reduction of localized venous pressure in the affected vascular beds.[1,3,5] Selective transhepatic embolization of the bleeding ectopic varices offers an effective alternative to TIPS in the management of jejunal or ileal varices.[14] For transhepatic embolization, a catheter is advanced percutaneously through the liver parenchyma into a portal venous branch under ultrasound and fluoroscopic guidance. Contrast is then injected to delineate the portal system, allowing selective catheterization of the mesenteric venous branch supplying the variceal plexus for embolization.

Anastomotic or stomal varices are often treated definitively by surgical resection rather than endoscopy or intervention by interventional radiology. Surgical resection of native small bowel segments containing varices may be considered for refractory bleeding in patients with preserved liver function. A comparison of management of varices based upon

Variceal Location	Typical Access/ Diagnosis	First-line Therapy	Interventional Options	Limitations
Esophagogastric Varices	Standard upper endoscopy (EGD)	Non-selective beta-blockers, Endoscopic Band Ligation	TIPS for refractory bleeding	Well-established algorithms but rebleeding risk persists
Duodenal Varices	EGD (duodenal bulb or second portion)	Endoscopic therapy with banding, glue, sclerosant, or clips	TIPS ± embolization, ATO/RTO	Access may be difficult depending on varix location
Jejunal/Ileal Varices	Device-Assisted Enteroscopy (DAE), VCE, CT Enterography	DAE with endoscopic therapy (if accessible)	Selective transhepatic embolization	TIPS is often ineffective due to peripheral drainage
Anastomotic /Stomal Varices	Device-Assisted Enteroscopy (DAE), VCE, CT Enterography, Direct examination of stoma	Surgical resection if focal and accessible	Transhepatic embolization vs sclerotherapy	Frequently refractory; surgical resection often definitive but high-risk in cirrhosis

Table 1. Management of varices based upon anatomic location.

anatomic location is included in **Table 1**.

Conclusion

Small bowel varices should be considered as a potential source of blood loss in patients with overt bleeding or iron deficiency anemia and a history of cirrhosis, portal vein thrombosis, or prior abdominal surgery. Bleeding from small bowel varices is associated with a high rate of mortality (20%-40%), particularly in patients with advanced liver disease.[12] Currently available diagnostic modalities, including VCE, DAE, and CTE, are effective in diagnosing SBV and providing information necessary for treatment planning. Management of SBV differs from management of esophagogastric varices and varies based upon anatomic location. Management is also influenced by additional patient factors as well as the experience of the treating gastroenterologist, interventional radiologist, and surgeon.

References

1. Hashimoto N, Akahoshi T, Yoshida D, et al. The efficacy of balloon-occluded retrograde transvenous obliteration on small intestinal variceal bleeding. Surgery. 2010;148(1):145-50.
2. N Norton ID, Andrews JC, Kamath PS. Management of ectopic varices. Hepatology. 1998;28(4):1154-8.
3. Helmy A, Al Kahtani K, Al Fadda M. Updates in the pathogenesis, diagnosis and management of ectopic varices. Hepatol Int. 2008;2(3):322-34. Erratum in: Hepatol Int. 2008;2(3):395-6.
4. Jansson-Knodell CL, Calderon G, Weber R, Ghabril M. Small intestine varices in cirrhosis at a high-volume liver transplant center: A retrospective database study and literature review. Am J Gastroenterol. 2021 Jul 1;116(7):1426-1436.
5. Sarin SK, Lahoti D, Saxena SP, Murthy NS, Makwana UK. Prevalence, classification and natural history of gastric varices: a long-term follow-up study in 568 portal hypertension patients. Hepatology. 1992;16(6):1343-9.
6. Lee EW, Eghtesad B, Garcia-Tsao G, et al. AASLD Practice Guidance on the use of TIPS, variceal embolization, and retrograde transvenous obliteration in the management of variceal hemorrhage. Hepatology. 2024;79(1):224-250.
7. Akhter N, Haskal Z. Diagnosis and management of ectopic varices. Gastrointestinal Intervention. 2012;1(1): 3–10.
8. Khor V, Soon Y, Aung L. A case report of bleeding from a duodenal varix: Rare cause of upper gastrointestinal bleeding. Int J Surg Case Rep. 2018;49:205-208.
9. Tang SJ, Zanati S, Dubcenco E, et al. Diagnosis

of small-bowel varices by capsule endoscopy. Gastrointest Endosc. 2004;60(1):129-35.
10. Figueiredo P, Almeida N, Lérias C, et al. Effect of portal hypertension in the small bowel: an endoscopic approach. Dig Dis Sci. 2008;53(8):2144-50.
11. Vangeli M, Patch D, Terreni N, et al. Bleeding ectopic varices--treatment with transjugular intrahepatic porto-systemic shunt (TIPS) and embolisation. J Hepatol. 2004;41(4):560-6
12. Jonnalagadda SS, Quiason S, Smith OJ. Successful therapy of bleeding duodenal varices by TIPS after failure of sclerotherapy. Am J Gastroenterol. 1998;93(2):272-4.
13. Xiao NJ, Chu JG, Ning SB, Wei BJ, Xia ZB, Han ZY. Successful management of bleeding ectopic small bowel varices secondary to portal hypertension: A retrospective study. World J Gastrointest Surg. 2025;17(3):102589.
14. Sato T. Treatment of ectopic varices with portal hypertension. World J Hepatol. 2015; 28;7(12):1601-5

Case Study Number 2

Presented by Brooke F. Mishkin and Daniel S. Mishkin, MD, CM, FRCP(C), FACG

Pre-capsule Findings (included in capsule study)

A 41-year-old woman presents for further evaluation of chronic anemia which has been severe in recent months. She has a pre-existing diagnosis of iron deficiency anemia attributed to blood loss due to menorrhagia as well as intermittent epistaxis. Her hemoglobin had remained stable ~10 gm/dl with parenteral iron therapy. Over the past 3 months, she has required transfusion of packed RBCs on 2 separate occasions for symptomatic anemia with a hemoglobin <7gm/dl. Prior evaluation of her anemia has included standard upper endoscopy and colonoscopy which were unrevealing. A repeat upper endoscopy with push enteroscopy was performed 2 weeks ago with endoscopic ablation of a suspected Dieulafoy lesion in the mid jejunum.

A capsule endoscopy study is performed to evaluate for small bowel bleeding. Review the capsule endoscopy study and report your findings, including: gastric passage time, small bowel passage time, and observed abnormalities. Be prepared to discuss your findings and management plan with your staff prior to reviewing the diagnosis and case discussion.

Fresh red blood is observed in the gastric body upon entry into the stomach. Although an active bleeding focus is not observed, the exam is revealing for multiple, small (5 mm) vascular ectasias (**Figure 1:** 00h 06min 05sec). Multiple additional angioectasias are found distributed throughout the small bowel accompanied by particles of bright red blood (**Figure 2:** 00h 12 min 28 sec; **Figure 3:** 00h 35m 17s). A submucosal India Ink tattoo is identified in the jejunum corresponding with the site of prior endoscopic therapy (**Figure 4**: 00h 22min 21sec).

Capsule Endoscopy Findings
First Gastric Image = 0h 0min 33sec
First Duodenal Image = 0h 11min 16sec
Gastric passage time = 0h 10min
First Cecal Image = 1h 6min 21sec
Small bowel passage time = 56min

Follow-up

This patient was elected for an antegrade DBE to facilitate endoscopic ablation of all identifiable vascular ectasias in the stomach, duodenum, jejunum and proximal ileum. This exam was successful in treating multiple (~20) vascular ectasias distributed evenly throughout the small bowel. Upon further investigation, this patient was found to have cutaneous telangiectasias on her hands and a family history of hereditary hemorrhagic telangiectasia (HHT).

Figure 1

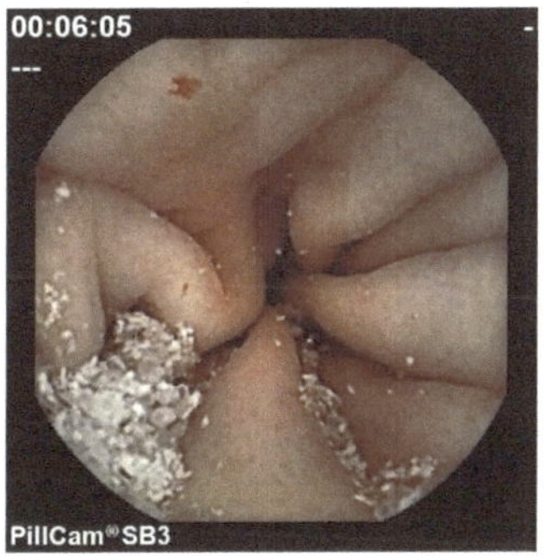

Figure 2

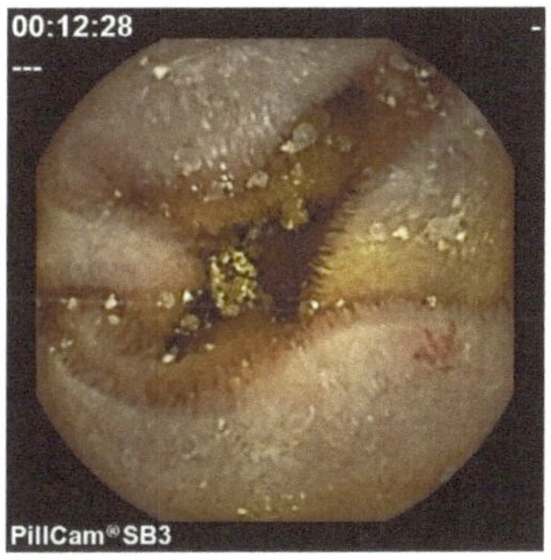

Figure 3

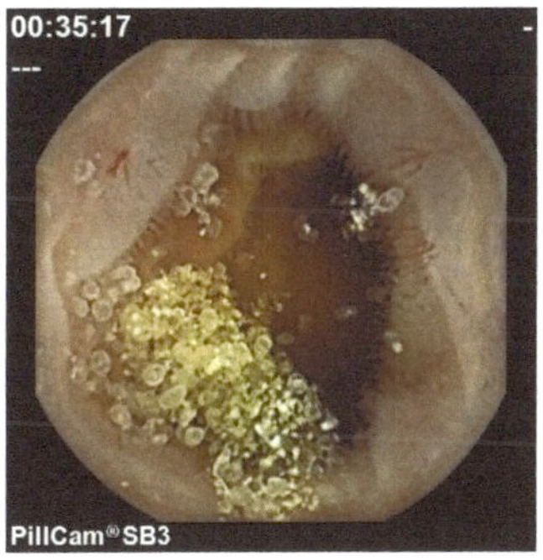

Figure 4

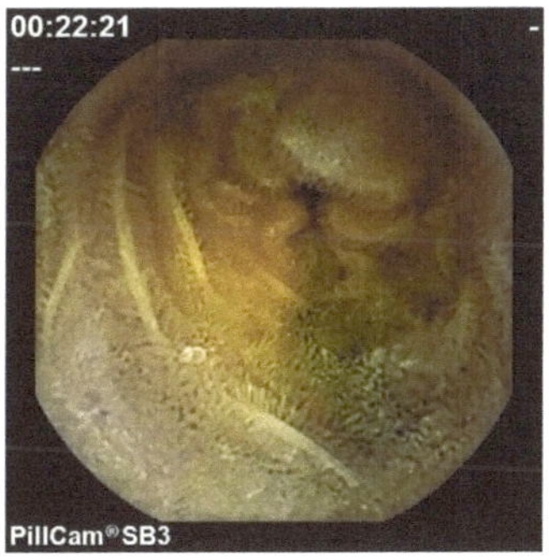

Chapter 2: Hereditary Hemorrhagic Telangiectasia (HHT)

Brooke F. Mishkin and Daniel S. Mishkin, MD, CM, FRCP(C), FACG

Introduction

Hereditary hemorrhagic telangiectasia (HHT), also known as Osler-Weber-Rendu syndrome, is a relatively common but often underrecognized vascular disorder that affects individuals across all ethnic and racial groups, with an incidence of 1 in 5,000 to 8,000 people.[1] The first definitive description was published in 1864 by Sutton,[2] but it was not until 1909 that Hanes coined the term "Osler-Weber-Rendu."[3] HHT manifests as small vessel telangiectasias and large vessel arteriovenous malformations (AVMs). Telangiectasias are formed by dilated arterioles and venules connected by arteriovenous shunts. These lesions may appear as 1-2 mm red spots on the skin and disappear with slight pressure. Telangiectasias of the nasopharynx and gastrointestinal lumen are often complicated by bleeding. Visceral AVMs are comprised of larger vascular structures with shunts bypassing capillary beds. Patients with HHT develop large vessel pulmonary, hepatic, cerebral or spinal AVMs.

Pathophysiology

HHT is primarily caused by mutations in genes involved in the TGF-β/BMP9 signaling pathway, which is crucial for maintaining vascular integrity. HHT is an autosomal dominant disorder with variable penetrance and expression, making the disorder genetically heterogeneous. The 2 most common mutations account for the majority of clinical cases, though additional genetic abnormalities are being identified.[4] HHT type 1 results from mutations in the endoglin gene (*ENG*) on chromosome 9 and is associated with pulmonary and cerebral manifestations. HHT type 2 results from mutations in the activin receptor-like kinase 1 gene (*ALK1*) on chromosome 12 and is linked to hepatic manifestations. Mutations in these genes disrupt endothelial cell (EC) signaling, resulting in malformed blood vessels that are prone to rupture, a hallmark of the disease.[4-6] Additional genetic mutations, such as in *SMAD4* gene, have been documented in patients with juvenile polyposis-HHT overlap syndrome. Pathogenic variants in *GDF2* have also been described in rare cases.[6,7]

Recent research has highlighted the importance of canonical BMP9/10 signaling in the formation of AVMs. Studies using murine models have shown that abnormal signaling through the *ALK1* and *ENG* receptors leads to defects in endothelial cell differentiation, smooth muscle actin coverage, and vessel wall integrity, contributing to the formation of arteriovenous malformations (AVMs). Furthermore, loss of the BMP9/10 signaling pathway in endothelial cells impairs pericyte coverage, exacerbating the formation and growth of AVMs, especially in high-flow vascular areas such as the lungs and GI tract.[6,7]

Clinical Features

Telangiectasias can occur throughout the body, including the skin (face, lips, tongue, trunk, arms, fingers), mucosa (oral mucosa, gums, conjunctiva), nasal passages, and gastrointestinal tract. Cutaneous lesions tend to appear early in life and progress with age, with most presenting by age 30 **(Figure 1)**.[8,9] Although cutaneous telangiectasias are cosmetically bothersome, they are known to cause only minor bleeding which is easily controlled. Epistaxis is the most common and often the earliest manifestation of HHT, occurring in 50%-80% of patients, frequently beginning before age 10.

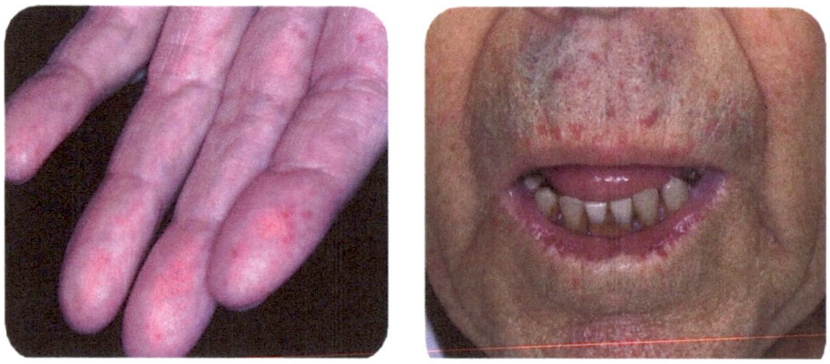

Figure 1: Telangiectasias of the fingers and face seen in HHT.

Telangiectasias of the GI tract develop in adult HHT patients with a prevalence of 13%-30%.[8,9] These malformed vessels are prone to rupture, leading to episodes of bleeding that can range from mild to life-threatening. Symptomatic bleeding from GI telangiectasias typically occurs after the fifth or sixth decade, although severe phenotypes may present much earlier. Telangioectasias may be indistinguishable from sporadic angioectasias **(Figure 2)**. Patients with HHT may develop numerous telangiectasias which are distributed diffusely throughout the gastrointestinal tract **(Figure 3)**. By contrast, sporadic angioectasias are primarily distributed in the stomach, duodenum,

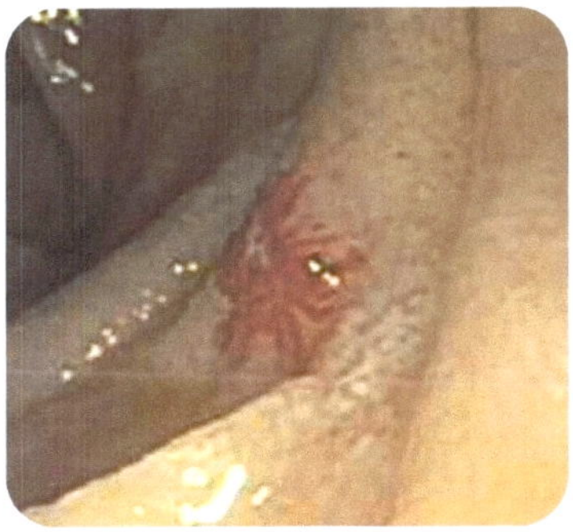

Figure 2: Jejunal telangiectasia with classic "fern-like" appearance.

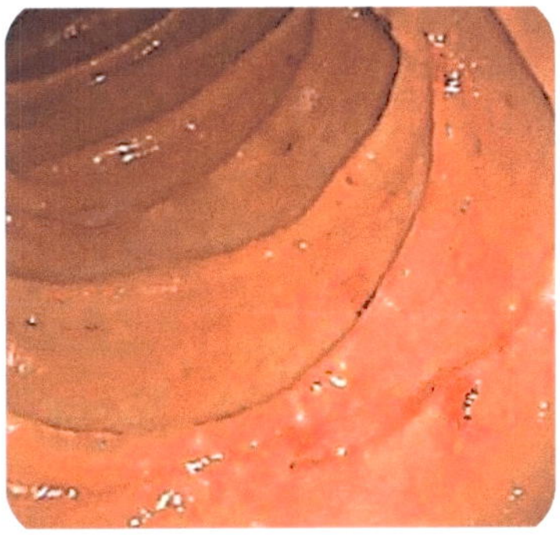

Figure 3: Multiple telangiectasias clustered in the ileum.

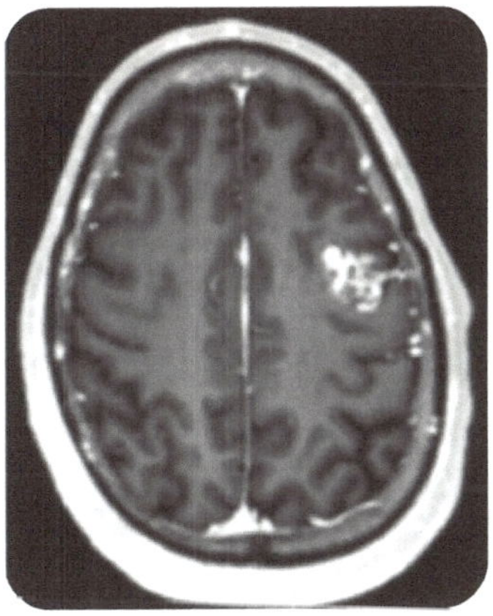

Figure 4: Cerebral arterio-venous malformation (AVM) identified by CT imaging with IV contrast.

proximal jejunum and right colon.[10-12] The number of telangiectasias may correlate with severity of GI bleeding in patients with HHT.

Large vessel AMVs may form in the lungs, liver, and central nervous system, including the brain and, more rarely, the spinal cord **(Figure 4)**. While AVMs may remain clinically silent, there is a risk of complication due to embolus, thrombosis, or high flow shunting. Pulmonary involvement is observed in 5%-30% of adults and is more common in HHT type 1. Pulmonary AVMs may remain asymptomatic or present with hemoptysis, hypoxemia, orthodeoxia, or even pulmonary hypertension.[13] These lesions may result in stroke or brain abscess due to paradoxical emboli. Hepatic involvement is observed in up to 70% of patients and is more common in HHT type 2. Hepatic AVMs may include arteriovenous, arterioportal, and portovenous shunts. These lesions may result in clinical complications such as high-output cardiac failure, portal hypertension, and biliary ischemia.[14] AVMs of the CNS occur in 10%-15% of patients with HHT. These lesions are thought to be congenital.

Diagnosis

The diagnosis of HHT relies on a detailed clinical examination combined with medical and family history. The HHT Foundation International developed the Curaçao criteria (**Table 1**) in 2000 to help clinicians determine the probability of HHT.[15] The Curaçao diagnostic criteria have been validated through molecular testing. In a cohort of probands who met these criteria, 148/152 out of 141 (97.4%) were found to have a pathogenic variant in either *ENG* (44.1%), *ACVRL1* (52.0%) or *SMAD4* (1.3%).[16] Genetic testing is now more accessible to identify specific pathogenic variants in *ENG*, *ACVRL1*, SMAD4, or *GDF2*. Identification of a specific HHT genetic mutation in an individual may be useful for screening of other family members. However, the absence of a known mutation does not exclude a diagnosis of HHT except in cases in which an individual tests negative for an established mutation identified within his/her family.[17]

Critera	
Epistaxis: Spontaneous, recurrent nosebleeds	
Telangiectasias: Multiple at characteristic sites (lips, oral cavity, fingers, nose)	
Visceral lesions: GI telangectasias (with or without bleeding) or arteriovenous malformations (pulmonary, hepatic, cerebral, spinal)	
Family history: a first-degree relative with HHT	
HHT Diagnosis	
Definite	3 criteria present
Possible or suspected	2 criteria present
Unlikely	< 2 criteria present

Table 1. Curaçao Diagnostic Criteria.

Several studies support the use of VCE in the HHT population.[18] One study of 38 patients with HHT and 55 patients without HHT found that identification of ≥5 telangiectases by VCE to be highly (86%) predictive of HHT. In addition, VCE helped upgrade the certainty of diagnosis by Curaçoa criteria in 13% of those with suspected HHT.[19,20] Another study of VCE in 30 patients with HHT complicated by severe anemia reported a diagnostic yield of 87%.[21]

Management

The goals for management in HHT are to control symptoms, monitor known lesions, and prevent complications associated with AVMs.[10,11] Treatment of epistaxis requires collaboration with otolaryngology. Management of chronic GI blood loss in patients with HHT involves a combination of interventions. Endoscopic ablation of telangiectasias in the small bowel and other segments of the GI tract is a key intervention but not curative. Aggressive iron supplementation including parenteral iron therapy is often necessary and may be missing in the current therapy plan. In patients who continue to require periodic packed red blood cell transfusion despite endoscopic ablation sessions and adequate parenteral iron supplementation, options for medical therapy have included depot octreotide injections and thalidomide.[21,22]

Recently, antiangiogenic therapies such as bevacizumab and pazopanib, in addition to thalidomide, have shown promise in reducing gastrointestinal bleeding. For example, bevacizumab, an anti-VEGF antibody, has demonstrated efficacy in reducing GI bleeding and improving hemoglobin levels. Thalidomide and pazopanib have also been used off-label with promising results. A 2023 study of thalidomide in bleeding angioectasias reported a 69% reduction in bleeding episodes with thalidomide 100 mg daily.[23] The use of antifibrinolytic agents, such as tranexamic acid, can help reduce bleeding. Hormonal therapy has been used in some cases, although its efficacy is limited and variable.[24]

Therapies targeted to specific genetic mutations hold promise for more effective management of this disease. The use of gene therapy or small molecules to correct endothelial dysfunction or inhibit abnormal vessel formation are currently under study. *BMP9* and *BMP10* signaling have recently been show to play a crucial role in the vascular homeostasis of various organs, including the GI tract. Restoring this signaling pathway could potentially reduce the formation of AVMs and control bleeding.

Patients with HHT should be screened for cerebral AVMs by MRI of the brain (once in adulthood) and pulmonary AVM's by echocardiography with bubble study to detect arteriovenous shunts (every 5 years). Patients with known pulmonary shunts should receive prophylaxis for infective endocarditis prior to dental and surgical procedures.[10,11]

Conclusions

HHT is more common than previously recognized. This diagnosis should be considered in all patients diagnosed with gastrointestinal bleeding due to vascular ectasias which may represent telangiectasias rather than sporadic angioectasias. Advances in genetic testing have improved our ability to diagnose HHT and manage its complications. As our understanding of the disease improves, new therapeutic options, particularly pharmacologic treatments, are emerging, offering hope for better management in the future.

References

1. Kjeldsen AD, Vase P, Green A. Hereditary haemorrhagic telangiectasia: a population-based study of prevalence and mortality in Danish patients. J Intern Med 1999;245:31-39.
2. Hanes F. Multiple hereditary telangiectasias causing hemorrhage (hereditary haemorrhagic telangiectasias). Bull Johns Hopkins Hosp 1909;20:63-73.
3. Sharathkumar AA, Shapiro A. Hereditary haemorrhagic telangiectasia. Haemophilia 2008;14:1269-1280.
4. Yuan J, Wu X, Zhao J, et al. Molecular mechanisms and clinical manifestations of hereditary hemorrhagic telangiectasia. Thromb Res. 2024;241:109117.
5. Govani FS, Shovlin CL. Hereditary haemorrhagic telangiectasia: A clinical and scientific review. Eur J Hum Genet 2009;17:860-871
6. Balachandar S, Graves TJ, Shimonty A, et al. Identification and validation of a novel pathogenic variant in *GDF2* (*BMP9*) responsible for hereditary hemorrhagic telangiectasia and pulmonary arteriovenous malformations. Am J Med Genet A. 2022;188:959-964.
7. Farhan A, Yuan F, Partan E, Weiss CR. Clinical manifestations of patients with *GDF2* mutations associated with hereditary hemorrhagic telangiectasia type 5. Am J Med Genet A. 2022;188:199-209.
8. Ola R, Hessels J, Hammill A, et al. Executive summary of the 14th HHT international scientific conference. Angiogenesis. 2023;26(Suppl 1):27-37.
9. Jackson SB, Villano NP, Benhammou JN, et al. Gastrointestinal manifestations of hereditary

hemorrhagic telangiectasia (HHT): A systematic review of the literature. Dig Dis Sci. 2017;62(10):2623-2630.
10. Hammill AM, Wusik K, Kasthuri RS. Hereditary hemorrhagic telangiectasia (HHT): A practical guide to management. Hematology Am Soc Hematol Educ Program. 2021;2021(1):469-477.
11. Faughnan ME, Mager JJ, Hetts SW, et al. Second international guidelines for the diagnosis and management of hereditary hemorrhagic telangiectasia. Ann Intern Med. 2020;173:989-1001.
12. Bollinger E, Raines DL, Saitta P. Distribution of bleeding gastrointestinal angioectasias in a Western Population. World J Gastroenterol. 2012;18(43):6235-9.
13. Garcia-Tsao G. Liver involvement in hereditary hemorrhagic telangiectasia (HHT). J Hepatol 2007;46:499-507
14. Anderson E, Sharma L, Alsafi A, Shovlin CL. Pulmonary arteriovenous malformations may be the only clinical criterion present in genetically confirmed hereditary haemorrhagic telangiectasia. Thorax. 2022;77:628-630.
15. Shovlin CL, Guttmacher AE, Buscarini E, et al. Diagnostic criteria for hereditary hemorrhagic telangiectasia (Rendu-Osler-Weber syndrome). Am J Med Genet 2000;91:66-67.
16. McDonald J, Bayrak-Toydemir P, DeMille D, Wooderchak-Donahue W, Whitehead K. Curaçao diagnostic criteria for hereditary hemorrhagic telangiectasia is highly predictive of a pathogenic variant in *ENG* or *ACVRL1* (HHT1 and HHT2). Genet Med. 2020;22(7):1201-1205.
17. Joyce KE, Onabanjo E, Brownlow S. Whole genome sequences discriminate hereditary hemorrhagic telangiectasia phenotypes by non-HHT deleterious DNA variation. Blood Adv. 2022; 6:3956-3969.
18. Ingrosso M, Sabba C, Pisani A, et al. Evidence of small-bowel involvement in hereditary hemorrhagic telangiectasia: A capsule-endoscopic study. Endoscopy 2004;36:1074-1079.
19. Mora-Luján JM, Iriarte A, Alba E, et al. Gastrointestinal bleeding in patients with hereditary hemorrhagic telangiectasia: Risk factors and endoscopic findings. J Clin Med. 2019;9(1):82.
20. Chamberlain SM, Patel J, Carter Balart J, Gossage JR Jr, Sridhar S. Evaluation of patients with hereditary hemorrhagic telangiectasia with video capsule endoscopy: a single-center prospective study. Endoscopy. 2007 Jun;39(6):516-20.
21. Greve E, Moussata D, Gaudin JL, et al. High diagnostic and clinical impact of small-bowel capsule endoscopy in patients with hereditary hemorrhagic telangiectasia with overt digestive bleeding and/or severe anemia. Gastrointest Endosc 2010;71:760-767
22. Houghton KD, Umar B, Schairer J. Successful treatment of hereditary hemorrhagic telangiectasia with octreotide. ACG Case Rep J. 2019;6:e00088.
23. Harrison L, Kundra A, Jervis P. The use of thalidomide therapy for refractory epistaxis in hereditary haemorrhagic telangiectasia: Systematic review. J Laryngol Otol. 2018;132:866-871
24. Al-Samkari H. Systemic antiangiogenic therapies for bleeding in hereditary hemorrhagic telangiectasia: A practical, evidence-based guide for clinicians. Semin Thromb Hemost. 2022;48:514-528.
25. Chen H, Wu S, Tang M, et al. Thalidomide for recurrent bleeding due to small-intestinal angiodysplasia. N Engl J Med. 2023;389(18):1649-1659.

Case Study Number 3

Presented by Muna Okafor MD, Brian Pae, Shirley Paski MD, and Michelle Kang Kim MD, PhD

Pre-capsule Findings (included in capsule study)

A 48-year-old man with no significant past medical history is transferred to your hospital for continued evaluation of overt gastrointestinal bleeding of suspected small bowel origin. He initially presented to a local ER with multiple (6) episodes of bloody stool with large clots over the preceding 24 hours. Initial serologic testing was remarkable for a hemoglobin of 6.9 gm/dl. An emergent CT angiogram was performed and negative for sources of active bleeding. Two units of packed red blood cells were transfused prior to endoscopic evaluation by standard EGD and colonoscopy. Colonoscopy demonstrated dark red blood throughout the colon and lumen of the terminal ileum ~20cm proximal to the ileocecal valve.

You complete an independent assessment upon the patient's arrival at your facility. The patient admits to ongoing episodes of hematochezia but denies any history of abdominal pain, fever, vomiting, or weight loss. He does not consume NSAIDs in any form. His physical exam is benign with a soft, non-tender abdomen.

An inpatient capsule endoscopy study is performed to evaluate for small bowel bleeding. Review the capsule endoscopy study and report your findings, including gastric passage time, small bowel passage time, and observed abnormalities. Be prepared to discuss your findings and management plan with your staff prior to reviewing the diagnosis and case discussion.

Capsule Endoscopy Findings
First Gastric Image = 0h 0min 34sec
First Duodenal Image = 2h 52min 34sec
Gastric passage time = 2h 52min
First Cecal Image = 3h 52min 36sec
Small bowel passage time = 1hr 0min

Visualization of the gastric mucosa is somewhat obscured by food and/or medication residue within the lumen. Following entry into the duodenum, the capsule transits quickly through the small bowel (1hr). In the distal ileum, a submucosal lesion associated with small amounts of red blood is observed (**Figure 1 and 2**: 3hr 48min 19sec). The lesion is characterized by a central cleft.

Figure 1

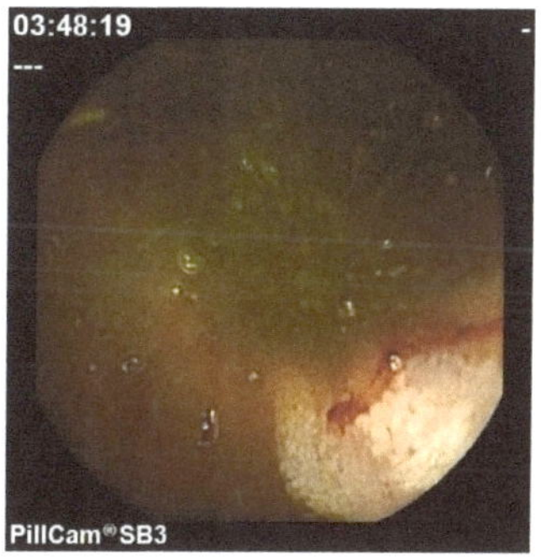

Figure 2

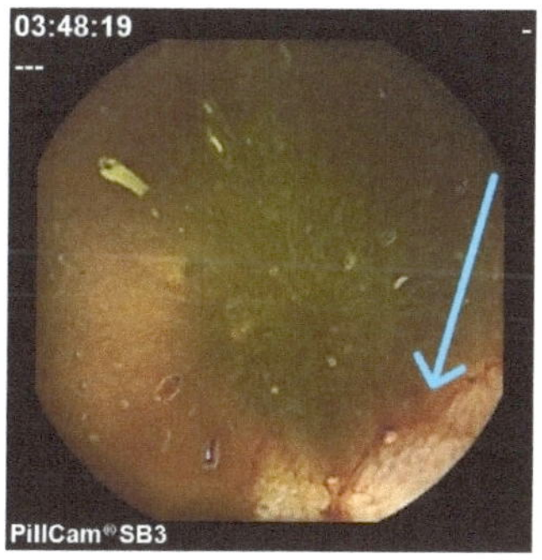

Follow-up

A retrograde double balloon enteroscopy (DBE) exam is performed the following day after completion of a full lavage bowel preparation. The submucosal lesion observed in the distal ileum is found ~50 cm proximal to the ileocecal valve **(Figure 3)**. The lesion is biopsied and marked with an submucosal India Ink tattoo. DBE examination of the mid and proximal ileum up to 250 cm proximal to the ileocecal valve is negative for additional pathology. Histology confirms a diagnosis of well-differentiated neuroendocrine tumor (carcinoid) with a Ki-67 score of 2%.

Figure 3.

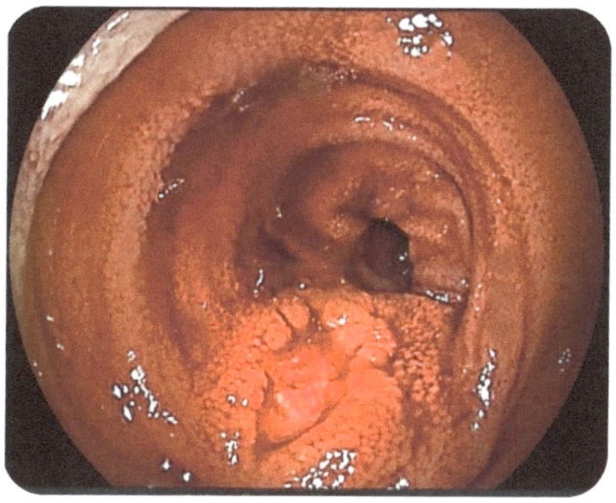

Chapter 3: Midgut Neuroendocrine Tumors

Muna Okafor, MD, Brian Pae, Shirley Paski, MD, and Michelle Kang Kim, MD, PhD

Introduction

Neuroendocrine tumors (NETs) are an increasingly common cancer and are particularly common in the small bowel. The incidence of all NETs has increased substantially in recent decades, from 1.6 per 100,000 people in 1975 to 9.6 per 100,000 people in 2022, with a 6-fold increase in the small bowel NETs.[1] The favorable long-term survival outcomes of NET patients resuls in a high 20-year prevalence (99,678 estimated cases),[2] exceeding the prevelance of esophageal, gastric, and pancreatic cancers combined.[3]

NETs arise from pluripotent stem cells that differentiate into enterochromaffin (EC) cells, which are primarily located within the gut wall, but can also be found in the bronchus, lungs, pancreas, and ovaries.[4] NETs are classified into foregut, midgut, and hindgut subtypes based on their embryologic origin. Midgut NETs arise from the distal duodenum, jejunum, ileum, appendix, and right colon—where EC cells are most concentrated.[5] Although NETs may be associated with a wide range of biologic behavior, they are often slow-growing, and less than 10% present as functionally active tumors.[6] Many NETs remain clinically indolent and asymptomatic for years, sometimes presenting with advanced or metastatic disease.

Clinical Presentation

When symptomatic, midgut NETs typically present with nonspecific gastrointestinal symptoms such as intermittent abdominal pain, changes in bowel habits, bloating, or unintentional weight loss.[7] Patients frequently experience longstanding gastrointestinal symptoms and undergo multiple evaluations by primary care providers before referral to a gastroenterologist, often leading to a misdiagnosis of irritable bowel syndrome (IBS).[7] These symptoms may persist for years, delaying diagnosis. A high index of suspicion is warranted in patients with persistent, unexplained IBS-like symptoms who do not respond to conventional management. Midgut NETs may often present with GI bleeding or obstructive symptoms.[7]

Some midgut NETs are associated with carcinoid syndrome, a condition characterized by secretory diarrhea, episodic flushing, bronchospasm, and in advanced cases, right-sided valvular heart disease.[8] Carcinoid syndrome develops when serotonin-producing NETs metastasize to the liver, allowing serotonin to bypass hepatic metabolism and enter the systemic circulation.[9]

Diagnosis

Diagnosis of NETs involves the use of a variety of studies, including serologic testing, imaging, endoscopy, and histology. These studies are often used in combination for assessment of prognosis and staging in addition to initial diagnosis.

Biomarkers

Biomarkers which are useful in the evaluation of midgut NETs include serum chromogranin A (CgA), urinary or serum 5-hydroxyindoleacetic acid (5-HIAA), and serum pancreastatin. CgA is commonly used to estimate tumor burden, but it is nonspecific and can be affected by factors like proton pump inhibitor (PPI) use or renal dysfunction.[10] PPIs can falsely elevate CgA levels by inducing hypergastrinemia; discontinuing PPIs for at least 2 weeks before testing is recommended when feasible.[11] 5-HIAA is a metabolite of serotonin used to assess the tumor's amine production and the likelihood of carcinoid syndrome.[12] Patients undergoing 24-hour urine collection for 5-HIAA should avoid serotonin-rich foods such as bananas, avocados, tomatoes, eggplant, pineapples, kiwi, melons, and nuts for at least 24 hours prior to and during collection, as these can falsely elevate results.[13] Serotonergic medications like acetaminophen, guaifenesin, caffeine, and alcohol should also be withheld when possible to improve test accuracy.[14] Pancreastatin levels have been shown to correlate with tumor burden, prognosis, and disease progression in midgut NETs. Compared to CgA, pancreastatin levels are less likely to be affected by PPI use. Caution should be taken when using biomarkers to exclude a diagnosis of midgut NET, but they may be helpful in tracking disease in patients with known disease.

Imaging

Imaging with triple-phase contrast-enhanced CT of the chest, abdomen, and pelvis should be performed as the initial modality to assess disease extent[15] **(Figure 1)**. While CT is preferred for assessing

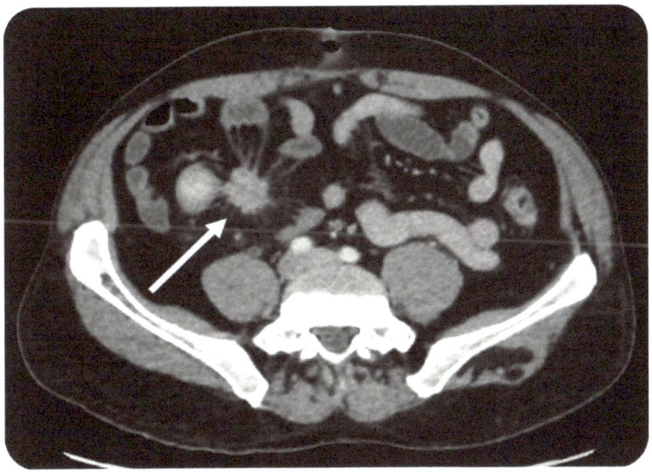

Figure 1. CT scan showing mesenteric mass in a patient with midgut NET.[26]

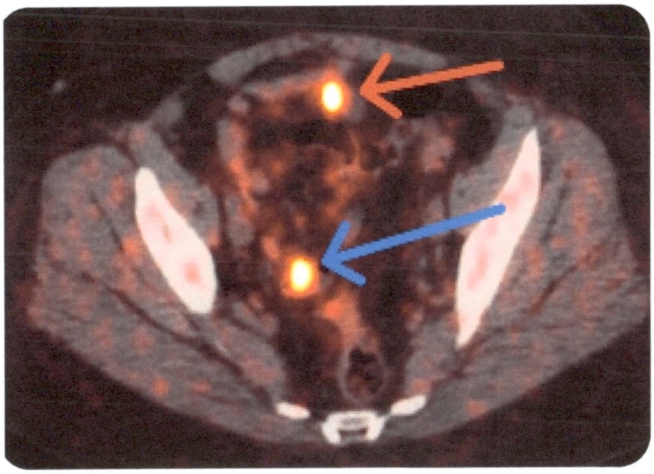

Figure 2. 64Cu-DOTATATE PET/CT scan demonstrating somatostatin receptor–avid midgut neuroendocrine tumor (red arrow) and associated nodal metastasis (blue arrow)

extrahepatic disease, liver metastases are best evaluated using MRI with gadoxetate disodium (Eovist).[16] Somatostatin receptor–based functional imaging is an essential component of NET evaluation. Gallium-68 (^{68}Ga)-DOTATATE and Copper-64 (^{64}Cu)-DOTATATE PET/CT are preferred due to their high sensitivity, improved spatial resolution, and reduced radiation exposure compared to conventional somatostatin receptor scintigraphy (OctreoScan)[16] (**Figure 2**). These radiotracers bind somatostatin receptor subtypes 2 and 5, facilitating more accurate detection of primary tumors, nodal involvement, and distant metastases. Careful interpretation is required to distinguish physiologic uptake from true tumor activity, as colonic tracer retention is a source of false-positive result.

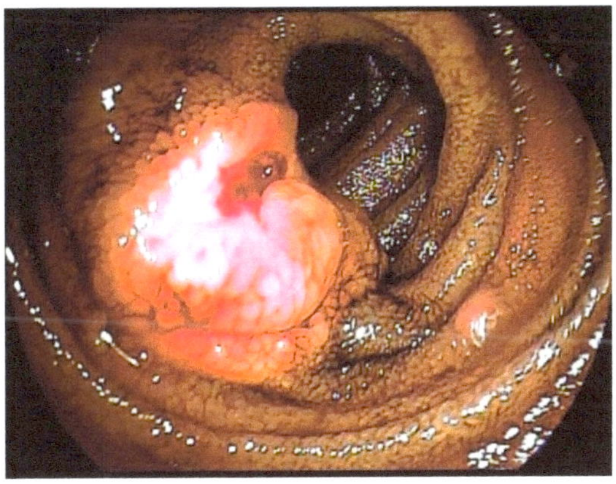

Figure 3. Endoscopic visualization of a midgut NET by retrograde DBE.

Endoscopy

Midgut NETs are often submucosal and can be detected by video capsule endoscopy and device-assisted enteroscopy[18] (**Figure 3**). Endoscopy is also useful in evaluating synchronous or metachronous lesions to guiding surgical planning for resection. These tumors may appear as solitary submucosal nodules or multifocal lesions (**Figure 4a & b**).[19]

Oncologic Assessment

Tumor Staging

Staging of midgut NETs is performed using the American Joint Committee on Cancer, Tumor, Node, Metastasis (TNM) staging system, which incorporates tumor size, nodal involvement, and presence of distant metastases.[20] The regional lymph nodes and liver are the most common sites of metastasis in midgut NETs. While tumor size may be an important predictor of regional or metastatic disease, it is notable that even small (≤1 cm), well-differentiated (G1) neuroendocrine tumors in these locations carry a substantial risk of regional lymph node metastasis, warranting a surgical resection with systematic lymph node evaluation.[5]

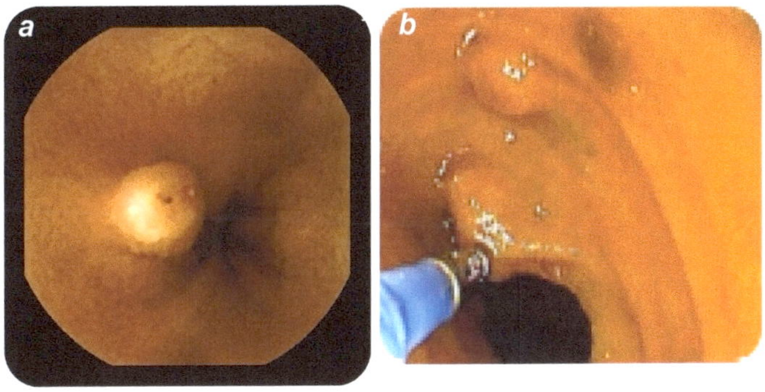

Figure 4. Multiple primary NETs identified by video capsule endoscopy (a) then device-assisted enteroscopy (b).

Metastasis to less typical locations, such as breast and thyroid, have been reported and may lead to diagnostic confusion with more common primary malignancies.[21] Given that a substantial number of patients present with advanced-stage disease, specifically with hepatic metastases, accurate staging at diagnosis is critical for determining therapeutic strategies and longitudinal surveillance.

Tumor Grading

Tumor grading is based on 2 histopathologic criteria: the degree of differentiation and the proliferative rate (**Table 1**). Most midgut NETs are well-differentiated and have a low proliferative index, placing them in the low-grade category. Accurate grading begins with visual examination of the tumor histology, noting features such as mitotic figures (reported as the number of mitoses per 10 high-power fields), lymphatic or neural invasion, and overall architectural differentiation.[22] Immunohistochemical (IHC) staining for Ki-67 using the MIB-1 antibody is used to quantify the proliferative index and is reported as the percentage of tumor cells with nuclear staining.[21] The Ki-67 index is an important determinant of tumor grade and correlates with clinical behavior. Additional IHC staining for neuroendocrine markers, such as CgA, helps confirm neuroendocrine differentiation and supports accurate classification.

Treatment

Treatment decisions require a holistic evaluation of the patient, including comorbidities, symptom severity, tumor stage, and tumor grade. Current guidelines emphasize the importance of integrating tumor grade, functional status, and overall disease burden when formulating a management plan. The mainstay of treatment for primary ileal, jejunal, or other small bowel NETs is surgical resection with extended lymph node dissection.[2] In patients with multiple jejunal or ileal primaries, the key surgical objective is to preserve bowel length while maximizing the chance of long-term survival. Surgical resection of the primary, even in the presence of liver metastases, may be considered in select patients.[23]

The North American Neuroendocrine Tumor Society recommends somatostatin analogs (SSAs), such as octreotide or lanreotide depot injections, for well-differentiated, unresectable, or metastatic midgut NETs to delay tumor progression. For patients with progressive disease despite SSAs, peptide receptor radionuclide therapy (PRRT) may be considered for somatostatin receptor–positive tumors.[24]

Surveillance

Patients with midgut NETs require long-term surveillance using serial plasma CgA, urinary or serum 5-HIAA, and cross-sectional imaging such as triple-phase CT and liver MRI with gadoxetate disodium.[25] Functional imaging with somatostatin receptor–based PET/CT, using either Gallium-68 or Copper-64 DOTATATE, offers superior sensitivity for detecting metastatic or recurrent disease and is increasingly used for routine follow-up.

Grade	Histologic Criteria	Mitotic Count (per mm3)	Ki-67 index (%)	Differentiation	Clinical Behavior
1	NET G1	< 2	< 3%	Well-differentiated	Usually indolent
2	NET G2	2-20	3 - 20%	Well-differentiated	Intermediate behavior
3	NET G3	> 20	> 20%	Well-differentiated	Aggressive, but retains NET morphology
3	NEC	> 20	> 20%	Poorly-differentiated	Highly aggressive, rapid progression

Table 1. World Health Organization NET Grading Classification[12]
NEC, neuroendocrine carcinoma; NET, neuroendocrine tumor.

References

1. Unpublished data analysis using SEER 8 (1975–2022). Surveillance, Epidemiology, and End Results (SEER) Program. National Cancer Institute. Accessed [July 2025]. SEER*Stat software, version [9.0.40.1].
2. Unpublished data analysis using SEER 12 (1998–2017). Surveillance, Epidemiology, and End Results (SEER) Program. National Cancer Institute. Accessed [July 2025]. SEER*Stat software, version [9.0.40.1].
3. Kunz PL. Understanding Neuroendocrine Tumors-A NET Gain. JAMA Oncol. 2017 Oct 1;3(10):1343-1344.
4. Niederle B, Pape UF, Costa F, et al. ENETS Consensus Guidelines Update for Neuroendocrine Neoplasms of the Jejunum and Ileum. Neuroendocrinology. 2016;103(2):125-38.
5. Boudreaux JP, Klimstra DS, Hassan MM, et al. The NANETS consensus guideline for well-differentiated neuroendocrine tumors of the jejunum, ileum, appendix, and cecum. Pancreas. 2010;39(6):753–766
6. Dasari A, Shen C, Halperin D, et al. Trends in the incidence, prevalence, and survival outcomes in patients with neuroendocrine tumors in the United States. JAMA Oncol. 2017;3(10):1335–1342
7. Basuroy R, Bouvier C, Ramage JK, Sissons M, Srirajaskanthan R. Delays and routes to diagnosis of neuroendocrine tumours. BMC Cancer. 2018;16;18(1):1122.
8. Modlin IM, Sandor A. An analysis of 8305 cases of carcinoid tumors. Cancer. 1997;15;79(4):813-29.
9. Ito T, Lee L, Jensen RT. Carcinoid-syndrome: recent advances, current status and controversies. Curr Opin Endocrinol Diabetes Obes. 2018;25(1):22-35.
10. Tseng CM, Cheng TY, Chen TB, et al. Low accuracy of chromogranin A for diagnosing early-stage pancreatic neuroendocrine tumors. Oncol Lett. 2018;15(6):8951-8958.
11. Arnold R, Wilke A, Rinke A, et al. Plasma chromogranin A as marker for survival in patients with metastatic endocrine gastroenteropancreatic tumors. Clin Gastroenterol Hepatol. 2008 Jul;6(7):820-7.
12. Nagtegaal ID, Odze RD, Klimstra D, et al. The 2019 WHO classification of tumours of the digestive system. Histopathology. 2020;76(2):182-188.
13. Gedde-Dahl M, Thiis-Evensen E, Tjølsen AM, Mordal KS, Vatn M, Bergestuen DS. Comparison of 24-h and overnight samples of urinary 5-hydroxyindoleacetic acid in patients with intestinal neuroendocrine tumors. Endocr Connect. 2013;2(1):50-4.
14. Pavel M, Jann H, Prasad V, Drozdov I, Modlin IM, Kidd M. NET Blood Transcript Analysis Defines the Crossing of the Clinical Rubicon: When Stable Disease Becomes Progressive. Neuroendocrinology. 2017104(2):170-182.
15. Singh S, Poon R, Wong R, Metser U. ^{68}Ga PET imaging in patients with neuroendocrine tumors: A systematic review and meta-analysis. Clin Nucl Med. 2018;43(11):802-810.
16. Barrio M, Czernin J, Fanti S. The Impact of Somatostatin Receptor-Directed PET/CT on the Management of Patients with Neuroendocrine Tumor. J Nucl Med. 2017;58(5):756-761.
17. Deprez PH, Moons LMG, O'Toole D, et al. Endoscopic management of subepithelial lesions including neuroendocrine neoplasms: European Society of Gastrointestinal Endoscopy (ESGE) Guideline. Endoscopy. 2022;54(4):412-429.
18. Standards of Practice Committee; Faulx AL, Kothari S, Acosta RD, et al. The role of endoscopy in subepithelial lesions of the GI tract. Gastrointest Endosc. 2017;85(6):1117-1132.
19. MB Amin, SB Edge, FL Greene, et al, eds. AJCC Cancer Staging Manual. 8th ed. New York: Springer; 2017.
20. Norlén O, Stålberg P, Öberg K, et al Long-term results of surgery for small intestinal neuroendocrine tumors at a tertiary referral center. World J Surg. 2012;36(6):1419-31.
21. Howe JR, Cardona K, Fraker DL, et al. The surgical management of small bowel neuroendocrine tumors: Consensus Guidelines of the North American Neuroendocrine Tumor Society. Pancreas. 2017;46(6):715-731.
22. Shah MH, Goldner WS, Benson AB, et al. Neuroendocrine and adrenal tumors, version 2.2021, NCCN Clinical Practice Guidelines in Oncology. J Natl Compr Canc Netw. 2021;19(7):839-868.
23. Gangi A, Manguso N, Gong J, et al. Midgut neuroendocrine tumors with liver-only metastases: Benefit of primary tumor resection. Ann Surg Oncol. 2020;27(11):4525-4532. Erratum in: Ann Surg Oncol. 2021 Dec;28(Suppl 3):872.
24. Strosberg JR, Halfdanarson TR, Bellizzi AM, et al. The North American Neuroendocrine Tumor Society consensus guidelines for surveillance and medical management of midgut neuroendocrine tumors. Pancreas. 2017;46(6):707-714.
25. Turner GB, Johnston BT, McCance DR, McGinty A, Watson RG, Patterson CC, Ardill JE. Circulating markers of prognosis and response to treatment in patients with midgut carcinoid tumours. Gut. 2006;55(11):1586-91.
26. Hofland J, de Herder WW. Gastrointestinal neuroendocrine tumors and the carcinoid syndrome. In: Feingold KR, Ahmed SF, Anawalt B, et al. (eds). Dartmouth, MA; Endotext [Internet]. MDText.com, Inc.; 2020. Updated Aug 25, 2023.

Case Study Number 4

Presented by David R. Cave, MD, PhD, FACG

Pre-capsule Findings (included in capsule study)

An 80-year old man with a history of coronary artery disease, ischemic stroke and osteoarthritis presents for additional evaluation of a 2-year history of iron deficiency anemia associated with heme-positive stool. The patient has no complaints other than fatigue associated with his anemia. He denies any history of abdominal pain, diarrhea, change in bowel habits, melena or weight loss. He has no family members who have been diagnosed with celiac disease or inflammatory bowel disease. Review of systems is unremarkable except for chronic bilateral knee pain and anemia. Evaluation by EGD and colonoscopy are unrevealing for sources of gastrointestinal blood loss.

A capsule endoscopy study is performed to evaluate for small bowel bleeding. Review the capsule endoscopy study and report your findings, including: gastric passage time, small bowel passage time, and observed abnormalities. Be prepared to discuss your findings and management plan with your staff prior to reviewing the diagnosis and case discussion.

Study recording begins in the stomach. The capsule encounters an abnormal segment in the deep small bowel, around 2 hours into the recording. Within this segment, multiple circular stenoses are observed. Several stenoses are associated with thin marginal ulceration (**Figure 1:** 2hr 15min 54sec; **Figure 2:** 2hr 16min 11sec; **Figure 3:** 2hr 45min 7sec). The capsule is held in this segment for nearly 2 hours until passing into the distal bowel around 3hrs 52min into the recording. Visualization of the distal small bowel limited due to luminal residue; however, entry into the cecum is clearly identified at 7 hours 3 minutes.

Follow-up

Capsule Endoscopy Findings
First Duodenal Image = 0h 7min 2sec
First Cecal Image = 7h 3min 33sec
Small bowel passage time = 6hr 56min

Figure 1

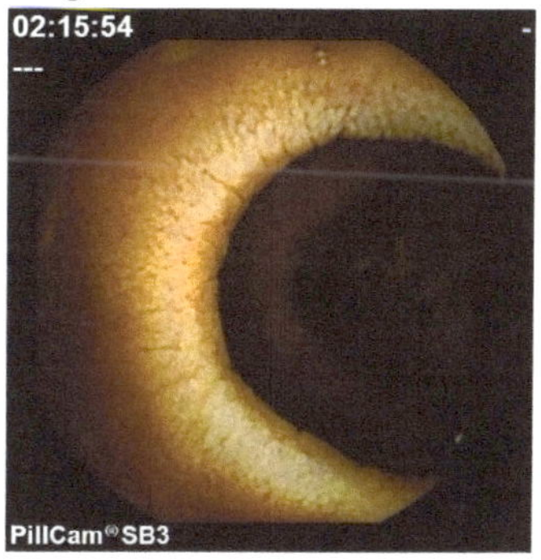

Figure 2

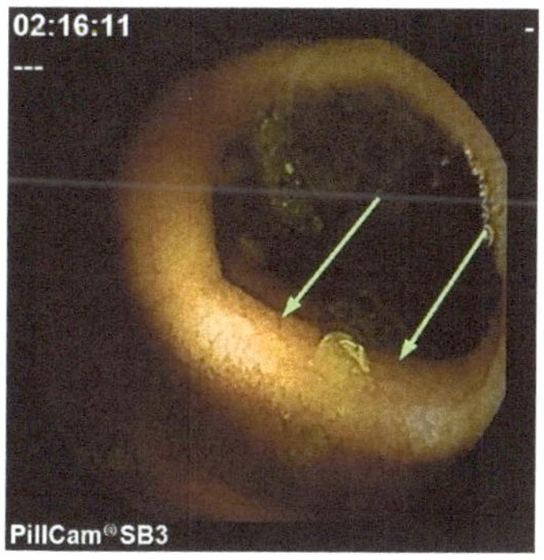

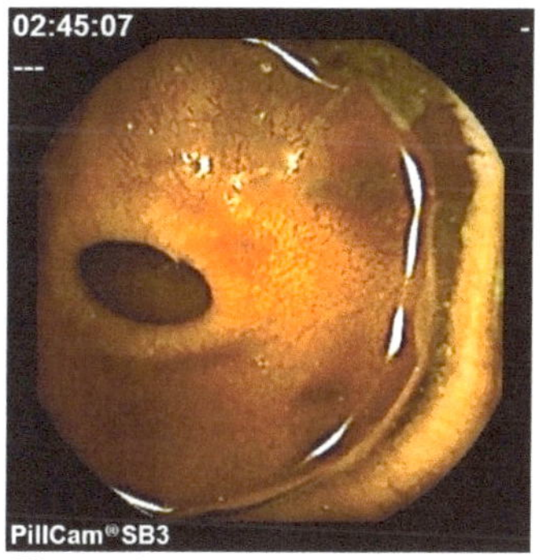

Figure 3

The patient underwent a retrograde double balloon enteroscopy (DBE) exam to further investigate the lesions identified on video capsule endoscopy (VCE). DBE confirmed the presence of multiple thin diaphragm-like strictures in the mid ileum, each associated with well-defined ulceration along the rim (**Figure 4**) . Endoscopic biopsies were obtained, and the most distal lesion was marked with an India ink tattoo. Histopathologic review was consistent with a diagnosis of NSAID inury and negative for features of Crohn's disease. Management included discontinuation of NSAIDs and initiation of misoprostol 200 mcg orally 4 times per day for 8 weeks. At 6-month follow-up, the patient's repeat hemoglobin returned to normal (14 g/dL) with improvement in iron stores.

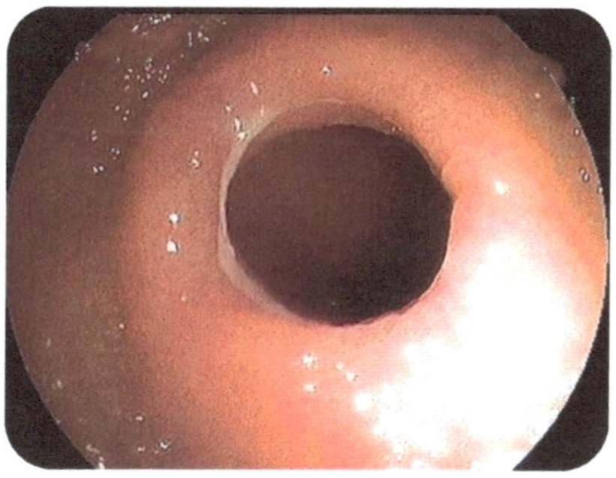
Figure 4

Chapter 4: NSAID-Induced Enteropathy

David R. Cave, MD, PhD, FACG

Epidemiology

Nonsteroidal anti-inflammatory drug (NSAID) ingestion has been known to cause injury of the gastrointestinal tract for many years. Of the 14 million people in the United States who use an NSAID on a regular basis, up to 60% will have gastrointestinal side effects related to these drugs. Vulnerability to these lesions increases with age, particularly in those over 65 years of age, due to the diminution of constitutive prostaglandin production.[1,2] While the gastro-duodenal aspects of the injury are well understood and widely reported, relatively little attention has been paid to the small intestine, largely due to its inaccessibility.

Since 2001, wireless VCE and deep enteroscopy have allowed much better visual access to the small bowel mucosa and direct visualization of "diaphragm disease" associated with NSAID injury. This condition is probably idiosyncratic for NSAID injury and was described in the pre-VCE era in patients requiring surgery for severe anemia and symptoms of intestinal obstruction.[3] After the advent of VCE, the prevalence of more subtle but more frequent types of NSAID-induced small bowel injury was investigated in several prospective studies.

In a large prospective study, Goldstein et al compared small bowel injury caused by a conventional NSAID (naproxen) and a Cox 2 inhibitor (celecoxib) versus placebo.[4] About 400 volunteers not on aspirin or NSAIDs underwent baseline VCE then were randomized to 3 groups taking naproxen, celecoxib or placebo for 2 weeks followed by repeat capsule study. The prevalence of small bowel mucosal breaks was significantly higher in the naproxen group (55%) compared to the celecoxib group (16%) or placebo group (7%).

A second smaller study by Graham et al[5] used capsule endoscopy to assess the extent of small bowel mucosal injury among 41 patients who were chronic NSAID users (3 months duration) and found that 71% of them had evidence of small-bowel injury compared with 10% of controls. Maiden et al[6] showed that of 68 healthy volunteers, 75% had small bowel injury after ingestion of diclofenac for 2 weeks. This study also demonstrated that concurrent administration of proton pump inhibitors was an ineffective strategy in protecting the small bowel from NSAID injury. These 3 studies demonstrate that NSAID injury in the small bowel is common; however, the clinical significance of these findings is still unclear.

Pathogenesis of NSAID Injury

The etiology of the injury caused by NSAIDs in the small intestine is believed to be the same as that which causes gastro-duodenal injury, through cyclo-oxygenase (Cox) enzyme inhibition. The Cox 1 enzyme is constitutive, and is known to increase mucus production, epithelial cell turnover, blood flow, and bicarbonate secretion. These effects have only been studied in the stomach and duodenum but are assumed to translate to the small intestine. The Cox 2 enzyme is inducible and associated with cytokine production and inflammation. It is likely that inhibition of the Cox 1 enzyme in the small intestine reduces the ability of the small bowel mucosa to repair itself, which in turn can lead to a spectrum of injury including mucosal breaks, villous denudation, erosions and ulceration. The distribution of these lesions along the length of small bowel seems to vary between individuals; however Fujimori et al showed that the impact of short-term NSAID medication on the site of small bowel injury differed according to type of lesion, with most denuded areas identified in the proximal part and all ulcers in the distal part.[7] Diaphragm disease, the extreme version of this injury, primarily occurs in the distal ileum but can occur throughout the small intestine. Multiple small bowel diaphragms may be seen in some cases with one previous report of 23 diaphragms in a single patient.[8] There are limited reports of the induction of diaphragms in the colon as well.

Pathological Findings

Minor injuries to the small intestine are very non-specific and most of the pathological changes of NSAID-induced enteropathy have been described in association with diaphragm disease. Macroscopically, these diaphragms are usually short in length and may be diaphanous. They are usually ulcerated on the inner aspect of the ring. On the serosal surface of the small intestine, there may be evidence of dimpling at the site of the rings but there is no advancement of the mesenteric fat as seen in Crohn's disease. It should be noted that thin rings may collapse when the surgical specimen is opened so gross specimens should be fixed in formalin prior to being incised.

NSAID injury is limited to the mucosa and may start as a mucosal break with nonspecific inflammatory changes. The mucosal break is associated with varying degrees of lymphocyte and plasma cell infiltration with subsequent ulceration which is superficial but clearly demarcated. Focal expansion of the smooth muscle of the muscularis mucosae is a significant pathologic characteristic that is followed by fibrotic changes and ensuing ulceration of the tip of the diaphragm.[3,9] Concentric or isolated ulcers are typically associated with oozing of blood rather than massive hemorrhage that may be seen in association with peptic ulcer disease.[10]

Clinical Presentation

The majority of small bowel injuries associated with NSAID injury are minor and asymptomatic. In cases of more significant disease, patients typically present with iron deficiency anemia due to chronic blood loss associated with mucosal ulceration. Obstructive symptoms in conjunction with iron deficiency anemia due to diaphragm-like strictures in the small intestine are less common. Finally, protein losing enteropathy may develop in rare cases.[11]

Advanced age is a recognized risk factor for NSAID enteropathy and risk increases due to reduction in prostaglandin production, particularly after 65 years of age.[1,2] Use of 2 or more NSAIDs is also associated with increased risk of injury. For example, adding aspirin to any other nonselective NSAID results in an 8-fold increase in the risk of injury compared to not adding aspirin. Other risk factors include: higher doses of NSAIDs, a history of gastro-duodenal ulcer or gastrointestinal bleeding, concomitant use of corticosteroids, serious coexisting conditions, and concomitant use of anticoagulants. The quantity of NSAID consumption appears to be quite variable for the development of diaphragm disease, but generally, long-term usage is required. Interestingly, the relative risk of injury associated with aspirin is not reduced for enteric coated products.[2]

Diagnosis

The most important aspect of the diagnosis of small bowel injury by NSAIDs is a good history. In the gastroenterologist's clinic setting, this diagnosis is worth considering in an older patient who walks into the office using a cane and reports a history of iron deficiency anemia. NSAID use is commonly underreported. Sidhu et al showed that, of patients who undergo CE, 13.6% took NSAIDs but most did not declare using these medications.[11] Patients should be questioned about use of over-the-counter medications, and urinalysis for NSAID metabolites may be helpful.[12] The use of NSAIDs does not have to be current, but may have stopped many months prior to presentation. This is particularly true of diaphragm disease where the ulceration is subtle and it may take a long time for a severe iron deficiency anemia to develop.

The use of small bowel barium studies in the diagnosis of diaphragm disease has proved very disappointing as has the use of CT enterography. The reason for this is that the diaphragms are usually circumferential and short so that they cannot be distinguished from the normal valvulae conniventes. Thus, the most effective way of detecting these diaphragms or any of the more subtle mucosal injuries in association with NSAIDs is VCE or deep enteroscopy. In someone who has taken large amounts of NSAIDs over a long period, it is appropriate to use a patency capsule prior to the deployment of a regular video capsule, since retention of the video capsule is likely to occur. The inner diameter of a diaphragm lesion may as small as 5 mm before it becomes symptomatic while the video capsule is 11 mm in diameter. Diaphragm lesions which obstruct the bowel may be amenable to dilation if accessible by DBE.[12,13]

Differential Diagnosis

The differential diagnosis of ulcerative disease of the small intestine is quite extensive and listed in **Table 1**.

It is important to note that clinical presentation can be just as important as endoscopic findings in differentiating NSAID injury from other small bowel disorders. The most common cause of confusion is Crohn's disease which can cause ulceration, stenosis, erosion, aphthoid ulceration and villous denudation. The ulcers associated with Crohn's disease tend to be deep and serpiginous, surrounded by edematous villi, whereas NSAID ulcers tend to have clearly demarcated edges without surrounding edema (**Figure 1**). The stenoses in Crohn's disease also tend to be much longer, and because the inflammation is transmural, there is associated wall thickening that is not seen with NSAID injury. Another pair of diseases termed chronic multifocal ulcerative stenosing enteritis [CMUSE] or chronic nonspecific stenosing ulcerative enteritis [CNSU][14,15] —and more recently in the U.S. chronic stenosing enteritis[16] — produce large, superficial ulcers and stenoses in the small bowel which recur after surgery. These 3 conditions, which probably have a common etiology, present with iron deficiency anemia and/or abdominal pain. Radiation enteritis tends to cause irregular stenoses and may involve a considerable length of small intestine with diffuse lymphangiectasia with sparse, white, deformed villi as a prominent feature. Drug-induced strictures, such as those caused by enteric coated potassium tablets are now rarely seen since the offending agents have been removed from the market.[17]

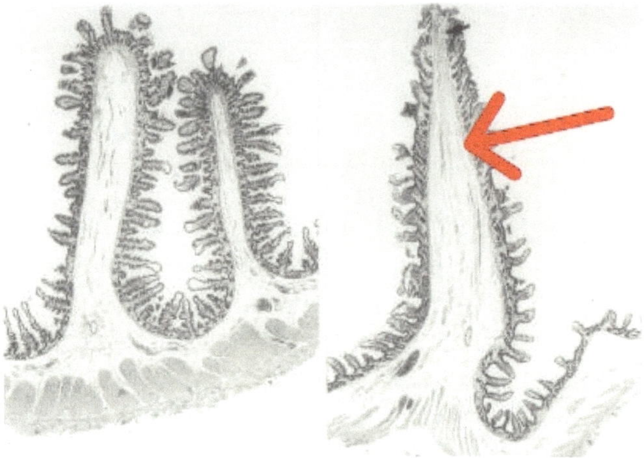

Figure 1. Normal plicae circulares are seen left. On the right, a cross section of a mucosal diaphragm caused by NSAID. Distinction is made by observing submucosal fibrosis in diaphragm lesion (red arrow).

Treatment

Treatment of the NSAID injury in the small intestine depends very much on the extent and severity of the lesion.[18,19] In those with iron deficiency or possible protein losing enteropathy, simply discontinuing NSAIDs may be sufficient for the condition to resolve spontaneously. However, once the diaphragms have become established the circumferential ulceration may remain as a persistent cause of iron deficiency anemia (**Figure 2**).

The effectiveness of misoprostol therapy for NSAID injury was demonstrated in a 2018 randomized, double-blind, placebo-controlled trial.[20] Patients received misoprostol 200 μg orally 4 times daily for 8 weeks or placebo and examined by VCE. The trial demonstrated that 54% of patients in the misoprostol group achieved complete healing of small bowel ulcers at 8 weeks, compared to 17% in the placebo group. Side effects of abdominal pain, diarrhea, and nausea occurred in 8% of the misoprostol group, but no serious adverse events were reported. These

Drug induced	Inflammatory conditions	Neoplasia
NSAID Injury	Crohn's Disease	Lymphoma
Asprin	Chronic stenosing enteritis (CSE)	Carcinoma
	Chronic multifocal ulcerative stenosing enteritis (CMUSE)	
	Chronic nonspecific stenosing ulcerative enteritis (CNSU)	
Enteric coated potassium tabs	Radiation enteritis	
	Bechet's disease	
	Eosinophilic gastroenteritis	
	Idiopathic	

Table 1. Differential diagnosis of ulcerative disease of the small intestine.

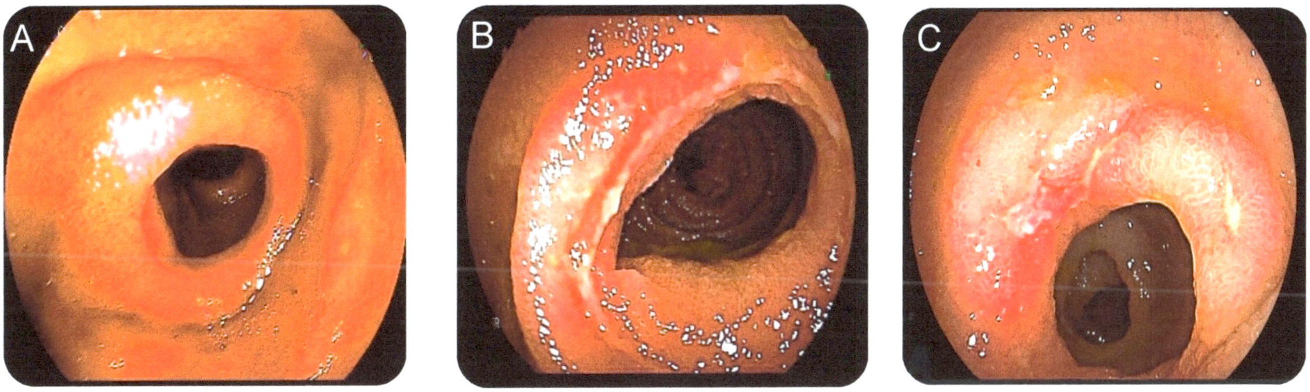

Figure 2. Serial examination of an NSAID diaphragm lesion of the mid ileum. Upon initial diagnosis (A), the diaphragm is sharply demarcated with a clean rim ulcer. Following withdrawal of NSAIDs, the diaphragm lesion heals partially at year 2 (B) and year 4 (C). However, it fails to completely heal despite avoidance of NSAIDs.

findings indicate that misoprostol therapy, if tolerated, is effective in promoting healing of small bowel ulcers related to NSAID injury.

If surgical resection is considered, it should be accompanied by use of intra-operative enteroscopy, since the strictures may be inapparent by inspection of the serosal surface of the small intestine.[14,15] As an alternative to intraoperative enteroscopy, proximal and distal margins of the diseased segment may be accessed by DBE and marked with an India Ink tattoo prior to segmental small bowel resection.

References

1. Cryer B, Redfern JS, Goldschmiedt M, Lee E, Feldman M. Effect of aging on gastric and duodenal mucosal prostaglandin concentrations in humans. Gastroenterology. 1992 ;102:1118-23.
2. Wolfe MM, Lichtenstein DR, Singh G. Gastrointestinal toxicity of nonsteroidal antiinflammatory drugs. N Engl J Med. 1999;340(24):1888-99.
3. Lang J, Price AB, Levi AJ, Burke M, Gumpel JM, Bjarnason I. Diaphragm disease: pathology of disease of the small intestine induced by non-steroidal anti-inflammatory drugs. J Clin Pathol. 1988;41(5):516-26.
4. Goldstein JL, Eisen GM, Lewis B, Gralnek IM, Zlotnick S, Fort JG; Investigators. Video capsule endoscopy to prospectively assess small bowel injury with celecoxib, naproxen plus omeprazole, and placebo. Clin Gastroenterol Hepatol. 2005;3(2):133-41.
5. Graham DY, Opekun AR, Willingham FF, Qureshi WA. Visible small-intestinal mucosal injury in chronic NSAID users. Clin Gastroenterol Hepatol. 2005;3(1):55-9.
6. Maiden L, Thjodleifsson B, Theodors A, Gonzalez J, Bjarnason I. A quantitative analysis of NSAID-induced small bowel pathology by capsule enteroscopy. Gastroenterology. 2005;128(5):1172-8.
7. Fujimori S, Gudis K, Takahashi Y, et al Distribution of small intestinal mucosal injuries as a result of NSAID administration. Eur J Clin Invest. 2010;40(6):504-10.
8. D'Agostino JA, Petros JG, Semegran AB, Cave DR, Lopez MJ. Complete intraoperative Sonde enteroscopy in the evaluation of recurrent partial small-bowel obstruction. Gastrointest Endosc. 1997;46(6):577-8.
9. De Petris G, López JI. Histopathology of diaphragm disease of the small intestine: A study of 10 cases from a single institution. Am J Clin Pathol. 2008;130(4):518-25.
10. Weil J, Langman MJ, Wainwright P, et al. Peptic ulcer bleeding: accessory risk factors and interactions with non-steroidal anti-inflammatory drugs. Gut. 2000 Jan;46(1):27-31.
11. Sidhu R, Brunt LK, Morley SR, Sanders DS, McAlindon ME. Undisclosed use of nonsteroidal anti-inflammatory drugs may underlie small-bowel injury observed by capsule endoscopy. Clin Gastroenterol Hepatol. 2010;8(11):992-5.
12. Hayashi Y, Yamamoto H, Kita H, et al. Non-steroidal anti-inflammatory drug-induced small bowel injuries identified by double-balloon endoscopy. World J Gastroenterol. 2005;11(31):4861-4.
13. Lopez MJ, Cooley JS, Petros JG, Sullivan JG, Cave DR. Complete intraoperative small-bowel endoscopy in the evaluation of occult gastrointestinal bleeding using the sonde enteroscope. Arch Surg. 1996;131(3):272-7.
14. Matsumoto T, Nakamura S, Esaki M, et al. Endoscopic features of chronic nonspecific multiple ulcers of the small intestine: Comparison with nonsteroidal anti-inflammatory drug-induced enteropathy. Dig Dis Sci 2006,51:1357-1363.
15. Matsumoto T, Kudo T, Esaki M, et al. Prevalence of non-steroidal anti-inflammatory drug-induced enteropathy determined by double-balloon endoscopy: a Japanese multicenter study. Scand J Gastroenterol. 2008;43(4):490-6.
16. Cave DR, Hanscom M, Bledsoe J, et al. Chronic stenosing enteritis: A variant of chronic non-specific stenosing ulceration (CNSU) that is distinct from Crohn's disease. Dig Dis Sci. 2025;70(4):1449-1456.
17. Baker DR, Schrader WH, Hitchcock CR. Small bowel

ulceration apparently associated with thiazide and potassium therapy. JAMA 1964,190:586-590.
18. Higuchi K, Umegaki E, Watanabe T, et al. Present status and strategy of NSAIDs-induced small bowel injury. J Gastroenterol. 2009;44(9):879-88.
19. Marlicz W, Loniewski I, Grimes DS, Quigley EM. Nonsteroidal anti-inflammatory drugs, proton pump inhibitors, and gastrointestinal injury: Contrasting interactions in the stomach and small intestine. Mayo Clin Proc. 2014;89(12):1699-709.
20. Taha AS, McCloskey C, McSkimming P, McConnachie A. Misoprostol for small bowel ulcers in patients with obscure bleeding taking aspirin and non-steroidal anti-inflammatory drugs (MASTERS): A randomised, double-blind, placebo-controlled, phase 3 trial. Lancet Gastroenterol Hepatol. 2018;3(7):469-476.

Case Study Number 5

Presented by Jose Aponte-Pieras, MD

Pre-capsule Findings (included in capsule study)

A 26-year-old man with a history of asthma is admitted to your hospital due to severe shortness of breath associated with anemia. The patient describes a 5-day history of shortness of breath with dyspnea upon exertion and associated fatigue. He denies wheezing or any recent flares of asthma. Laboratory studies obtained in the emergency room are notable for a hemoglobin of 6 gm/dl with a serum ferritin of 13 ng/ml (normal = 30-300 ng/ml). Following resuscitation with IVF's and 2 units of packed red blood cells, an upper endoscopy is performed and negative. A colonoscopy is completed the following day with small amounts of dark red blood identified in the colonic lumen. Intubation of the ileocecal valve for examination of the terminal ileum was attempted but unsuccessful.

An inpatient capsule endoscopy study is performed to evaluate for small bowel bleeding. Review the capsule endoscopy study and report your findings, including gastric passage time, small bowel passage time, and observed abnormalities. Be prepared to discuss your findings and management plan with your staff prior to reviewing the diagnosis and case discussion.

Capsule Endoscopy Findings
First Gastric Image = 0h 0min 38sec
First Duodenal Image = 0h 13min 3sec
Gastric passage time = 0h 13min
First Cecal Image = 3h 45min 25sec
Small bowel passage time = 3hr 32min

Figure 1

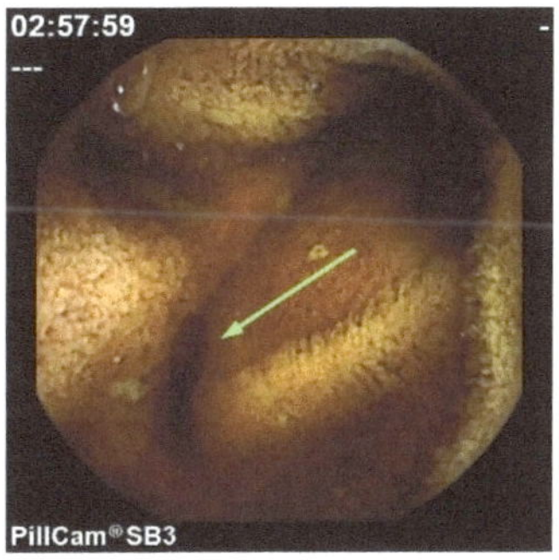

Figure 2

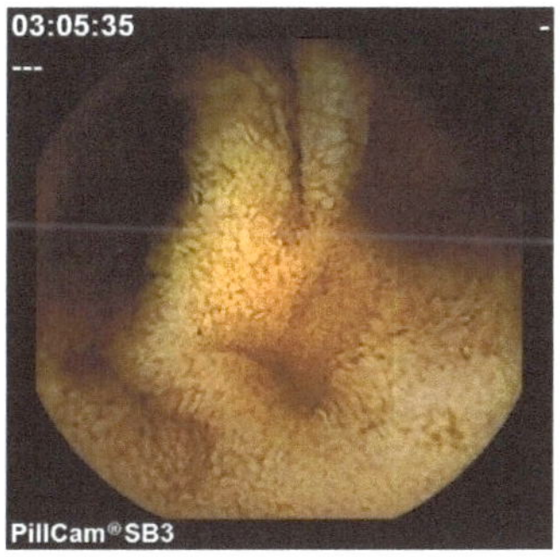

Figure 3

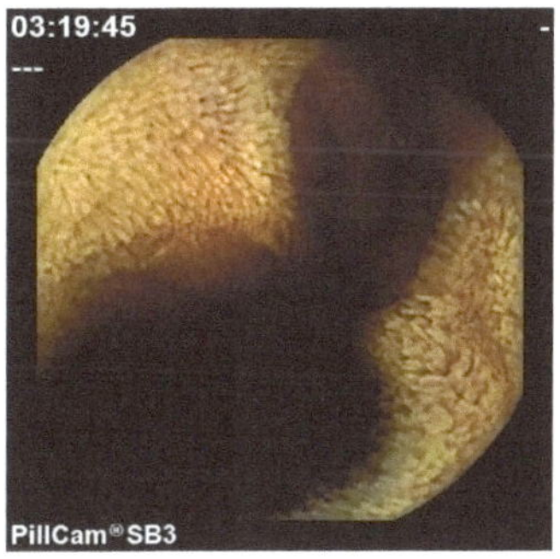

The video capsule passes through the stomach quickly to enter the duodenum in 13 minutes. Transit appears to be delayed within the mid small bowel (capsule hold-up) beginning ~1hr 45min. The capsule passes back and forth in the same segment prior to entry into the distal bowel, which contains dark fluid and small blood clots (**Figure 1**: 2hrs 57min 59sec). Capsule hold-up is also observed in this segment while multiple frames identify 2 distinct luminal openings divided by a mucosal isthmus (**Figure 2**: 3hrs 5min 35sec). Additional blood clots are observed in the distal small bowel lumen (**Figure 3:** 3hrs 19min 45sec) prior to entry into the cecum at 3hrs 45min.

Follow-up

Examination of the distal small bowel by retrograde double balloon enteroscopy (DBE) is diagnostic for a large diverticulum ~80cm proximal to the ileocecal valve (**Figure 4**). The margins of the diverticulum are ulcerated. The base of the diverticulum is lined with variant mucosa (**Figure 5**). A laparoscopic small bowel resection is performed for definitive treatment of a Meckel's diverticulum complicated by gastrointestinal bleeding. Gastric heterotopia is confirmed by histology.

Figure 4

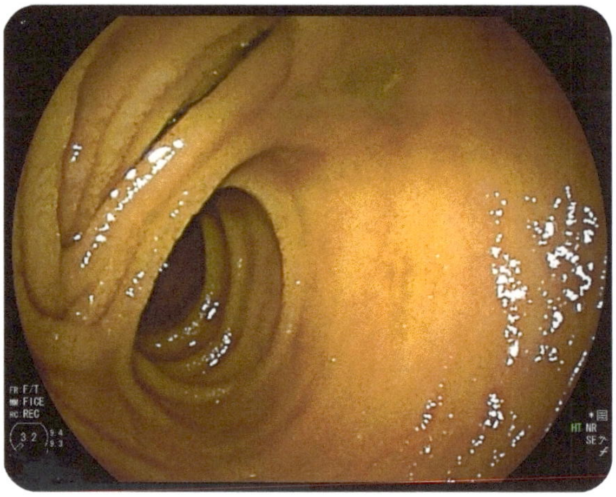

Figure 5

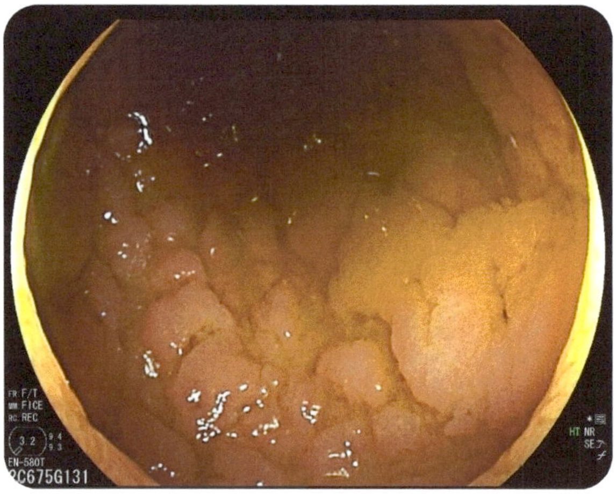

Chapter 5: Meckel's Diverticulum

Presented by Jose Aponte-Pieras, MD

Introduction

Meckel's diverticulum (MD) is the most common congenital anomaly of the gastrointestinal tract.[1] Wilhelm Fabricius Hildanus first identified this anomaly in 1598 but Johann Friedrich Meckel established its embryonic origin in 1806.[2] MD is a true diverticulum, comprised of all intestinal layers, resulting from incomplete involution of the omphalomesenteric or vitelline duct.[1,3,4,5] It is most commonly found within 100 cm of the ileocecal valve (range of 7 cm-200 cm) on the antimesenteric portion of the ileum.[1,4,6,7,8,9] The length of the diverticulum has been reported to range from 2 cm to 11 cm with a diameter of up to 7 cm.[2,8] Ectopic tissue is found in ~50% of Meckel's cases and is associated with an increased risk of complication, namely gastrointestinal bleeding.[1,4] Ectopic gastric mucosa is most common (23%-50%), followed by pancreatic heterotopia (5%). Cases of MD containing ectopic colonic, hepatobiliary, and endometrial mucosa have been reported in the medical literature.[1,3,8,10]

Epidemiology

The incidence of MD ranges from 0.3% to 2.9 % of the general population with a male: female predominant ratio of 1.5:1 to 4:1.[1,2,8,9,11] Up to 60% of symptomatic MD present before age 2, but diagnosis of MD may occur much later in life. Pediatric patients most commonly present with small bowel obstruction (47%-60% of patients) followed by gastrointestinal bleeding (25%-37%), and diverticulitis (8%-20%). Gastrointestinal bleeding is typical presenting symptom in adults although small bowel obstruction and diverticulitis are also common.[2,8,10,12] Symptomatic MD should be considered in the differential diagnosis of adults with unexplained episodes of melena, particularly when abdominal pain is present.[1,6,13] Abdominal pain may be secondary to ulceration, bowel obstruction, diverticulitis, or perforation.[7,14] Mucosal ulceration is typically related to secretion of hydrochloric acid by ectopic gastric mucosa but also occurs with secretion alkaline pancreatic fluid by ectopic pancreatic tissue.[1,8] Less frequent presentations of MD reported in the medical literature include: intussusception, volvulus, ileo-umbilical fistula, and entrapment of MD within an internal hernia sac (Littre's hernia).[2,7,8,12,14,15]

Lastly, Meckel's diverticulum is considered as a "hot spot" for small bowel malignancy with a reported 70-fold increased risk of cancer in comparison to normal ileal mucosa.[16] Malignancies known to complicate MD include neuroendocrine tumors (63%), gastrointestinal stromal tumor (GIST), and adenocarcinoma.[2,8,17] Lag time to diagnosis of MD in adults following the onset of symptoms averages 3 years, hinting at the diagnostic complexity of this clinical condition.[4,9]

Diagnosis

The diagnosis of Meckel's diverticulum requires a high index of suspicion in adults with overt bleeding which is unexplained after standard EGD/colonoscopy. Computed tomography (CT) imaging is often cited as a diagnostic tool but has low sensitivity for MD (0%-24%) with most positive results observed when diverticulitis is present.[2] Small bowel obstruction or intussusception observed on CT serve as diagnostic clues.[7] Administration of oral contrast with CT or magnetic resonance enteroclysis may increase the diagnostic yield up to 44%.[4,1] Identification of a branching vitelline artery by CT or conventional angiography is virtually pathognomonic for MD with a reported sensitivity of 33% to 59%.[1,8] Transabdominal ultrasound examination of the right lower abdomen may reveal a tubular or cyst-like structure in select cases.[2] The use of radionuclide 99m-technetium pertechnetate or "Meckel's scan" was classically considered as the diagnostic test of choice for detection of Meckel's prior to the widespread availability of video capsule endoscopy (VCE) and the advent of DBE. This study relies on the accumulation of intravenous radiotracer within gastric mucosa, including ectopic mucosa (**Figure 1**). The sensitivity of Meckel's scan in cases of gastrointestinal bleeding is high in pediatric cases (80%-90%) but lower in adults (62.5%). The frequency of false negative studies observed in adult populations may be related to limited experience of adult radiologists, positioning of MD posterior to the stomach/kidneys/bladder, or reduction in mucosal uptake of tracer with active bleeding.[2,3,8,12]

VCE is the procedure of choice for evaluation of overt or occult bleeding of suspected small bowel origin. The positive predictive value of VCE for MD has been reported to be as high as 85%. For identification of obscure bleeding, the diagnostic accuracy of

VCE compared to Meckel's scan is 36% vs 9%, respectively.[1,12] The most commonly reported finding suggestive of Meckel's is the presence of a 'double lumen' sign with or without an intraluminal septum ('diaphragm sign').[1,4,9,13,14] Additional features of MD observed on VCE include fresh blood, focal ulceration, stricture, and/or inflammatory mucosal changes[4,7,9,13,18] (**Figure 2**). Retention of the video capsule within a MD is rare (2%) and can facilitate diagnosis when DBE or surgery are performed for retrieval.[19] Examination of the ileum by retrograde DBE is highly effective in detecting MD and should be considered in patients with suspected small bowel bleeding which is undefined after standard EGD/colonoscopy, imaging, and VCE[1,8,20,21] (**Figure 3**).

Management

Definitive treatment of MD includes laparoscopy or laparotomy with either diverticulectomy or segmental small bowel resection. Segmental resection is favored to ensure removal of the entire diverticulum and all associated ectopic mucosa.[2,7] The management of asymptomatic MD diagnosed incidentally is controversial. Resection is favored in cases in which the diverticulum is >2 cm in length and/or associated with ectopic mucosa as these features confer an increased risk of complication (70%).[2,10] Additional features which may favor resection include the presence of fibrous bands and an inflamed/thickened diverticulum.[2,7,8,10] Citing a lifetime risk of 4.2% of becoming symptomatic, one epidemiologic study from Washington, USA recommended against resection of incidental MD considering a number needed to treat of 800 to prevent 1 fatality.[22] Proton pump inhibitor therapy may be prescribed as an adjunctive therapy to heal ulceration and control bleeding in MD complicated by ectopic gastric mucosa.[5] Proton pump inhibitor therapy may also serve as an alternative to surgery when the diagnosis is uncertain or in patients who are not surgical candidates.

Conclusion

Meckel's diverticulum is classically characterized in textbooks using the 'rule of 2s', which still holds mostly true[5,8] (**Table 1**). A diagnosis of MD may be missed or delayed in many cases due to non-specific symptoms and suboptimal diagnostic testing. Suspicion for Meckel's should be heightened in cases of overt, obscure gastrointestinal bleeding or unexplained

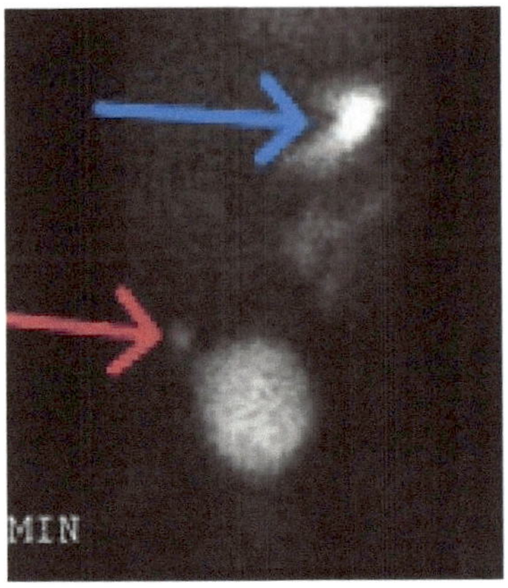

Figure 1. Positive Meckel's scan with radiotracer uptake in gastric body (blue arrow) and ectopic focus of small bowel (red arrow).

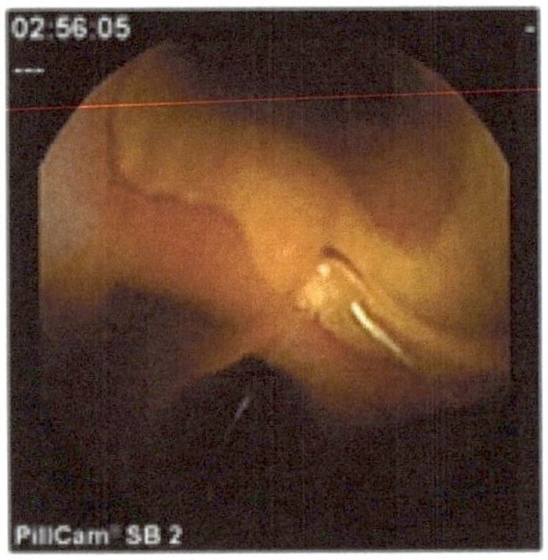

Figure 2. Meckel's diverticulum with ulceration observed by VCE.

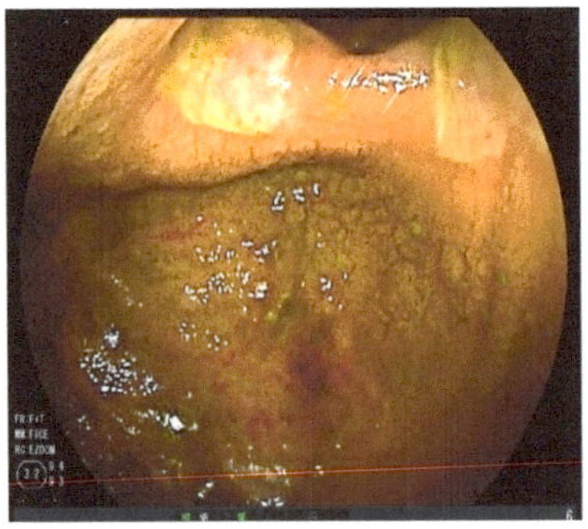

Figure 3. Meckel's diverticulum identified by retrograde DBE.

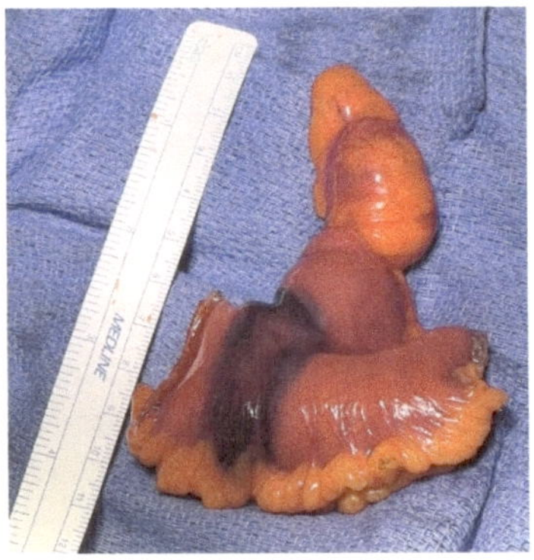

Figure 4. Meckel's diverticulum gross surgical specimen.

Meckel's Diverticulum Rule of Two's
2% prevalence in the general population
2 to 1 male:female ratio
2 feet proximal to the ileocecal valve
2 inch diverticulum length
Symptomatic presentation prior to age 2

Table 1. Meckel's Diverticulum rule of two's.

small bowel obstruction. Examination of the small bowel lumen by VCE and DBE allows for a high rate of diagnosis of MD. Segmental small bowel resection is recommended for patients with symptomatic MD as well as incidental MD with risk factors for complication. Cases of asymptomatic MD without associated risk factors may be managed conservatively. Advances in endoscopy over time may allow for endoscopic resection of MD as an alternative to laparotomy in the future.

References

1. Day NJ, Fultz P, Marino D. Recurrent small-bowel obstruction caused by a Meckel's diverticulum diagnosed on video capsule endoscopy. Clin Gastroenterol Hepatol. 2016; 14(6):A21-A22.
2. Nakatani S, Inoki K, Tashiro T, et al. Small intestinal bleeding and stricture caused by Meckel's diverticulum. Clin Case Rep. 2022; 10(8):e6144.
3. Krstic SN, Martinov JB, Sokic-Milutinovic AD, Milosavljevic TN, Krstic MN. Capsule endoscopy is useful diagnostic tool for diagnosing Meckel's diverticulum. Eur J Gastroenterol Hepatol. 2016;28(6):702-7.
4. Lin L, Liu K, Liu H, Wu J, Zhang Y. Capsule endoscopy as a diagnostic test for Meckel's diverticulum. Scand J Gastroenterol. 2019 Jan 54(1):122-127.
5. Lindeman RJ, Søreide K. The many faces of Meckel's diverticulum: update on management in incidental and symptomatic patients. Curr Gastroenterol Rep. 2020; 22(1):3.
6. Baltes P, Dray X, Riccioni DX, et al. Small bowel capsule endoscopy in patients with Meckel's diverticulum: clinical features, diagnostic workup, and findings. A European multicenter I-CARE study. Gastrointest Endosc. 2023; 97(5):917-926.e3.
7. Dias de Castro F, Magalhaes J, Moreira MJ, Cotter J. Ulcerated Meckel's diverticulum. Gastroenterol Hepatol. 2014; 37(2):69-71.
8. El Hajra Martínez I, Calvo M, Martínez-Porras JL, Gomez-Pimpollo Garcia L, Rodriguez JL, Leon C, Calleja Panero JL. Inverted Meckel's diverticulum diagnosed using capsule endoscopy: a case report. World J Gastroenterol. 2021; 27(36):6154-6160.
9. Hansen CC, Søreide K. Systematic review of epidemiology, presentation, and management of meckel's diverticulum in the 21st century. Medicine (Baltimore). 2018; 97(35):e12154.
10. Li L, Zhan X, Chen Y, Li J, Wang Y. Application of small bowel capsule endoscopy in children with meckel's diverticulum. Eur J Gastroenterol Hepatol. 2024; 36(7):845-849.
11. García-Compeán D, Jiménez-Rodríguez AR, Del Cueto-Aguilera ÁN, Herrera-Quiñones G, González-González JA, Maldonado-Garza HJ. Meckel's diverticulum diagnosis by video capsule endoscopy: a case report and review of literature. World J Clin Cases. 2018; 6(14):791-799.
12. Silva M, Cardoso H, Peixoto A, Lopes S, Santos AL, Gomes S, Macedo G. The role of capsule endoscopy in urgent evaluation of obscure gastrointestinal bleeding: a case series of Meckel diverticulum . Arq Bras Cir Dig. 2018; 31(4):e1409.
13. Wu J, Huang Z, Wu H, Ji M, Wang Y, Tang Z, Huang Y. The diagnostic value of video capsule endoscopy for Meckel's diverticulum in children. Rev Esp Enferm Dig. 2020;112(6):429-433
14. Park JJ, Wolff B, Tollefson M, et al. Meckel Diverticulum: The Mayo Clinic experience with 1476 patients (1950–2002). Ann Surg. 2005; 241(3): 529-533.
15. Parvanescu A, Bruzzi M, Voron T. et al. Complicated meckel's diverticulum: presentation modes in adults. Medicine (Baltimore). 2018; 97(38): e12457.
16. Thirunavukarasu P, Sathaiah M, Sukumar S, et al. Meckel's Diverticulum—A High-risk region for malignancy in the ileum: Insights from a population-based epidemiological study and implications in surgical management. Ann Surg. 2011;253(2):223-230.
17. Krstevski G, Isahi U, Andreevski V. Bleeding meckel's diverticulum in a 33-year-old female diagnosed with video capsule endoscopy and a technetium-99 m pertechnetate scan with a favorable response to H2 blocker and PPI. Case Rep Gastrointest Med 2021;1381395
18. Yu H, Song H, Cai J. Laparoscopic treatment of hemorrhagic meckel diverticulum after diagnosis with wireless capsule endoscopy and double-balloon enteroscopy. Rev Esp Enferm Dig. 2017;109(4):315.
19. Alemayehu H, Hall M, Desai AA, St Peter SD, Snyder CL. Demographic disparities of children presenting with symptomatic meckel's diverticulum in children's hospitals. Pediatr Surg Int. 2014; 30(6):649-53.

20. van Malderen K, Vijayvargiya P, Camilleri M, Larson DW, Cima R. Malignancy and Meckel's diverticulum: A
21. systematic literature review and 14-year experience at a tertiary referral center. United European Gastroenterol J. 2018; 6(5):739-747.
22. Zani A, Eaton S, Rees CM, Pierro A. Incidentally detected meckel diverticulum: to resect or not to resect? Ann Surg. 2008; 247(2):276-281.
23. He Q, Zhang YL, Xiao B, Jiang B, Bai Y, Zhi FC. Double-balloon enteroscopy for diagnosis of meckel's diverticulum: Comparison with operative findings and capsule endoscopy. Surgery. 2013;153(4):549-54.
24. Soltero MJ, Bill AH. The natural history of meckel's diverticulum and its relation to incidental removal. A study of 202 cases of diseased Meckel's Diverticulum found in King County, Washington, over a fifteen-year period. Am J Surg. 1976;132(2):168-173.

CAPSULE ENDOSCOPY BY CASE STUDY
Case Study Number 6

Presented by Matthew Rice, MD

Pre-capsule Findings (included in capsule study)

A 38-year-old man with no significant past medical history presents for further evaluation of unexplained iron deficiency anemia. He was initially diagnosed with symptomatic anemia 12 weeks ago after an emergency room evaluation for symptoms of pre-syncope, fatigue, and dyspnea on exertion. A standard outpatient endoscopic evaluation, including EGD and colonoscopy, were completed but failed to reveal a cause of anemia. Duodenal biopsies were found to be negative for villous atrophy. Upon interview today, the patient complains of fatigue as well as recent symptoms of early satiety and epigastric pain.

A capsule endoscopy study is performed to evaluate for small bowel bleeding. Review the capsule endoscopy study and report your findings, including: gastric passage time, small bowel passage time, and observed abnormalities. Be prepared to discuss your findings and management plan with your staff prior to reviewing the diagnosis and case discussion.

Following entry into the duodenum, a retrograde view of the pylorus is observed (**Figure 1:** 0hr 19min 15sec). Red blood is encountered soon after transition into the proximal small bowel (**Figure 2**: 0hr 20min 44sec; **Figure 3:** 0hr 21min 0sec). Abnormal mucosa is observed in this segment (**Figure 4:** 20min, 48sec) which appears to be smooth, lacking the villous architecture of normal small bowel. Dark blood in the lumen limits visualization of the remaining small bowel.

Figure 1

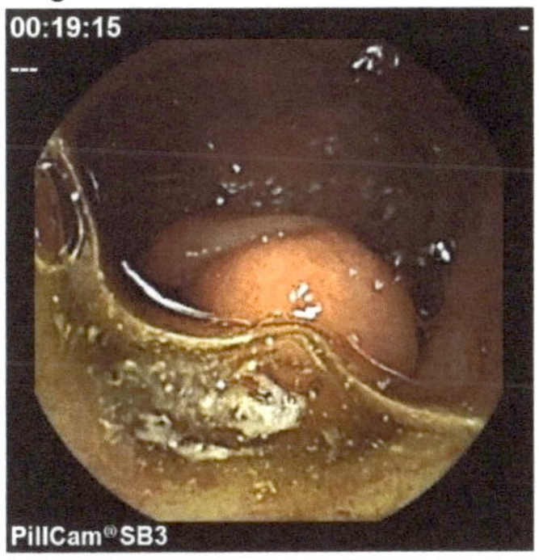

Figure 2

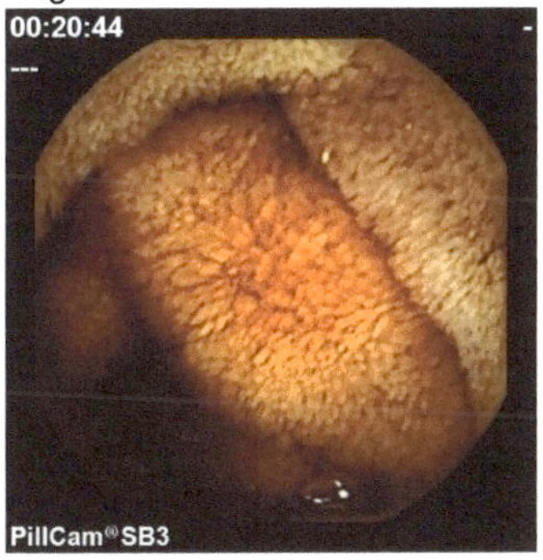

Figure 3

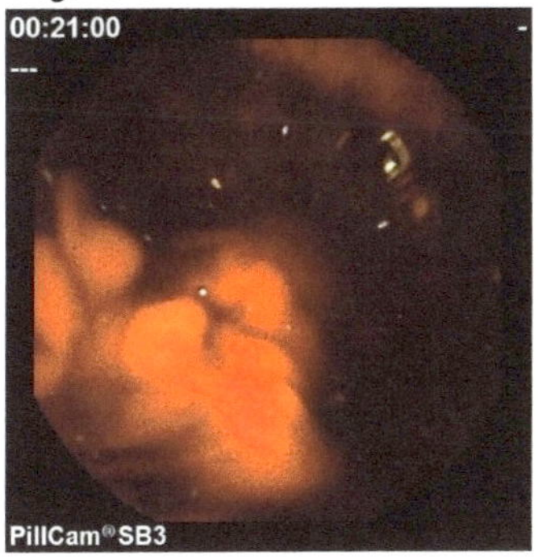

Figure 4

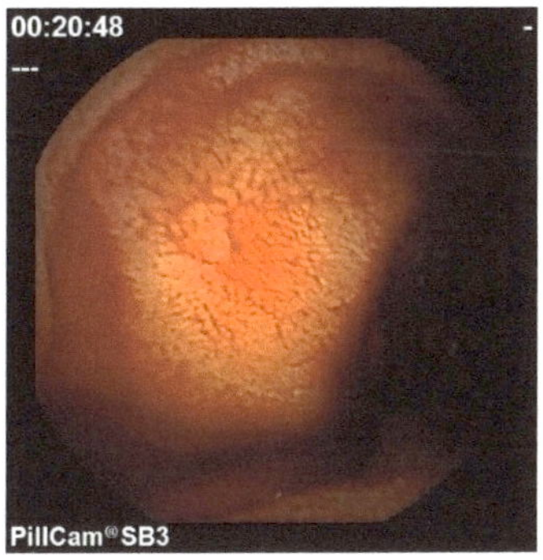

Capsule Endoscopy Findings
First Gastric Image = 0hr 3min 34sec
First Duodenal Image = 0h 18min 39sec
Gastric passage time = 0h 14min
First Cecal Image = 4h 58min 02sec
Small bowel passage time = 4hr 40min

Follow-up

An upper single balloon enteroscopy was performed to further evaluate the abnormal segment of bowel identified by VCE. This exam was revealing for a stricture of the proximal jejunum associated with malignant-appearing tissue (**Figure 5**). The mass was 3 cm in length and circumferential. It was traversed with the enteroscope then biopsied and marked with a submucosal ink tattoo. A diagnosis of adenocarcinoma was confirmed by pathology. Complete CT imaging of the chest/abdomen/pelvis identified a mass in the proximal jejunum and lacked evidence of regional or distant metastasis. The patient was elected for laparotomy with segmental small bowel resection and local lymph node dissection. Surgical pathology results revealed a primary adenocarcinoma invading the subserosa (T3) and lymph nodes which were negative for malignant cells. (Stage IIA) This patient was elected by oncology for a course of systemic chemotherapy (FOLFOX) as an adjunctive therapy due to his young age.

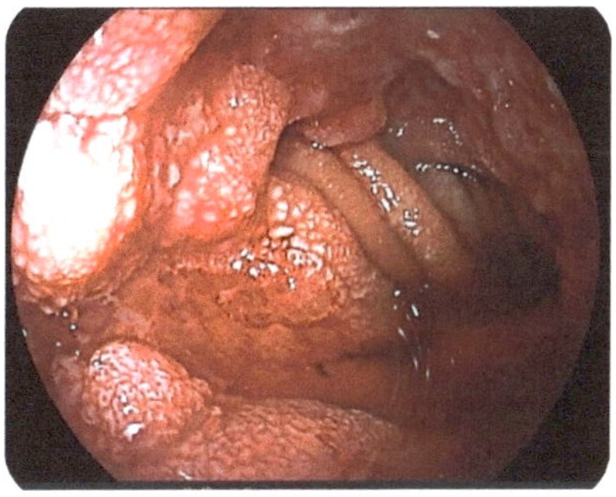

Figure 5

Chapter 6: Small Bowel Adenocarcinoma

Matthew Rice, MD

Introduction

Small bowel adenocarcinoma (SBA) is a rare malignancy, representing less than 5% of all gastrointestinal malignancies, and only 0.6% of all cancers in the United States.[1,2] It accounts for approximately 30%-40% of all primary small bowel cancers. Despite its rarity, the incidence of SBA has been steadily increasing in the U.S. and globally, almost doubling over the last 50 years.[3] An average of 0.67 cases/100,000 SBA cases were reported annually from 2000-2019.[4] In 2024, there were an estimated 12,440 new cases of small intestine cancer in the U.S., translating into approximately 5,000 new SBA cases annually.[5] Despite the significant increases in cases, overall survival outcomes have remained stable over the last 20 years.[4]

Most cases of SBA are diagnosed in the sixth decade of life.[4,6,7]. Men and African Americans in the U.S. are disproportionally affected, with African Americans experiencing nearly double the incidence rates.[1,2] Geographic differences have been identified as well. Higher incidences of small intestinal cancer were seen in countries with higher human development index, gross domestic product, prevelance of unhealthy lifestyle habits, and metabolic disorders. These rates were highest in North America.[8] Anatomically, SBA most frequently arises in the duodenum (approximately 60% of cases), followed by the jejunum (25-29%) and ileum (10%-13%).[7] There is an exception in patient with Crohn's disease (CD) where the most common distribution is in the distal small bowel.[9]

Risk Factors

Several risk factors for SBA have been identified. Chronic inflammatory conditions such as CD and celiac disease significantly increase its risk. Patients with CD have a relative risk of developing SBA, which is 30 times higher than the general population. This risk increases with disease duration, more than tripling over the span of 20 years after diagnosis.[7,9] Additional risk factors identified in CD include disease severity, location of disease (highest in disease confined to the small bowel), abdominal surgery, stricturoplasty, and bypassed bowel segments.[9,10] Celiac disease predisposes individuals to SBA with an estimated relative risk up to 34 times that of the general population.[7] Celiac patients are more likely to present at a younger age resulting in better overall survival.[7,11]

Genetic predispositions play a crucial role in SBA development. Hereditary syndromes such as familial adenomatous polyposis (FAP), Lynch syndrome (hereditary nonpolyposis colorectal cancer), and Peutz-Jeghers syndrome (PJS) are strongly associated with SBA.[2,7] SBA develops in approximately 5% of patient with FAP and is the primary cause of death in patients post-colectomy.[2,11] Lynch syndrome is associated with 100-fold increase in risk for SBA, with a lifetime risk of 1%-4%. PJS is linked to a 520-fold increased risk compared to unaffected persons.[7,11]

Environmental and lifestyle factors have been identified as potential risk factors for SBA. Smoking, alcohol consumption, and metabolic disease are associated with increased risk.[7,8] Diets high in refined carbohydrates, red meat, smoked foods, and/or saturated fats have been suggested as risk factors for SBA based upon limited, and sometimes conflicting, evidence. Conversely, diets rich in coffee and vegetables may offer protective effects.[2,7]

Diagnosis

SBA typically presents nonspecific, insidious symptoms resulting in an average delay of 7-8 months for diagnosis and a 33% rate of distant metastases upon diagnosis.[6,7] The most common presenting symptom is abdominal pain (66% of patients) which is described as intermittent and crampy.[6,12] Other symptoms include nausea, vomiting, unintentional weight loss, iron deficiency anemia, and jaundice.[12] Approximately 22%–26% of patients with jejunal or ileal tumors present acutely with overt GI bleeding, intestinal obstruction, or perforation.[6,7]

Historically, small bowel follow-through (SBFT) was used to evaluate the small intestine, but its sensitivity for diagnosing small bowel cancer is limited is low (30%-44%) especially for tumors <10 mm in size.[13] Modern techniques such as video capsule endoscopy (VCE) and CT enterography have largely surpassed small bowel follow-through in diagnostic performance.[13,14] VCE allows for non-invasive visualization of the entire small bowel lumen with a sensitivity of 80% for all small bowel tumors (miss rate of 17%-19%).[12,13,14,15,16] The miss rate of VCE for SBA is estimated to lower than for all tumors as adenocarcinomas are characterized by bleeding, ulcerated tissue which grows into the small bowel lumen, resulting in delay in capsule passage. Examination of the proximal small bowel by upper endoscopy with push enteroscopy is often diagnostic in cases of SBA involving the duodenum or proximal jejunum (**Figure 1**). In cases of unexplained gastrointestinal blood loss or suspected small bowel malignancy, device-assisted enteroscopy (DAE) may be required to definitely exclude SBA of the jejunum or ileum.[17] Cross-sectional imaging of the small bowel by CT enterography or MR enterography may be performed for the initial diagnosis of SBA or as an additional test in cases of suspected small bowel bleeding with negative VCE.[18,19] Positron emission tomography (PET-CT) can be used for staging and detecting recurrence but is not routinely utilized as an initial diagnostic test due to cost and limited availability[12] (**Figure 2**).

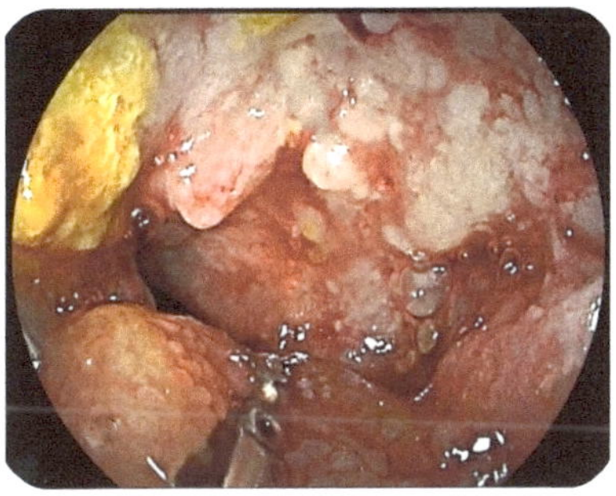

Figure 1. SBA of the proximal jejunum diagnosed by push enteroscopy.

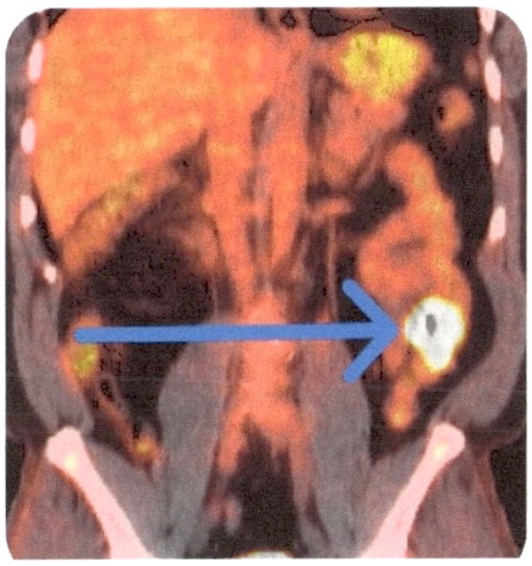

Figure 2. SBA identified by PET-CT (sagittal view).

Staging

SBA is staged according to the American Joint Committee on Cancer (AJCC) tumor, node, and metastasis (TNM) system (**Table 1**). The 5-year survival rates for SBA vary significantly depending on stage at diagnosis. Unfortunately, the majority of cases of SBA are advanced upon initial diagnosis, with 60% of cases at stages III or IV.[3] Approximately 10% of patients present with stage I disease, 30% with stage II, 25% with stage III, and 35% with stage IV disease.[12]

For stage I SBA, the 5-year overall survival rate ranges from 55% to 66%. In stage II, the 5-year overall survival rate decreases to between 43% and 50%. Stage III SBA has a poorer prognosis, with overall survival rates ranging from 31% to 42%. For stage IV or metastatic SBA, the prognosis is particularly poor, with a 5-year overall survival rate of only 5% to 19%.[12,21]

Adverse prognostic indicators include advanced age > 75, primary duodenal location, and the presence of regional or distant metastasis.[20] According to SEER data, patients with localized SBA confined to the small intestine have a relative 5-year survival rate of approximately 84%, while those with regional spread to nearby tissues or lymph nodes have a survival rate of about 79%. For patients with distant metastases, the relative survival rate drops significantly to around 45%. These statistics underscore the critical importance of early diagnosis in improving outcomes for this malignancy.[22]

Management

Surgical resection remains the cornerstone of treatment for localized disease. Complete tumor removal with negative margins, along with adequate lymph node dissection is essential. The type of surgery depends on the tumor's location. For jejunal and ileal tumors, segmental resection with mesentery removal is standard, while duodenal tumors may require pancreaticoduodenectomy if the second part of the duodenum or surrounding structures are involved. Right hemicolectomy is performed for ileocecal tumors to ensure proper lymphatic clearance. Recurrence of SBA after surgery is common, especially for advanced stage disease.[12,21]

Adjuvant chemotherapy is recommended for stage III SBA (node-positive disease) and is typically based on regimens used for colorectal cancer, such as FOLFOX (5-fluorouracil, leucovorin, and oxaliplatin) or CAPOX (capecitabine and oxaliplatin). Stage II

Stage	TMN criteria	Description
0	Tis, N0, M0	Preinvasive cancer in mucosa[14]
I	T1-2, N0, M0	Localized to bowel wall layers[14]
IIA	T3, N0, M0	Reaches subserosa[18]
IIB	T4, N0, M0	Invades serosa/adjacent structures[18]
IIIA	Any T, N1, M0	1-2 lymph nodes involved[23]
IIIB	Any T, N2, M0	≥3 lymph nodes affected[23]
IV	Any T, Any N, M1	Distant metastasis present

Table 1. Staging of small bowel adenocarcinoma[20]

patients with high-risk features, such as T4 tumors or poor differentiation, may also benefit from adjuvant therapy. Microsatellite instability-high (MSI-H) or mismatch repair-deficient (dMMR) tumors have a better prognosis and may not require chemotherapy, whereas microsatellite-stable (MSS) tumors are more likely to benefit from oxaliplatin-based regimens. The ongoing BALLAD trial aims to clarify the role of adjuvant chemotherapy in SBA.[12]

For advanced or metastatic SBA, systemic therapy is the primary treatment option. First-line regimens include FOLFOX or CAPOX, while second-line options involve FOLFIRI (5-fluorouracil, leucovorin, and irinotecan) or taxane-based chemotherapy. Immunotherapy with pembrolizumab is an option for patients with microsatellite instability-high/ mismatch repair-deficient tumors, resulting in 42% rate of response rate in trials. Palliative radiation therapy may be used in some cases to manage symptoms such as obstruction or pain.[12]

Conclusion

Small bowel adenocarcinoma is rare but increasing in incidence significantly over time, nearly doubling over the past 50 years. Despite advancements in diagnostic tools and treatment strategies, overall prognosis remains poor, with 5-year survival rates ranging from 20% to 50%, Surgical resection remains the cornerstone of treatment for localized disease. Due to the rarity of SBA, the efficacy of systemic chemotherapy is unclear and largely extrapolated from colorectal cancer research. Future investments in focused research with international collaboration are needed to refining treatment specific to this disease.

References

1. Pan SY, Morrison H. Epidemiology of cancer of the small intestine. World J Gastrointest Oncol. 2011;3(3):33-42.
2. Barsouk A, Rawla P, Barsouk A, Thandra KC. Epidemiology of cancers of the small intestine: trends, risk factors, and prevention. Med Sci (Basel). 2019;7(3):46. doi:
3. Bilimoria KY, Bentrem DJ, Wayne JD, Ko CY, Bennett CL, Talamonti MS. Small bowel cancer in the United States: changes in epidemiology, treatment, and survival over the last 20 years. Ann Surg. 2009;249(1):63-71.
4. Sears JJ, Xu Y, Fiala MA, McWilliams RR, Overman MJ, Pedersen KS. Incidence and survival trends in small bowel adenocarcinoma (SBA) from 2000-2019 in the United States. J Clin Oncol. 2025;43(S4): Abstract 801.
5. National Cancer Institute. Cancer Stat Facts: Small Intestine Cancer. SEER*Explorer: An interactive website for SEER cancer statistics [Internet]. Updated November 5, 2024. Accessed April 6, 2025. Available from: https://seer.cancer.gov/statfacts/html/smint.html
6. Aparicio T, Zaanan A, Svrcek M, et al. Small bowel adenocarcinoma: Epidemiology, risk factors, diagnosis and treatment. Dig Liver Dis 2014;46:97–104.
7. Huang J, Chan SC, Fung YC, et al. Incidence, Risk Factors, and Temporal Trends of Small Intestinal Cancer: A Global Analysis of Cancer Registries. Gastroenterology. 2023;165(3):600-612.
8. Pedersen KS, Raghav K, Overman MJ. Small Bowel Adenocarcinoma: Etiology, Presentation, and Molecular Alterations. J Natl Compr Canc Netw. 2019 Sep 1;17(9):1135-1141
9. Faggiani I, D'Amico F, Furfaro F, et al. Small bowel cancer in Crohn's disease. Cancers (Basel). 2024; 16(16):2901.
10. Cahill C, Gordon PH, Petrucci A, Boutros M. Small bowel adenocarcinoma and Crohn's disease: any further ahead than 50 years ago? World J Gastroenterol. 2014;20(33):11486-95.

11. Delaunoit T, Neczyporenko F, Limburg PJ, Erlichman C. Pathogenesis and risk factors of small bowel adenocarcinoma: a colorectal cancer sibling? Am J Gastroenterol. 2005;100(3):703-10.
12. Khosla D, Dey T, Madan R, et al. Small bowel adenocarcinoma: An overview. World J Gastrointest Oncol. 2022;14(2):413-422.
13. Han JW, Hong SN, Jang HJ, et al. Clinical Efficacy of Various Diagnostic Tests for Small Bowel Tumors and Clinical Features of Tumors Missed by Capsule Endoscopy. Gastroenterol Res Pract. 2015;2015:623208.
14. Hara AK, Leighton JA, Sharma VK, Fleischer DE. Small bowel: preliminary comparison of capsule endoscopy with barium study and CT. Radiology. 2004;230(1):260-5.
15. Schwartz GD, Barkin JS. Small-bowel tumors detected by wireless capsule endoscopy. Dig Dis Sci. 2007;52(4):1026-30.
16. Lewis BS, Eisen GM, Friedman S. A pooled analysis to evaluate results of capsule endoscopy trials. Endoscopy. 2005;37(10):960-5. Erratum in: Endoscopy. 2007 Mar;39(4):303.
17. Ross A, Mehdizadeh S, Tokar J, et al. Double balloon enteroscopy detects small bowel mass lesions missed by capsule endoscopy. Dig Dis Sci. 2008;53(8):2140-3.
18. Paulsen SR, Huprich JE, Fletcher JG, et al. CT enterography as a diagnostic tool in evaluating small bowel disorders: Review of clinical experience with over 700 cases. Radiographics. 2006;26(3):641-57.
19. Hakim FA, Alexander JA, Huprich JE, Grover M, Enders FT. CT-enterography may identify small bowel tumors not detected by capsule endoscopy: Eight years experience at Mayo Clinic Rochester. Dig Dis Sci. 2011;56(10):2914-9.
20. Howe JR, Karnell LH, Menck HR, Scott-Conner C. The American College of Surgeons Commission on Cancer and the American Cancer Society. Adenocarcinoma of the small bowel: review of the National Cancer Data Base, 1985-1995. Cancer. 1999;86(12):2693-706.
21. Chen EY, Vaccaro GM. Small Bowel Adenocarcinoma. Clin Colon Rectal Surg. 2018 Sep;31(5):267-277. doi: 10.1055/s-0038-1660482. Epub 2018 Sep 4. PMID: 30186048; PMCID: PMC6123009.
22. American Cancer Society. Survival Rates for Small Intestine Cancer (Adenocarcinoma). American Cancer Society. Updated January 17, 2025. Accessed September 14, 2025. https://www.cancer.org/cancer/types/small-intestine-cancer/detection-diagnosis-staging/survival-rates.html

Case Study Number 7

Presented by Daniel Raines, MD FACG and Barry Rubin, MD

Pre-capsule Findings (included in capsule study)

A 64-year-old man with a past medical history significant for hypertension, coronary artery disease, and stage III chronic kidney disease presents for evaluation of acute on chronic anemia. He was initially diagnosed with mild anemia 4 years ago by his nephrologist. His hemoglobin had remained stable around 11.5 g/dL, until 2 months ago, when he was hospitalized for symptomatic anemia (hemoglobin 6.8 g/dL) associated with a ferritin of 11 ng/ml. He received 2 units of packed red blood cells prior to discharge for outpatient upper endoscopy and colonoscopy, which were reported as normal.

The patient currently admits to occasional constipation but denies diarrhea, hematochezia, abdominal pain, or weight loss. Medications include oral iron, enalapril, carvedilol, and dual antiplatelet therapy (aspirin & clopidogrel). Dual antiplatelet therapy was initiated 8 years ago after coronary stent placement. Social history is significant for smoking 1 pack per day for over 40 years. Family history is negative for colorectal cancer or inflammatory bowel disease. Physical examination is unremarkable.

A capsule endoscopy study is performed to evaluate for small bowel bleeding. Review the capsule endoscopy study and report your findings, including: gastric passage time, small bowel passage time, and observed abnormalities. Be prepared to discuss your findings and management plan with your staff prior to reviewing the diagnosis and case discussion.

Capsule Endoscopy Findings
First Gastric Image = 0hr 0min 32sec
First Duodenal Image = 0h 37min 14sec
Gastric passage time = 0h 36min
First Cecal Image = 3h 10min 18sec
Small bowel passage time = 2hr 34min

Figure 1

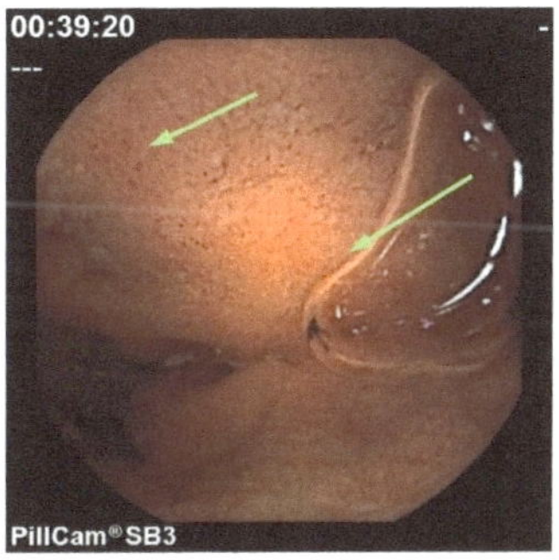

Figure 2

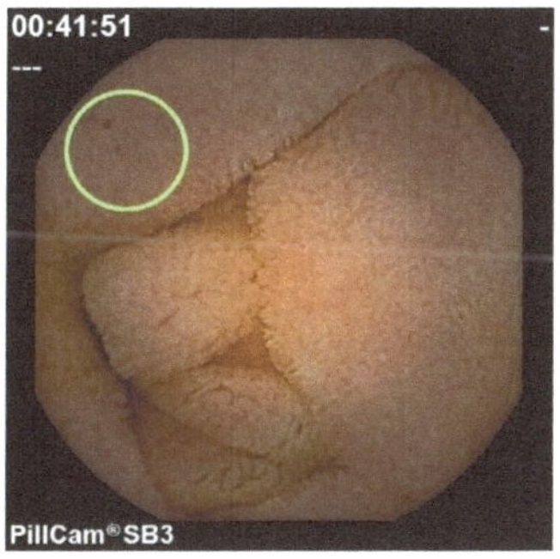

Figure 3

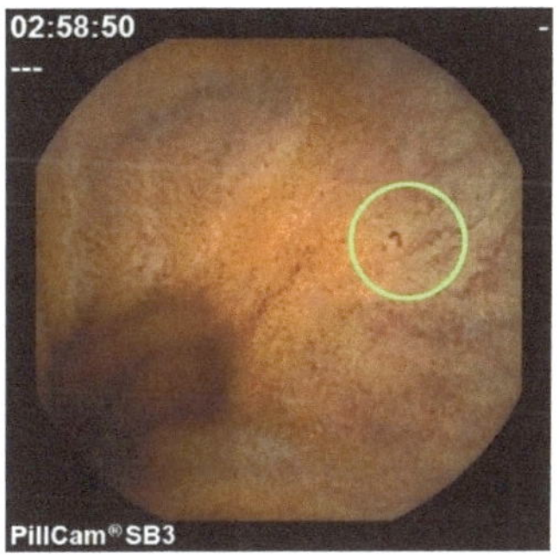

The study is challenging to interpret because it is negative for pathology which might cause iron deficiency anemia. Minor mucosal erythema is observed in the duodenal bulb (**Figure 1:** 0hr 39min 20sec). A few tiny red spots are observed in the proximal and distal small bowel (**Figure 2:** 0hr 41min 51sec; **Figure 3:** 2hr 58min 50sec). These minor findings do not explain the patient's recent presentation with severe iron deficiency anemia.

Follow-up

Following review of video capsule endoscopy results, the patient was monitored on oral iron supplementation. Over the subsequent 30 days, his hemoglobin level returned to his prior baseline of 11–12 g/dL. Clopidogrel therapy was discontinued given the absence of a clear indication for prolonged dual antiplatelet therapy and potential risk of gastrointestinal blood loss. The patient's hemoglobin remained stable across 5 years of long-term follow-up by nephrology.

CASE STUDY DISCUSSIONS — CASE NUMBER 7
Chapter 7: Unexplained Iron Deficiency Anemia

Daniel Raines, MD FACG and Barry Rubin, MD

Introduction

Iron deficiency anemia (IDA) is one of the most common conditions encountered by gastroenterologists. The prevalence of IDA in the United States is estimated at 2%–4% among adults, with rates up to 13% in women of reproductive age (12–49 years).[1,2] In cases of IDA with non-diagnostic standard upper and lower endoscopy, video capsule endoscopy (VCE) yields a diagnosis in a majority (57%–66%) but a substantial percentage of patients remain without an etiology.[3] Managing these cases can be challenging, as the physician must first attest that all VCE images are normal, then formulate a strategy to manage IDA in the absence of an identified cause.[4] This chapter provides a framework for evaluation of these patients, including a concise overview of iron physiology, a review of etiologies of unexplained IDA, and diagnostic testing tailored to individual patient factors.[4,5]

Iron Homeostasis

Iron is absorbed by intestinal enterocytes and exported into the circulation, where it binds to transferrin for transport. Transferrin delivers iron to the liver and spleen for storage as ferritin, or to the bone marrow as hemosiderin. Iron from senescent red blood cells is salvaged by macrophages then recycled through the reticuloendothelial system.[6] Cellular transfer of iron is mediated by ferroportin, the sole iron exporter. Hepcidin, a peptide hormone synthesized in the liver, plays a key role in regulation of systemic iron levels by binding to ferroportin, resulting in degradation. Degradation of ferroportin blocks iron efflux from key sites of iron transfer: duodenal enterocytes (which absorb dietary iron), hepatocytes (which store iron), and macrophages (which recycle iron from senescent erythrocytes). Hepcidin is upregulated in the setting of chronic inflammation, resulting in reduced levels of circulating iron available for erythropoiesis and leading to a state of functional, or relative, iron deficiency anemia.[7]

Absolute iron deficiency is defined as ferritin < 30 ng/mL and/or transferrin saturation (TSAT) < 20%. A ferritin level < 30 ng/mL is highly predictive of depleted bone marrow iron stores, with 98% specificity and 92% sensitivity. TSAT reflects bioavailable circulating iron and is particularly useful in chronic inflammatory states such as chronic kidney disease (CKD) or congestive heart failure (CHF).[8] Serum soluble transferrin receptor (sTfR) may be useful in differentiating absolute iron deficiency anemia and anemia of inflammation increase as sTfR levels are elevated in tissue iron deficiency but not with inflammation. An elevated serum platelet count may also support a diagnosis of absolute IDA, whereas thrombocytopenia may indicate hypersplenism from portal hypertension or cirrhosis. Although invasive, bone marrow biopsy remains the gold standard for evaluating body iron stores.[9]

Etiologies of IDA after Negative VCE

Gastroenterologists routinely encounter cases of IDA which is unexplained following standard evaluation by

Unidentified GI Bleeding Sources	Iron Malabsorption	Extraintestinal Etiologies
Angioectasias	Celiac disease	Menorrhagia
Dieulafoy lesion	Autoimmune chronic gastritis (AMAG)	Blood Donation
Cameron's erosion	*Helicobacter pylori* chronic gastritis	Chronic hemolysis
Portal hypertensive gastropathy (PHG)	Duodenal bypass	Hematuria
Gastric antral vascular ectasia (GAVE)	Strict vegan diet	Bedbugs
NSAID enteropathy		
Small bowel tumor		
Internal hemorrhoids		
Anastomotic ulceration		
Hookworm infection		

Table 1. Etiologies of unexplained iron deficiency anemia

EGD, colonoscopy, and VCE. Etiologies of IDA in these cases may be grouped into unidentified GI bleeding sources, disorders of intestinal iron absorption, and extraintestinal conditions (**Table 1**)

Unidentified GI bleeding

In patients over 50 years of age, angioectasias of the stomach, duodenum, jejunum, and right colon represent the most common source of obscure or undetected bleeding. Evanescent or diminutive lesions are often undetectable unless actively bleeding at the time of endoscopy. Even small (1-3 mm) angioectasias are capable of hemorrhaging in large volumes intermittently. Subtle or "missed" bleeding sources within reach of EGD include angioectasias, Cameron's erosions, portal hypertensive gastropathy (PHG), gastric antral vascular ectasia (GAVE), and Dieulafoy lesion (**Figures 1 and 2**). Bleeding sources which may be easily overlooked during colonoscopy include cecal angioectasias and flat neoplasms.[1,4,10] Small bowel tumors account for only 1.3% of cases of small bowel bleeding. Nonetheless, the possibility of a tumor escaping detection on VCE—whether overlooked by the reader or not captured in the recording—remains a source of unease for gastroenterologists. CT and MR enterography have demonstrated high sensitivity and specificity for the detection of submucosal tumors, such as gastrointestinal stromal tumors and carcinoid tumors, in research settings.[11,12,13,14,15] Non-steroidal anti-inflammatory drugs (NSAID) use is a well-established cause of GI bleeding, yet the mucosal breaks and erosions responsible for blood loss may not always be evident on VCE. In patients with unexplained IDA, clinicians should inquire not only about current NSAID use but also about prior use, as mucosal injury can persist long after the drug has been discontinued.[16] Additional sources of GI bleeding which may remain undetected or underappreciated include frequent hemorrhoidal bleeding, chronic ulceration of intestinal anastomoses, and hookworm infection.[1,4,17]

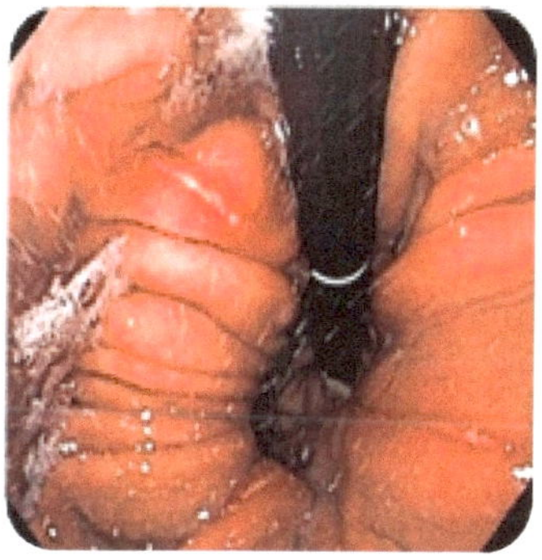

Figure 1. Cameron's erosions associated with a large hiatal hernia.

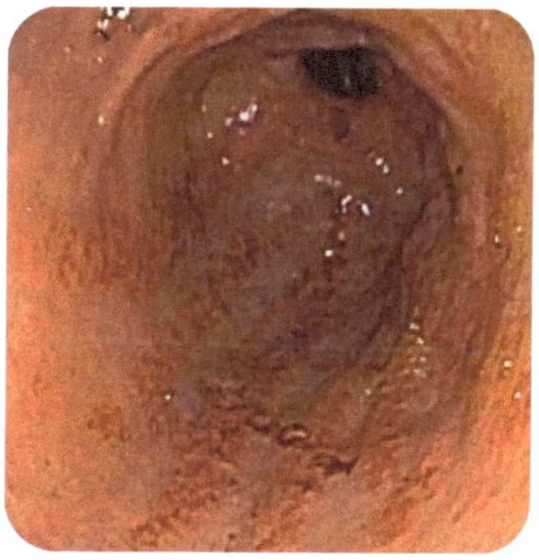

Figure 2. Stippled gastric antral vascular ectasia observed in the gastric antrum.

Malabsorption of iron

Enteric absorption of iron requires gastric acid (HCl), healthy duodenal mucosa, and adequate dietary intake. Gastric acid is necessary to denature dietary proteins, solubilize ferric iron (Fe^{3+}), and facilitate its conversion to ferrous iron (Fe^{2+}) for transport through duodenal enterocytes. Pepsin further contributes by cleaving denatured proteins to liberate iron. Lack of gastric acid production (achlorhydria) is a complication of autoimmune atrophic metaplastic gastritis (AMAG), chronic *Helicobacter pylori* gastritis, and radiation enteritis. Autoimmune metaplastic atrophic gastritis (AMAG) is a common cause of unexplained IDA which may be challenging to diagnose in clinical practice. Serologic testing has notable limitations. Anti–parietal cell antibodies are moderately sensitive (70%–80%) but may yield false positives in as many as 10% of cases, whereas anti-intrinsic factor antibodies are highly specific yet insensitive (< 30%). Gastric biopsy is considered the gold standard; however, inconsistent recognition by pathologists contributes to underdiagnosis. Histopathology reports often cite only "chronic gastritis," overlooking the loss of oxyntic glands or metaplasia (pseudopyloric or intestinal) that defines AMAG. Additional indicators of AMAG include a high gastric pH (6–7) on endoscopic aspirate and elevated serum gastrin levels.[18]

H. pylori infection is a recognized cause of chronic gastritis that may reduce or eliminate gastric acid secretion. The strongest evidence linking eradication to improvement in chronic IDA comes from a prospective study by Annibale et al.[19] Thirty patients with moderate to severe IDA refractory to oral iron, in whom other secondary causes were excluded, were treated for *H. pylori* infection while iron supplementation was discontinued. In the 27 patients with successful eradication, hemoglobin rose from 10.2 g/dL at baseline to 13 g/dL at 6 months and remained stable on long-term follow-up, whereas the 3 with persistent infection remained anemic. These findings suggest that *H. pylori* eradication can correct IDA in chronic gastritis, likely through reversal of achlorhydria. Celiac disease is a well-established cause of IDA and should be screened for using anti-tissue transglutaminase (TTG) antibodies and/or duodenal mucosal biopsy.[20] Proton pump inhibitor (PPI) therapy has been implicated as a cause of IDA based upon low quality data from observational studies. However, randomized controlled trials have not demonstrated a meaningful association.[21,22] PPIs suppress gastric acid production only partially (50%), whereas AMAG results in near-complete achlorhydria. Surgical bypass of the duodenum can result in IDA, often necessitating long-term intermittent parenteral iron therapy. Pure dietary deficiency of iron, such as in strict veganism, is rarely sufficient to cause IDA alone but may contribute when combined with other risk factors.[1,4,5]

Extraintestinal etiologies

Extraintestinal causes of IDA include heavy menstrual bleeding, frequent blood donation, chronic hemolysis, and chronic microscopic hematuria. Menstrual blood loss is by far the most common etiology of iron deficiency in women of reproductive age, particularly among those with heavy menstrual bleeding. Heavy menstrual bleeding is defined as menses lasting longer than 7 days, soaking more than 5 pads or tampons per day, and/or passage of large clots.[23] Obtaining a history of blood donation may identify frequent blood donation as a cause of IDA as well as patients with lifelong microcytic anemia—such as α- or β-thalassemia trait—who may have been declined for donation in the past. Chronic, low-grade hemolysis is a non-GI cause of iron deficiency anemia and may occur in conditions such as hereditary spherocytosis, sickle cell disease, glucose-6-phosphate dehydrogenase (G6PD) deficiency, autoimmune hemolytic anemia, prosthetic heart valves, and exercise-induced hemolysis.[24] Additional sources of extraintestinal blood loss include chronic hematuria and bedbug infestation.[25]

Management of IDA after Negative VCE

Evaluation of IDA after negative VCE is influenced by the chronicity and severity of anemia, patient age, and clinical course. Mild, chronic IDA persisting for years is reassuring against malignancy, whereas a new diagnosis of severe IDA raises greater concern. In older patients, the likelihood of blood loss from angioectasias may allow for expectant management with oral iron, particularly in those with risk factors such smoking, chronic obstructive pulmonary disease, or CKD. Asymptomatic patients may often be managed conservatively once a malignant process has been reasonably excluded. In this group, additional testing is indicated if anemia recurs, with an expected 20%–35% rate of recurrent IDA within 2-3 years.[26,27] While persistent or recurrent IDA is an indication for additional evaluation in patients over age 50, continued evaluation of IDA is indicated in most patients younger than 50 after negative VCE.

Continued evaluation begins with supplemental history, including screening for features of hereditary hemorrhagic telangiectasia (epistaxis, cutaneous telangiectasias), history of blood donation, prior radiation therapy, NSAID use, rectal bleeding, hematuria, and family history of celiac disease. Supplemental laboratory testing should include celiac serology (anti-TTG IgA with total IgA), markers of AMAG (anti–intrinsic factor and anti–parietal cell antibodies), and *H. pylori* testing. Serum lactate dehydrogenase (LDH), unconjugated bilirubin, and haptoglobin are useful in screening for chronic hemolysis, while urinalysis may detect hematuria.[1,24]

Given that VCE may fail to detect approximately 19% of small bowel tumors, CT or MR enterography can serve as a complementary study to aid in their exclusion. In research settings, CTE and MRE are highly sensitive (up to 93%) for small bowel tumors such as gastrointestinal stromal tumors or carcinoids, which enhance with IV contrast. However, CTE/MRE studies performed in clinical practice are less intensive, as reimbursement does not increase with number of images interpreted.[28-31] A research protocol CTE may include ~3,000 multiphase images, compared with ~80 images in a standard study. Consequently, diagnostic performance reported in research settings may not fully translate into clinical practice.

Push enteroscopy is often recommended as next step after negative VCE as this exam allows for reinspection of upper GI tract for subtle or "missed" lesions, examination of the proximal small bowel for angioectasias, sampling of gastric fluid to screen for achlorhydria, biopsies of the stomach for AMAG or

H. pylori infection, and duodenal biopsies for villous atrophy. Repeat colonoscopy may reveal missed flat neoplasms, right-sided angioectasias, or terminal ileal disease. Second-look capsule endoscopy can provide additional diagnostic value, particularly in older patients with suspected angioectasias, with a diagnostic yield of 33%–40%. In cases of progressive anemia, reported yields are higher, ranging from 35% to 65%.[4,32,33]

Co-management with hematology should be considered in patients with CKD, chronic inflammatory disorders, or hematologic disease. In those on antiplatelet or anticoagulant therapy, the risks and benefits of continuation should be reassessed, as anticoagulation is an independent risk factor for rebleeding, with hazard ratios approaching 5 in some cohorts.[27]

Conclusion

The management of unexplained IDA after negative VCE must be individualized, with patient age serving as a key determinant of strategy. In older patients, angioectasias represent the most common etiology, and when anemia is mild, chronic, and responsive to oral iron, a conservative approach with close monitoring may be appropriate. By contrast, younger patients warrant a definitive evaluation, as angioectasias are uncommon and other clinically significant causes must be excluded. Regardless of age, severe, recurrent, or progressive anemia demands repeated testing and continued investigation until a cause is identified or anemia resolves. This framework allows for both avoidance of unnecessary testing in lower-risk scenarios and prevention of missed diagnoses in patients at greater risk for clinically significant pathology.

References

1. Ko CW, Siddique SM, Patel A. AGA Clinical practice guidelines on the gastrointestinal evaluation of iron deficiency anemia. Gastroenterology 2020;159:1085–1094
2. Wen S, Nisenbaum R, Weyand AC, et al. High prevalence of iron deficiency and socioeconomic disparities in laboratory screening of non-pregnant females of reproductive age: A retrospective cohort study. Am J Hematol. 2024;9
3. Koulaouzidis A, Rondonotti E, Giannakou A, Plevris JN. Diagnostic yield of small-bowel capsule endoscopy in patients with iron-deficiency anemia: A systematic review. Gastrointest Endosc. 2012;76(5):983-92.
4. Gerson LB, Fidler JL, Cave DR, Leighton JA. ACG Guideline: Diagnosis and management of small bowel bleeding. Am J Gastroenterol. 2015;110:1265-87.
5. ASGE Standards of Practice Committee; Gurudu SR, Bruining DH, Acosta RD, et al. The role of endoscopy in the management of suspected small-bowel bleeding. Gastrointest Endosc. 2017;85(1):22-31.
6. Evstatiev R, Gasche C. Iron sensing and signalling. Gut. 2012;61(6):933-52.
7. Vogt AS, Arsiwala T, Mohsen M, Vogel M, Manolova V, Bachmann MF. On iron metabolism and its regulation. Int J Mol Sci. 2021;22(9):4591.
8. Auerbach M, DeLoughery TG, Tirnauer JS. Iron deficiency in adults: A review. JAMA. 2025;333(20):1813-23.
9. Camaschella C. Iron deficiency. Blood. 2019;133(1):30-39. Erratum in: Blood. 2023 Feb 09;141(6):682.
10. Gill SS, Heuman DM, Mihas AA. Small intestinal neoplasms. J Clin Gastroenterol. 2001;33(4):267-82.
11. Lewis BS, Kornbluth A, Waye JD. Small bowel tumours: yield of enteroscopy. Gut. 1991;32(7):763-65.
12. Boriskin HS, Devito BS, Hines JJ, Scarmato VJ, Friedman B. CT enterography vs. capsule endoscopy. Abdom Imaging. 2009;34(2):149-55.
13. Huprich JE, Fletcher JG, Fidler JL, Alexander JA, Guimarães LS, Siddiki HA, McCollough CH. Prospective blinded comparison of wireless capsule endoscopy and multiphase CT enterography in obscure gastrointestinal bleeding. Radiology. 2011;260(3):744-51.
14. Sengupta N, Kastenberg DM, Bruining DH, et al. The role of imaging for gastrointestinal bleeding: Consensus recommendations from the American College of Gastroenterology and Society of Abdominal Radiology. Am J Gastroenterol. 2024;119(3):438-449.
15. Spada C, Riccioni ME, Familiari P, Marchese M, Bizzotto A, Costamagna G. Video capsule endoscopy in small-bowel tumours: a single centre experience. Scand J Gastroenterol. 2008;43(4):497-505.
16. Taha AS, McCloskey C, McSkimming P, McConnachie A. Misoprostol for small bowel ulcers in patients with obscure bleeding taking aspirin and non-steroidal anti-inflammatory drugs (MASTERS): A randomised, double-blind, placebo-controlled, phase 3 trial. Lancet Gastroenterol Hepatol. 2018;3(7):469-476.
17. Lara LF, Bloomfeld RS, Pineau BC. The rate of lesions found within reach of EGD during push enteroscopy depends on the type of obscure gastrointestinal bleeding. Endoscopy. 2005;37(8):745-50.

18. Shah SC, Wang AY, Wallace MB, Hwang JH. AGA Clinical Practice Update on screening and surveillance in individuals at increased risk for gastric cancer in the United States: Expert review. Gastroenterology. 2025;168(2):405-416.e1.
19. Annibale B, Marignani M, Monarca B, et al. Reversal of iron deficiency anemia after *Helicobacter pylori* eradication in patients with asymptomatic gastritis. Ann Intern Med. 1999;131(9):668-72.
20. Mahadev S, Laszkowska M, Sundström J, et al. Prevalence of celiac disease in patients with iron deficiency anemia-A systematic review with meta-analysis. Gastroenterology. 2018;155(2):374-382.e1.
21. Attwood SE, Ell C, Galmiche JP, et al. Long-term safety of proton pump inhibitor therapy assessed under controlled, randomised clinical trial conditions: data from the SOPRAN and LOTUS studies. Aliment Pharmacol Ther. 2015;41(11):1162-74.
22. Moayyedi P, Eikelboom JW, Bosch J, et al. Safety of proton pump inhibitors based on a large, multi-year, randomized trial of patients receiving rivaroxaban or aspirin. Gastroenterology. 2019 Sep;157(3):682-691.e2
23. Munro MG, Mast AE, Powers JM, et al. The relationship between heavy menstrual bleeding, iron deficiency, and iron deficiency anemia. Am J Obstet Gynecol. 2023;229(1):1-9.
24. Phillips J, Henderson AC. Hemolytic anemia: Evaluation and dfferential diagnosis. Am Fam Physician. 2018;98(6):354-361.
25. Thomas C, Castillo Valladares H, Berger TG, Chang AY. Scabies, bedbug, and body lice infestations: A review. JAMA. 2024;332(14):1189-1199
26. Park JJ, Cheon JH, Kim HM, et al. Negative capsule endoscopy without subsequent enteroscopy does not predict lower long-term rebleeding rates in patients with obscure GI bleeding. Gastrointest Endosc. 2010;71(6):990-7.
27. Lai LH, Wong GL, Chow DK, Lau JY, Sung JJ, Leung WK. Long-term follow-up of patients with obscure gastrointestinal bleeding after negative capsule endoscopy. Am J Gastroenterol. 2006;101(6):1224-8.
28. Rondonotti E, Pennazio M, Toth E, et al. Small-bowel neoplasms in patients undergoing video capsule endoscopy: a multicenter European study. Endoscopy. 2008;40(6):488-95.
29. Yaghoobi M, Tan J, Alshammari YTATA, Scandrett K, Mofrad K, Takwoingi Y. Video capsule endoscopy versus computed tomography enterography in assessing suspected small bowel bleeding: a systematic review and diagnostic test accuracy meta-analysis. Eur J Gastroenterol Hepatol. 2023;35(11):1253-1262.
30. Hakim FA, Alexander JA, Huprich JE, Grover M, Enders FT. CT-enterography may identify small bowel tumors not detected by capsule endoscopy: Eight years experience at Mayo Clinic Rochester. Dig Dis Sci. 2011;56(10):2914-9.
31. Ross A, Mehdizadeh S, Tokar J, et al. Double balloon enteroscopy detects small bowel mass lesions missed by capsule endoscopy. Dig Dis Sci. 2008, 53(8):2140-2143.
32. Viazis N, Papaxoinis K, Vlachogiannakos J, Efthymiou A, Theodoropoulos I, Karamanolis DG. Is there a role for second-look capsule endoscopy in patients with obscure GI bleeding after a nondiagnostic first test? Gastrointest Endosc. 2009;69(4):850-6.
33. Bar-Meir S, Eliakim R, Nadler M, Barkay O, Fireman Z, Scapa E, Chowers Y, Bardan E. Second capsule endoscopy for patients with severe iron deficiency anemia. Gastrointest Endosc. 2004;60(5):711-3.

CAPSULE ENDOSCOPY BY CASE STUDY
Case Study Number 8

Presented by Oleh Haluzska, MD and Daniel Raines, MD, FACG

Pre-capsule Findings (included in capsule study)

A 47-year-old man presents as an inpatient transfer for management of recurrent small bowel bleeding. He initially presented to an outside hospital with symptomatic anemia, with a hemoglobin level of 6 g/dL. Evaluation prior to transfer included EGD, colonoscopy, and computed tomography angiography (CTA), which were revealing only for maroon blood in the right colon. Over the past 3 years, this patient has experienced 6 hospitalizations for acute anemia attributed to suspected small bowel bleeding. Testing performed to date includes 7 upper endoscopies, 8 colonoscopies, 8 CTA studies, 3 video capsule endoscopy (VCE) studies, 3 device-assisted enteroscopy (DAE) exams (anterograde & retrograde), a mesenteric angiogram, and an exploratory laparotomy. The bleeding site had been localized to the proximal jejunum by 2 VCE studies and 1 CTA. However, 2 complete small bowel evaluations by DAE failed to identify an active source.

On this admission, repeat upper endoscopy with push enteroscopy, colonoscopy, VCE, and CTA are again negative. Medical provocation is elected as the next step in management of a suspected Dieulafoy lesion of proximal jejunum. The patient is transferred to the ICU for close monitoring while clopidogrel 300 mg is administered orally (12hrs prior to endoscopy) and heparin 80 units/kg is given intravenously (IV; 6hrs prior to endoscopy). A lavage bowel preparation solution is administered 12hrs and 6hrs prior to endoscopy. A VCE is initiated 8hrs prior endoscopy with metoclopramide 10 mg IV.

A capsule endoscopy study is performed to evaluate for small bowel bleeding. Review the capsule endoscopy study and report your findings, including: gastric passage time, small bowel passage time, and observed abnormalities. Be prepared to discuss your findings and management plan with your staff prior to reviewing the diagnosis and case discussion.

Capsule Endoscopy Findings

First Gastric Image = 0h 2min 2sec

First Duodenal Image = 0h 32min 54sec

Gastric passage time = 0h 30min

First Cecal Image = 6h 23min 34sec

Small bowel passage time = 5hr 53min

Gross red blood is encountered in the proximal small bowel (likely proximal jejunum) around 39 minutes into the study (**Figure 1:** 0hr 39min 2sec). Visualization of the remaining small bowel is impaired due to accumulation of blood in the bowel lumen.

Follow-Up

An emergent antegrade DAE was performed, which revealed a 1 mm focus of active, pulsatile hemorrhage in the proximal jejunum (**Figure 2**). Hemostasis was achieved with argon plasma coagulation (25 watts, 1 L/min) followed by placement of 4 hemostatic clips. Prior to withdrawal of the enteroscope, the site was marked with a submucosal India ink tattoo for future reference. The patient subsequently achieved durable resolution of bleeding, with no recurrence at 5-year follow-up.

Figure 1

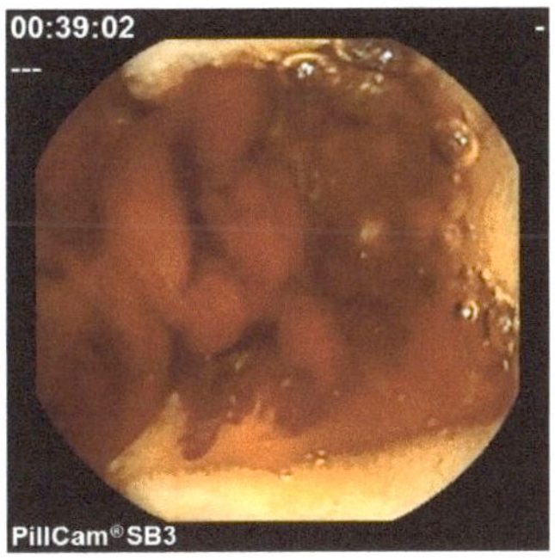

Figure 2

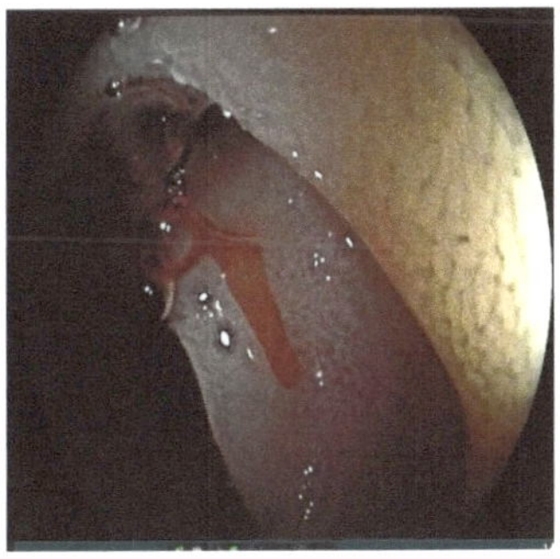

Chapter 8: The Dieulafoy Lesion

By Oleh Haluzska, MD and Daniel Raines, MD, FACG

Introduction

The Dieulafoy lesion (DL) represents one of the most problematic sources of gastrointestinal hemorrhage (GIH). It accounts for up to 5% of all cases of GIH and can result in life threatening blood loss.[1] Anatomically, DL consists of an abnormally large submucosal arteriole. While the majority of cases occur in the gastrointestinal tract these submucosal lesions have been described in other organs including the biliary tree, pancreatic duct, and pulmonary bronchi.[2] DL is currently estimated to account for 1.9% of all cases of upper GI bleeding, 0.09% of cases of lower GI bleeding, and 3.5% of cases of obscure GI bleeding.[3,4]

Anatomy and Epidemiology of Dieulafoy Lesion

The DL or "caliber persistent artery" is a submucosal artery that fails to demonstrate the standard diminution as it penetrates through the mucosa. The diameter of this artery is 1-3 mm, or almost 10 fold the diameter of normal arteries at the same level, and it erodes through a minute (2-5 mm) mucosa l defect devoid of any evidence of inflammation.[5,6] Following the initial description of this abnormality by Gallard in 1884, French surgeon Paul Georges Dieulafoy presented a series of cases which he surmised as an early presentation of a gastric ulcer, prompting him to coin the term "exulceratio simplex".[7,8] Subsequent pathologic study of DL has demonstrated common features including subintimal fibrosis, loss of elastic fibers adjacent to the necrotic wall of the artery, and a loss of circular fibers at the point of rupture. These findings suggest a slow weakening of the vessel wall with pressure erosion through the overlying epithelium.[1]

The majority of DL are found in the proximal half of the stomach (61%-82%) typically along the lesser curvature.[9] However, these lesions can be seen throughout the GI tract. The first case report of small bowel DL appeared in 1978 with 2 patients with jejunal bleeding identified and treated surgically.[10] One review of 90 DL identified in a single institution prior to the advent of video capsule endoscopy (VCE) found that 64% were gastric, 20% small intestinal, 10% colonic, and 2% esophageal.[11] The recent availability of methods of endoscopically visualizing the entire small bowel have made greater identification and recognition of these lesions possible and may well alter the reported distribution of DL as more data becomes available. DL appears to be more common in males, and although it is rarely described in childhood, it is more commonly associated with aging.[12] It may be more common in those with comorbid conditions such as cardiovascular disease, chronic renal disease, hypertension, and diabetes mellitus. It has also been associated with the use of NSAIDs, aspirin, and antiplatelet aggregation agents but not associated with the use of alcohol.[9,13]

Presentation of Dieulafoy Lesion

The typical presentation of DL is a patient with evidence of rapid blood loss presenting with hematemesis or melena, and hemodynamic instability.[13,14,15,16] Small bowel DL may present as intermittent bleeding necessitating repeated red blood cell transfusions, typically with negative bleeding scans, CTA, and angiography. One Japanese series utilizing both VCE and double balloon enteroscopy in evaluation of cases of overt and occult bleeding identified small bowel DL as a potential source of both patterns of bleeding.[17]

Diagnosis of Dieulafoy Lesion

Endoscopic criteria for the diagnosis of a DL include: (1) active arterial spurting or micropulsatile streaming from a minute (<3 mm) mucosal defect with otherwise normal surrounding mucosa (**Figure 1**); (2) visualization of a protruding vessel, with or without active bleeding, through a small defect in normal-appearing mucosa; or (3) a fresh, densely adherent clot with a narrow point of attachment to either a minute mucosal defect or to otherwise normal mucosa.[18] In the absence of active hemorrhage, this lesion can be easily overlooked. Meticulous technique is required during endoscopic evaluation, including irrigation to clear blood and adherent clot. Multiphasic contrast-enhanced CT has emerged as an increasingly valuable diagnostic tool for localization of DL in preparation for subsequent endoscopic therapy or angiographic embolization. On imaging, DL may appear as a tiny, round or linear enhancing submucosal focus abutting the lumen, occasionally with evidence of active contrast extravasation.[19]

Medical provocation of bleeding in DL may be considered in highly selected cases, with the

LSU Provocation Protocol representing the most widely studied and commonly applied approach.[20] Candidates should undergo comprehensive evaluation to exclude alternative sources of gastrointestinal bleeding, including upper endoscopy, colonoscopy, capsule endoscopy, DAE, and cross-sectional imaging (CTE/MRE). Optimal candidates are those in whom a bleeding segment has been previously localized. The protocol consists of oral clopidogrel (300 mg) combined with intravenous heparin (80 U/kg) to provoke recurrent bleeding, achieving a per procedure diagnostic yield of 71%, with DL as the most common etiology (**Figure 2a, 2b**). One subgroup receiving clopidogrel alone demonstrated a 53% yield. Subsequent protocol modifications exclude patients at increased risk for catastrophic hemorrhage, including those with risk factor for aortoenteric fistula, hemosuccus pancreaticus, hemobilia, or small bowel varices. Successful implementation requires advance planning and resources, including ICU monitoring, surgical and interventional radiology support, access to crossmatched packed red blood cells and reversal agents, and capability to examine the entire small bowel by DAE.[20]

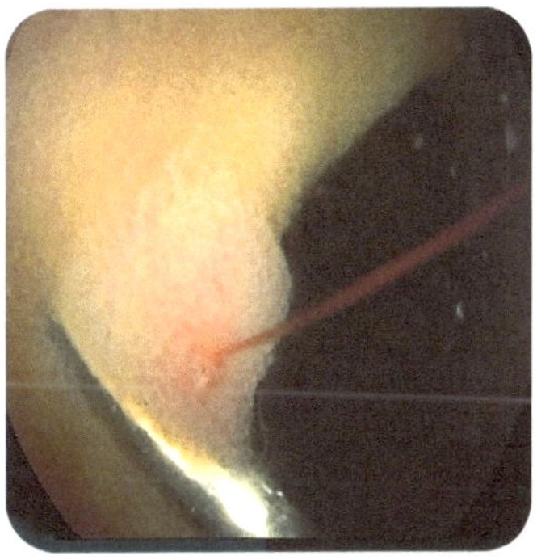

Figure 1. Active arterial spurting or micropulsatile streaming from a minute (<3 mm) mucosal defect with otherwise normal surrounding mucosa.

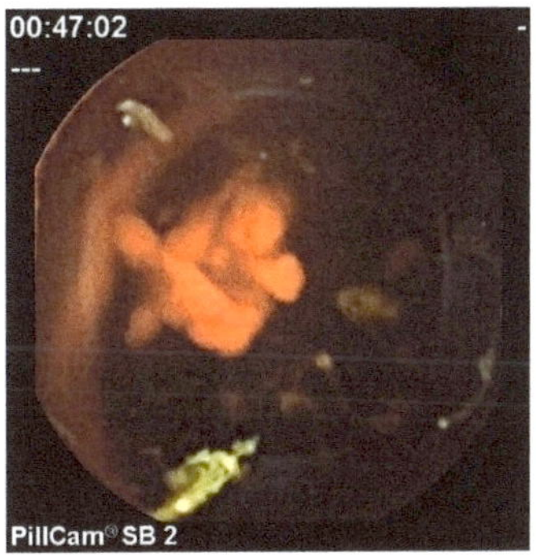

Figure 2a. Active small bowel hemorrhage from a jejunal DL, observed by VCE.

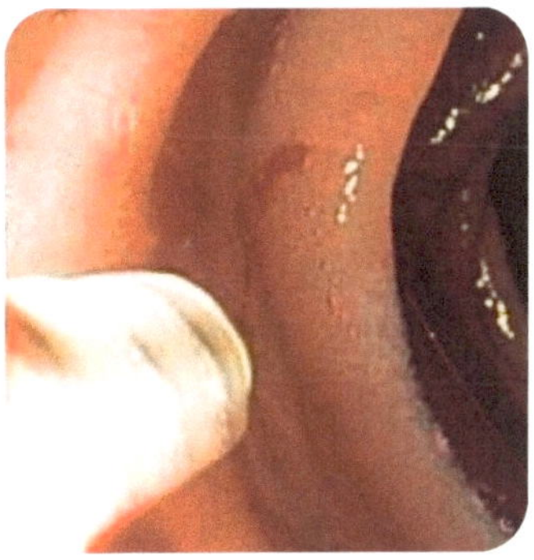

Figure 2b. The same jejunal DL identified by VCE is localized for endoscopic therapy using DAE.

Management of Dieulafoy Lesion

Prior to the development of therapeutic endoscopy, the only available therapy for DL was surgical ligation of the offending vessel or segmental resection. Reported experience with endoscopic therapy for DL suggests that endoscopic methods are highly effective within the range of 90%-95% success at initial hemostasis. A variety of methods have been used including heater probe contact coagulation, laser photoablation, argon plasma coagulation, and hemoclips.[21,22,23,24] Epinephrine injection is a useful adjunct to slow or stop bleeding prior to contact thermal ablation and/or endoscopic ligation with hemoclips. Combination therapy with both thermal ablation and clips is more likely to be successful than either therapy alone.[25] Given the difficulties in accessing the deeper regions of the small bowel, it is useful to mark the site with an India ink tattoo to facilitate localization by either repeat enteroscopy or surgery. Hemoclips may also guide angiography in the acute setting. Angiography with embolization is generally considered as secondary or salvage therapy for DL.[3,26]

Endoscopic band ligation has been reported as option for endoscopic therapy of DL. In one study by Ahn et al, endoscopic band ligation (EBL) was found to be equally effective as hemoclips for treatment of upper GI bleeding related to DL with active bleeding.[27] Utilization of a doppler endoscopic probe may also be useful in the management of DL, if available. This modality allows confirmation of obliteration of arterial flow following hemostasis. In a retrospective analysis of 82 patients with DL complicated by severe upper GI bleeding, treatment using doppler endoscopic probe as an adjunct was associated with a lower risk of rebleeding at 30 days (11%) compared to standard hemostasis (33%).[28]

Summary of Dieulafoy Lesion

Dieulafoy lesion is an uncommon but important cause of gastrointestinal hemorrhage that may be difficult to identify unless actively bleeding during examination.

Endoscopic therapy is highly effective, with clips, thermal coagulation, and band ligation all achieving high rates of initial hemostasis, particularly when used in combination. In select cases of recurrent, obscure bleeding, provocation of hemorrhage has been shown to improve diagnostic yield and facilitate targeted therapy. Overall, recognition of this lesion and persistence in evaluation are essential, as successful endoscopic therapy is often curative.

References

1. Lara LF, Sreenarishimhaiah J, Tag S, et al. Dieulafoy lesions of the GI tract: Localization and therapeutic outcomes. Dig Dis Sci 2010, 55:3436-3441.
2. Zhou P, Yu W, Chen K, Li X, Xia Q. A case report and review of literature of Dieulafoy's disease of bronchus: A rare life-threatening pathologic vascular condition. Medicine (Baltimore). 2019; 98(7):e14471.
3. Wang Y, Bansal P, Li S, Iqbal Z, Cheryala M, Abougergi MS. Dieulafoy's lesion of the upper GI tract: a comprehensive nationwide database analysis. Gastrointest Endosc. 2021;94(1):24-34.e5.
4. Nguyen DC, Jackson CS. The dieulafoy's lesion: An update on evaluation, diagnosis, and management. J Clin Gastroenterol. 2015; 49(7):541-9.
5. Lee YT, Walmsley RS, Leong RWL, et al. Dieulafoy's lesion. Gastrointest Endosc 2003, 58: 236-243.
6. Miko TL, Thomazy VA. The caliber persistent artery of the stomach: a unifying approach to gastric aneurysm, Dieulafoy's lesion, and submucosal arterial malformation. Hum Pathol 1988, 19:914-921.
7. Gallard MT. Anevrismes miliares de l'estomac donnant lieu à des hematemeses mortelles. Bull Soc Med Hop Paris. 1884;1:84–91.
8. Dieulafoy G. Exulceratio simplex. L'intervention chirurgicale dans les hématémèses foudroyantes consécutives à l'exulcération simple de l'estomac. Bull Acad Med. 1898;39:49–84.
9. Schmulewitz N, Baillie J. Dieulafoy lesions: A review of 6 years of experience at a tertiary referral center. Am J Gastroenterol. 2001; 96:1688-1694.
10. Matuchansky C, Babin P, Abadie JC, Payen J, Gasquet C, Barbier J. Jejunal bleeding from a solitary large submucosal artery. Report of two cases. Gastroenterology. 1978;75(1):110-3.
11. Norton ID, Petersen BT, Sorbi D, Balm RK, Alexander GL, Gostout CJ. Management and long-term prognosis of Dieulafoy lesion. Gastrointest Endosc. 1999; 50(6):762-7.
12. Lee YJ, Oh JM, Park SE, Park JH. Successful treatment of a gastric Dieulafoy's lesion with a hemoclip in a newborn infant. Gastrointest Endosc. 2003 Mar;57(3):435-6.
13. Stark ME, Gostout CJ, Balm RK. Clinical features and endoscopic management of Dieulafoy's disease. Gastrointest Endosc. 1992; 38(5):545-50.
14. Marchese M, De Cristofaro R, Federici AB, et al. Duodenal and gastric Dieulafoy's lesions in a patient with type 2A von Willebrand's disease. Gastrointest Endosc. 2005; 61(2):322-5.
15. Ding Yj, Zhao L, Luo HS. Clinical and endoscopic analysis of gastric Dieulafoy's lesion. World J Gastroenterol. 2010; 16:631-635.
16. Blecker D, Bansal M, Zimmerman RL, et al. Dieulafoy's lesion of the small bowel causing massive gastrointestinal bleeding: two case reports and literature review. Am J Gastroenterol. 2001;96(3):902-5.
17. Arakawa D, Ohmiya N, Nakamura M, et al. Outcome after enteroscopy for patients with obscure GI bleeding: diagnostic comparison between double-balloon endoscopy and videocapsule endoscopy. Gastrointest Endosc. 2009; 69(4):866-74.
18. Dy NM, Gostout CJ, Balm RK. Bleeding from the endoscopically-identified Dieulafoy lesion of the proximal small intestine and colon. Am J Gastroenterol. 1995;90(1):108-11.
19. Batouli A, Kazemi A, Hartman MS, Heller MT, Midian R, Lupetin AR. Dieulafoy lesion: CT diagnosis of this lesser-known cause of gastrointestinal bleeding. Clin Radiol. 2015;70(6):661-6.
20. Raines DL, Jex KT, Nicaud MJ, Adler DG. Pharmacologic provocation combined with endoscopy in refractory cases of GI bleeding. Gastrointest Endosc. 2017;85(1):112-120.
21. Chung IK, Kim EJ, Lee MS, et al. Bleeding Dieulafoy's lesions and the choice of endoscopic method: comparing the hemostatic efficacy of mechanical and injection methods. Gastrointest Endosc. 2000; 52(6):721-4.
22. Kasapidis P, Georgopoulis P, Delis V, et al. Endoscopic management and long-term follow-up of Dieulafoy's lesions in the upper GI tract. Gastrointest Endosc. 2002; 55:527-531.
23. Yamaguchi Y, Yamato T, Katsumi N, et al. Short-term and long-term benefits of endoscopic hemoclip application for Dieulafoy's lesion in the upper GI tract. Gastrointest Endosc. 2003 May;57(6):653-6.
24. Sone Y, Kumada T, Toyoda H, Hisanaga Y, Kiriyama S, Tanikawa M. Endoscopic management and follow up of Dieulafoy lesion in the upper gastrointestinal tract. Endoscopy. 2005;37(5):449-53.
25. Kanth R, Mali P, Roy PK. Outcomes in Dieulafoy's Lesion: A 10-Year Clinical Review. Dig Dis Sci. 2015;60(7):2097-103.
26. Loffroy R, Falvo N, Nakai M, Pescatori L, Midulla M, Chevallier O. When all else fails - Radiological management of severe gastrointestinal bleeding. Best Pract Res Clin Gastroenterol. 2019; 42-43:101612.
27. Ahn DW, Lee SH, Park YS, et al. Hemostatic efficacy and clinical outcome of endoscopic treatment of Dieulafoy's

lesions: comparison of endoscopic hemoclip placement and endoscopic band ligation. Gastrointest Endosc. 2012;75(1):32-8.
28. Nulsen B, Jensen DM, Kovacs TOG, et al. Outcomes in severe upper gi hemorrhage from dieulafoy's lesion with monitoring of arterial blood flow. Dig Dis Sci. 2021;66(10):3495-3504.

Case Study Number 9

Presented by Jason Stibbe, MD

Pre-capsule Findings (included in capsule study)

A 32-year-old woman with a history of hypertension and type II diabetes is admitted to the hospital with hematochezia. She reports multiple bowel movements with bright red blood over the past 12 hours. She admits to nausea and intermittent epigastric pain associated with these symptoms. Upon admission, her hemoglobin is 8 gm/dl compared to her baseline of 13 gm/dl. An urgent upper endoscopy is performed and negative. She is admitted to the Intensive Care Unit for monitoring and potential packed red blood cell transfusion. She completes a bowel prep overnight in preparation for colonoscopy the next day. A CT angiogram was ordered by the on-call team but cancelled due to a history of severe allergy to iodinated contrast. A colonoscopy is performed 24 hours after admission with findings of gross red blood throughout the colon and within the terminal ileum.

An inpatient capsule endoscopy study is performed to evaluate for small bowel bleeding. Review the capsule endoscopy study and report your findings, including gastric passage time, small bowel passage time, and observed abnormalities. Be prepared to discuss your findings and management plan with your staff prior to reviewing the diagnosis and case discussion.

Capsule transit through the stomach is somewhat delayed ~4hrs with first entry into the duodenum at 3hrs 46min 13sec, followed by reflux into the stomach. The capsule passes through the pylorus a second, and final time, at 3hrs 58min 20sec. A tiny red spot is observed in the duodenum at 3hrs 51min 49sec (**Figure 1**). Gross red blood is encountered in the distal duodenum but a source of bleeding is not identified (**Figure 2:** 4hrs 3min 0sec).

Capsule Endoscopy Findings
First Gastric Image = 0h 0min 8sec
First Duodenal Image = 3h 58min 20sec*
Gastric passage time = 3h 58min
First Cecal Image = 4h 40min
Small bowel passage time = 6hr 19min

*Last entry into the duodenum.

Figure 1

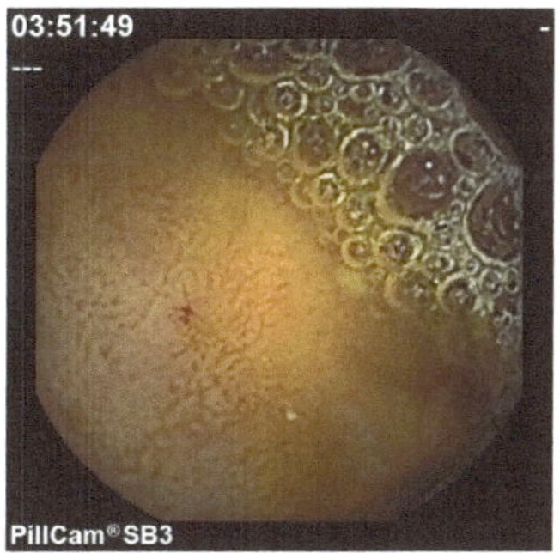

Figure 2

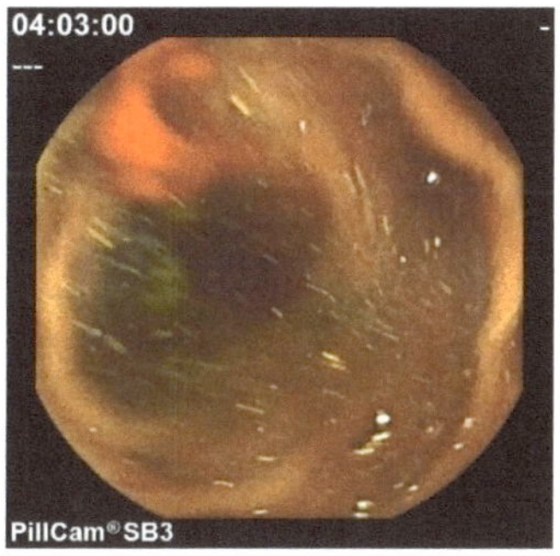

Follow-up

A repeat upper endoscopy is performed using a pediatric colonoscope for push enteroscopy. Inspection of the duodenum is revealing for active bleeding from the major papilla. (**Figure 3**) To further investigate this finding, an MRI of the abdomen is performed which demonstrates a 25 mm nodule within the gallbladder which enhances with IV contrast. (**Figure 4**) The patient is elected for surgery which is successful in removing the gallbladder with nodule intact. A large adenomatous polyp was diagnosed by pathology.

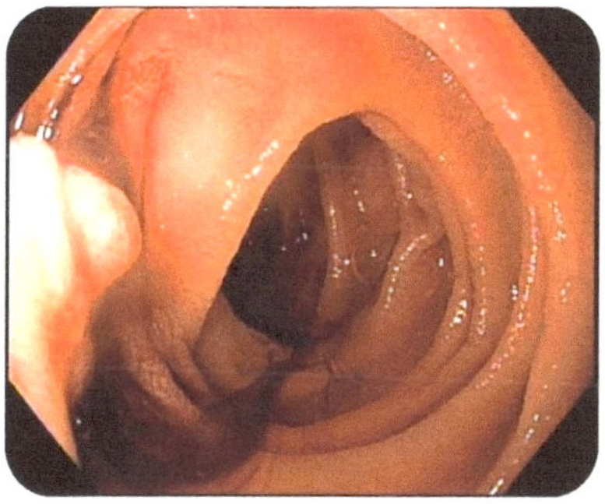

Figure 3

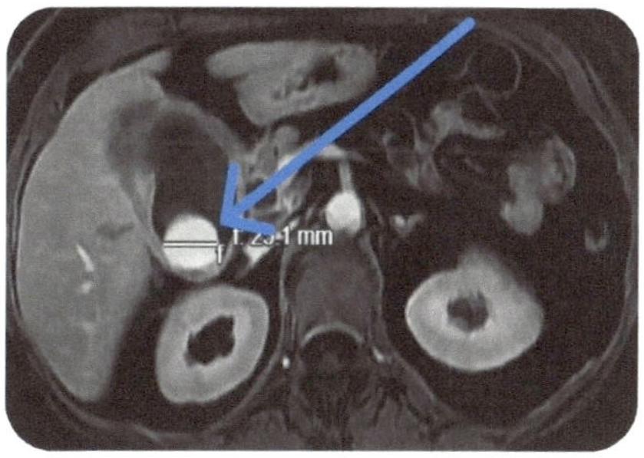

Figure 4

Chapter 9: Hemobilia & Hemosuccus

Jason Stibbe, MD

Introduction

Hemobilia is defined as gross bleeding within the biliary system[1] while hemosuccus pancreaticus is defined as bleeding within the pancreatic duct.[2] Endoscopic visualization of blood flowing from the major papilla is often required for diagnosis of hemobilia or hemosuccus. As active bleeding may occur sporadically in these cases, confirmation of the bleeding source is often challenging. Most cases of hemobilia and hemosuccus in the United States are iatrogenic, related to surgery or interventional radiology procedures.[3] However, a variety of pathologies may present with bleeding from the biliary tree or pancreatic duct.

Pathophysiology

Reported cases of hemobilia have been described for nearly 4 centuries although the moniker 'hemobilia' was not given until the 1940s. Over 3 major case series since the 1970s, etiologies have been broadly categorized into traumatic, iatrogenic, inflammatory, vascular, neoplastic, or miscellaneous. The first series of 355 cases published in 1973 by Sandblom et al[4] reported that the majority of cases of hemobilia were traumatic (38%) or iatrogenic (17%). Technological advancement in interventional procedures over the past few decades has resulted in iatrogenic hemobilia as the leading category. This trend was demonstrated in 1987 by Yoshida et al with 41% iatrogenic vs 19% traumatic (of 103 patients) then by Green et al in 2001 with 65% iatrogenic vs 6% traumatic (of 222 patients).[5,6] These publications illustrate how the incidence of iatrogenic hemobilia parallels the adoption of increasingly intricate hepatobiliary interventions. Etiologies of hemobilia and hemosuccus are presented in **Table 1**.[8-12]

Vascular communications with the biliary or pancreatic ducts may develop as the result of any chronic inflammatory process complicated by pseudoaneurysm formation or by a direct arterial or venous fistula. Hemobilia is observed in cases of chronic cholecystitis, chronic cholangitis, or intrahepatic abscess or tumor while pancreatic pseudocysts are a common cause of hemosuccus.[13,14] Hemobilia is a known complication of hepatic malignancies due to invasion of vessels and ductal systems by tumors while hemosuccus is a complication of pancreatic malignancies for the same reason. Cholangiocarcinoma and hepatocellular carcinoma are particularly prone to bleeding into the biliary tree.[15] In rare cases, bleeding may originate from a vascular lesion within or associated with pancreaticobiliary ductal epithelium (i.e., Dieulafoy, arteriovenous malformation, or vascular tumor). Specific etiologies of hemobilia are illustrated in **Figure 1.**

Clinical Presentation

Approximately one-third of cases of hemobilia present with a classic triad of clinical findings, including right-upper quadrant abdominal pain, jaundice, and melenic/bloody stools (Quincke's Triad).[16] The majority of patients present with 1 or 2 of these findings along with additional symptoms of hematemesis, symptomatic anemia, hypotension, or fever. A thorough history should assess for any history of surgery, trauma, or other hepatobiliary interventions. Findings of an acute drop in hemoglobin combined with an acute rise in AST, ALT, alkaline phosphatase, and/or total bilirubin are important clues. Imaging studies may show filling defects in the bile ducts due

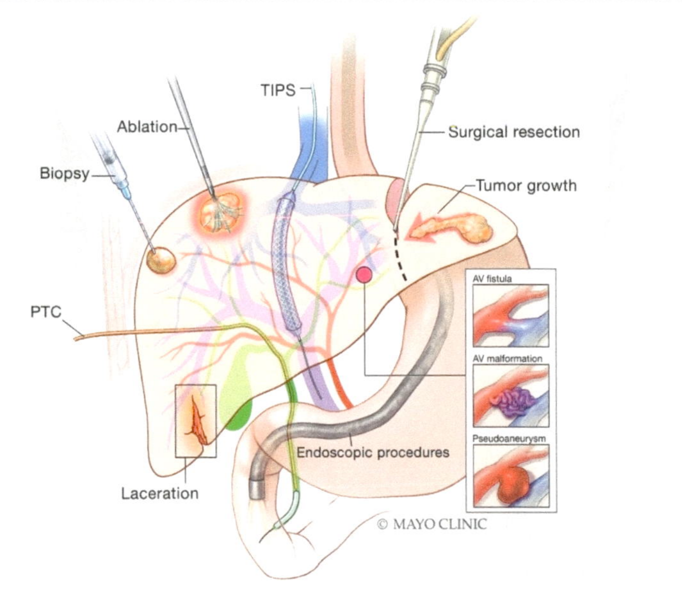

Figure 1. Common causes of hemobilia, including various hepatobiliary procedures as well as noniatrogenic trauma, neoplasm, and vascular disorders. AV, arteriovenous; PTC, percutaneous transhepatic cholangiography; TIPS, transjugular intrahepatic portosystemic shunt.

Reused with permission from the Mayo Clinic.

	Hemobilia	Hemosuccus Pancreaticus
Iatrogenic	*Surgical* • Cholecystectomy • Liver segment resection • Liver transplant *Radiologic* • Transjugular intrahepatic portosystemic shunt (TIPS) • Percutaneous liver biopsy • Percutaneous cholangiogram (PTC) or cholecystostomy • Radiofrequency ablation (RFA) *Endoscopic* • ERCP with sphincterotomy • ERCP with biliary instrumentation • EUS-guided liver biopsy	*Surgical* • Pancreatic resection • Panceaticointestinal anastamosis *Radiologic* • Percutaneous drainage of fluid collection *Endoscopic* • EUS-guided biopsy • EUS-guided cystgastrostomy • EUS-guided cyst or tumor ablation • ERCP with pancreatic duct instrumentation
Trauma	Motor vehicle collisions Liver lacerations	Blunt trauma Penetrating injury
Inflammatory	Hepatic artery pseudoaneurysm (secondary) Chronic cholecystitis Chronic cholangitis Hepatic abscess Parasitic inflammation (ex: Clonorchis, Ascaris, Fasciola hepatica)	Pseudoaneurysm with hemorrhage (secondary) • Splenic artery • Gastroduodenal artery • Pancreaticoduodenal artery Diffuse parenchymal hemorrhage with necrosis
Malignancy	Cholangiocarcinoma Hepatocellular carcinoma (HCC) Metastatic disease	Pancreatic adenocarcinoma Neuroendocrine tumor Metastatic disease
Vascular	Dieulafoy lesion of the bile duct AVM of the bile duct or communicating with the duct Vascular tumor communicating with the duct	Primary aneurysm • Splenic artery (congenital or acquired) • Celiac trunk aneurysm • Mycotic aneurysm (brucellosis, syphilis) Segmental arterial mediolysis (SAM) Intraparenchymal AVM

Table 1. Etiologies of hemobilia and hemosuccus.

AVM, arteriovenous malformation ERCP, endoscopic retrograde cholangiopancreatography; EUS, endoscopic ultrasound.

to blood clots. Hemosuccus pancreaticus presents with abdominal pain and melenic or bloody stools. Laboratory findings may show a combination of drop in hemoglobin with elevation of serum amylase and/ or lipase.[17]

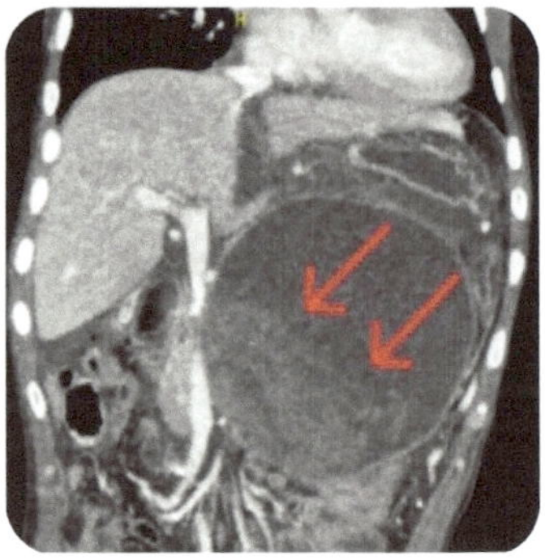

Figure 3a. CTA study of hemosuccus secondary to vascular hemorrhaging into pseudocyst with layering blood (red arrows).

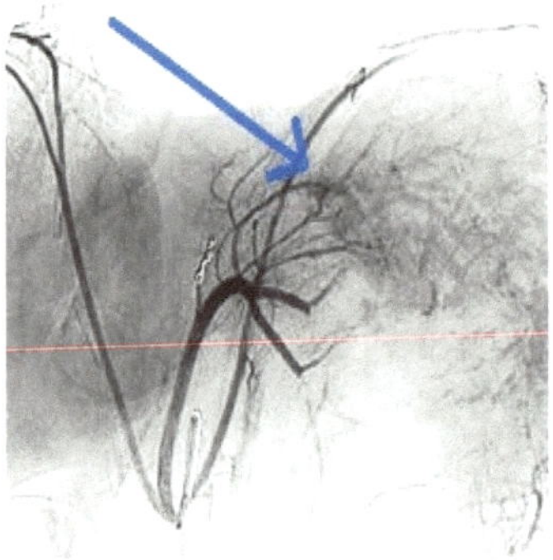

Figure 3b. Angiographic embolization of the left gastric artery in the same patient to treat the site of the hemorrhage (blue arrow).

Diagnosis

CT angiography is the diagnostic study of choice to document active bleeding from the biliary tree or pancreatic duct. In cases in which bleeding is inactive or intermittent, direct visualization of the major ampulla may support a diagnosis of hemobilia or hemosuccus pancreaticus. A side-viewing duodenoscope can be invaluable for clear visualization and close inspection of the papilla for active bleeding or visible clot. In cases of intermittent bleeding, a technique of prolonged (5-10 minutes) inspection of the papilla and intermittent suctioning may be useful in eliciting visible flow of red blood or blood clots.

Video capsule endoscopy (VCE) is the next step in evaluation of patients with gastrointestinal bleeding which is unexplained after standard upper and lower endoscopy. In cases of hemobilia or hemosuccus, VCE may successfully localize the source of bleeding to the duodenum. In some cases, a video capsule study may obtain images of active bleeding from the ampullary orifice (**Figure 2**).[18] Magnetic resonance cholangiopancreatography may also be useful in these cases by identifying filling defects suggestive of clots or blood in the pancreaticobiliary ducts.

Management

Angiography is the standard primary intervention for hemobilia and hemosuccus as it allows for precise localization and embolization of the bleeding source (**Figure 3a,b**).[19] In select cases, endoscopic intervention with endoscopic retrograde cholangiopancreatography may be considered with or without direct cholangioscopy. Endoscopic therapy may include balloon tamponade, stenting, ablation, and/or injection. In cases of hepatopancreaticobiliary bleeding that cannot be controlled using angiography or endoscopic intervention, surgery may be required to achieve hemostasis.

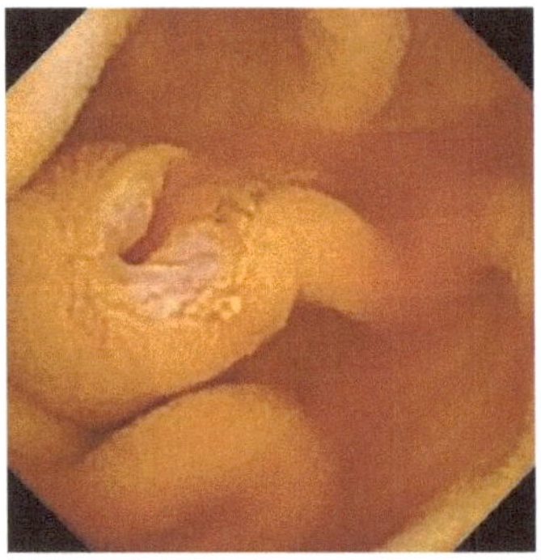

Figure 2. Capsule endoscopy showing fresh blood from an otherwise normal appearing ampulla of Vater.
Image reused from from Scarola et al[18] with permission from Oxford University Press.

Conclusion

Gastrointestinal bleeding which originates from the pancreatobiliary ducts should be considered in the differential of all cases of obscure gastrointestinal bleeding. The finding of gross blood in the duodenum by endoscopy is suggestive of pancreaticobiliary hemorrhage while direct visualization of blood flowing from the papilla is often necessary for confirmation. Video capsule endoscopy is an essential diagnostic tool for localizing bleeding sources in the GI tract. In the majority of cases, bleeding from the biliary tree or pancreatic duct can be effectively treated once the source has been established.

References

1. Khamaysi I, Suissa A. Hemobilia. Gastrointest Endosc. 2017;86(6):1176-1177
2. Anil Kothari R, Leelakrishnan V, Krishnan M. Hemosuccus pancreaticus: A rare cause of gastrointestinal bleeding. Ann Gastroenterol. 2013;26(2):175-177.
3. Zhornitskiy A, Berry R, Han JY, Tabibian JH. Hemobilia: Historical overview, clinical update, and current practices. Liver Int. 2019;39:1378-1388.
4. Sandblom P. Hemobilia. Surg Clin North Am. 1973;53(5):1191-1201.
5. Yoshida J, Donahue PE, Nyhus LM. Hemobilia: Review of recent experience with a worldwide problem. Am J Gastroenterol. 1987;82(5):448-453.
6. Green MH, Duell RM, Johnson CD, Jamieson NV. Haemobilia. Br J Surg. 2001;88(6):773-786.
7. Bloechle C, Izbicki JR, Rashed MY, el-Sefi T, Hosch SB, Knoefel WT, Rogiers X, Broelsch CE. Hemobilia: presentation, diagnosis, and management. Am J Gastroenterol. 1994;89(9):1537-40.
8. Lee S, Gavin M. Hemosuccus pancreaticus on endoscopy. ACG Case Rep J. 2022;9(9):e00814.
9. Cathcart S, Birk JW, Tadros M, Schuster M. Hemobilia: An uncommon but notable cause of upper gastrointestinal bleeding. J Clin Gastroenterolo. 2017;51(9):796-804.
10. Stabile BE, Wilson SE, Debas HT. Reduced mortality from bleeding pseudocysts and pseudoaneurysms caused by pancreatitis. Arch Surg. 1983;118(1):45-51
11. Balthazar EJ, Fisher LA. Hemorrhagic complications of pancreatitis: Radiologic evaluation with emphasis on CT imaging. Pancreatology. 2001;1(4):306-13
12. Han B, Song ZF, Sun B. Hemosuccus pancreaticus: A rare cause of gastrointestinal bleeding. Hepatobiliary Pancreat Dis Int. 2012;11(5):479-88.
13. Saad NE, Saad WE, Davies MG, Waldman DL, Fultz PJ, Rubens DJ. Pseudoaneurysms and the role of minimally invasive techniques in their management. RadioGraphics 2005;25(Suppl 1):S173–S189.
14. Liou TC, Ling CC, Pang KK. Liver abscess concomitant with hemobilia due to rupture of hepatic artery aneurysm: A case report. Hepatogastroenterology 1996;43(7):241–244.
15. Massarweh NN, El-Serag HB. Epidemiology of hepatocellular carcinoma and intrahepatic cholangiocarcinoma. Cancer Contr 2017;24(3):1073274817729245.
16. Parvinian A, Fletcher JG, Storm AC, Venkatesh SK, Fidler JL, Khandelwal AR. Challenges in diagnosis and management of hemobilia. RadioGraphics 2021; 41:802-813.
17. Liu B, Contreras FJ, Ward TJ. Hemosuccus pancreaticus. J Vasc Interv Radiol 2017;28(8):1194.
18. Scarola S, Sibia US, Gibson G. Gallbladder cancer presenting as hemobilia on capsule endoscopy. J Surg Case Rep. 2022(5):1-3
19. Saad WE, Davies MG, Darcy MD. Management of bleeding after percutaneous transhepatic cholangiography or transhepatic biliary drain placement. Tech Vasc Interv Radiol 2008;11(1):60–71.

Case Study Number 10

Presented by Erika Haviland, DO and Catherine Hudson, MD

Pre-capsule Findings (included in capsule study)

A 53-year-old male physician presents to your office for evaluation of a new diagnosis of iron deficiency anemia. There are no associated symptoms of weight loss, change in bowel habits, hematochezia, vomiting, or epistaxis. He reports no medical issues and maintains peak physical condition as a triathlete. Medications include melatonin for sleep and a testosterone supplement prescribed by his urologist. He denies any history of NSAID use. Physical examination is negative for any signs of pathology. Your colleague is scheduled for an endoscopic evaluation which includes upper endoscopy with duodenal biopsies and colonoscopy with inspection of the terminal ileum. When these exams fail to define a cause of his iron deficiency anemia, a video capsule endoscopy study is recommended.

A capsule endoscopy study is performed to evaluate for small bowel bleeding. Review the capsule endoscopy study and report your findings, including: gastric passage time, small bowel passage time, and observed abnormalities. Be prepared to discuss your findings and management plan with your staff prior to reviewing the diagnosis and case discussion.

Capsule Endoscopy Findings
First Gastric Image = 0h 0min 27sec
First Duodenal Image = 0h 6min 50sec
Gastric passage time = 0h 6min
First Cecal Image = 6h 25min 44sec
Small bowel passage time = 6hr 19min

The esophagus, stomach and duodenum appear normal. During transit through the deep small bowel, an inflammatory stricture is encountered with diffuse mucosal lymphangiectasia (white-tipped villi) (**Figure 1**: 1hr 26min 32sec; **Figure 2**: 2hr 5min 15sec) The video capsule identifies additional inflammatory strictures in the mid and distal small bowel including several lesions associated with ulceration and bleeding (**Figure 3**: 4h 53min 8sec).

Follow-up

The patient is scheduled for a follow-up visit to discuss his video capsule endoscopy study results. Upon re-evaluation, the patient reports that he had been treated with external beam radiation therapy for testicular cancer in his early 20's but forgot to mention this during his medical history. A retrograde device-assisted enteroscopy (DAE) exam is performed to obtain tissue biopsies from the ileum (**Figure 4**), which confirm a diagnosis of radiation enteritis.

Figure 1

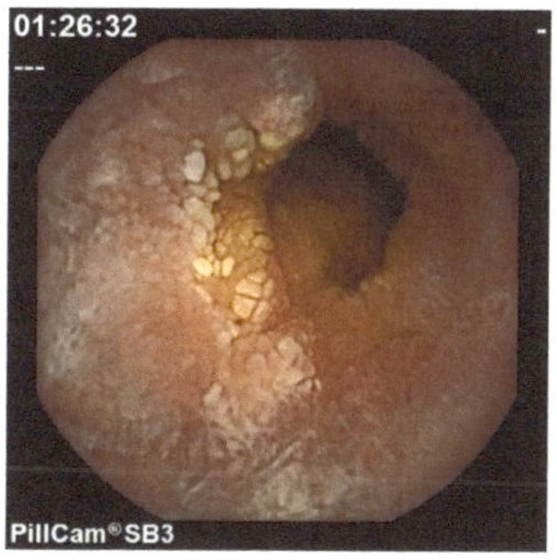

Figure 2

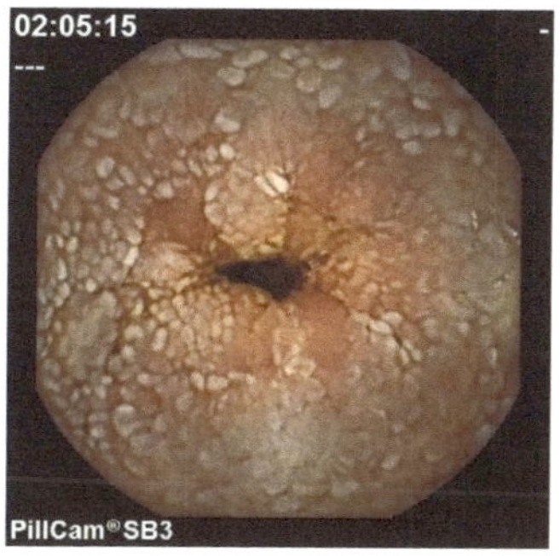

Figure 3

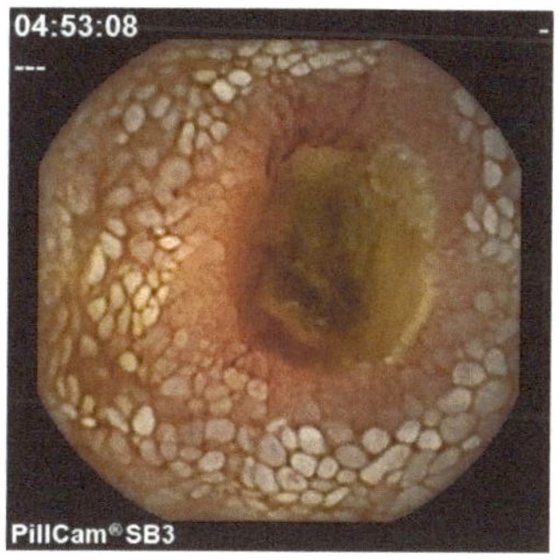

Figure 4

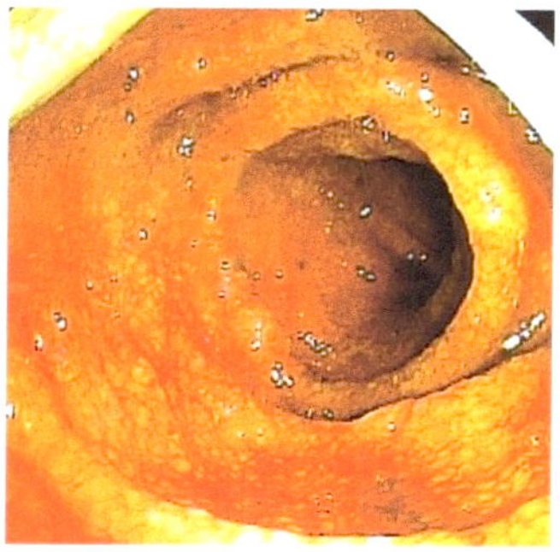

Chapter 10: Radiation Enteritis

Erika Haviland, DO, and Catherine Hudson, MD

Introduction

Radiation enteritis (RE) refers to inflammation and injury of the small intestine resulting from external beam radiation (XRT) used to treat abdominal and pelvic cancers. In the acute setting, patients treated with XRT may experience temporary abdominal discomfort, diarrhea, and/or nausea. Chronic radiation injury develops years after therapy, resulting in complications of malabsorption, chronic gastrointestinal blood loss, intestinal obstruction, and/or fistula formation. Current treatment options primarily focus on alleviating symptoms, while surgical interventions are reserved as a therapy of last resort.

Pathophysiology

Radiation therapy remains a cornerstone of treatment for a variety of malignancies. It is estimated that up to 70% of cancer patients will undergo radiotherapy at some point as part of their oncological regimen.[1] Patients who receive abdominopelvic radiation are at risk for RE. Specifically, those undergoing treatment for gastrointestinal, gynecological, urological, or other intraabdominal tumors.[2] A history of intraabdominal surgery is a major risk factor for RE, as adhesions may tether segments of bowel to a fixed location receiving XRT. At doses of 10-30 Gy, around 40% of patients will have gastrointestinal manifestations, while up to 90% of patients will be affected at doses of 30 Gy or beyond.[3] As a reference, a common prostate cancer treatment regimen consists of 75 Gy administered over 8 weeks.[4]

Multiple factors contribute to the pathogenesis of RE, including direct cellular injury, disruption of the gut microbiota, and ischemia resulting from microvascular injury. Direct cellular injury initiates a shift in the gut microbiota, which induces DNA damage, which in turn creates reactive oxygen species that trigger apoptosis in the intestinal epithelial and stem cells. This leads to a breakdown of the mucosal barrier through the loss of crypts, thereby increasing intestinal permeability. Consequently, luminal bacteria and endotoxins translocate across the damaged barrier, further altering microbiota composition and perpetuating a chronic inflammatory response. Intestinal blood flow is impaired in RE due to progressive intimal thickening and fibrosis of the microvasculature. Impaired blood flow leads to a reduction in capillary density (rarefaction), further contributing to tissue hypoxia and reduced healing capacity.[5,6]

Clinical Features

Acute radiation enteritis typically presents with nausea, vomiting, abdominal pain, diarrhea, and/or tenesmus. Symptoms may begin within hours of radiation exposure, but more commonly emerge by the second week of treatment. They are usually self-limiting and resolve with cessation of radiation therapy, with regeneration of the intestinal villi typically occurring within 6 months.[7] Treatment for acute RE is directed at symptomatic treatment.

Chronic radiation enteritis is highly variable concerning the timing of presentation and spectrum of symptoms. Chronic RE may present as early as 2 months after treatment or several decades later. The symptoms of chronic RE often mimic those of other common gastrointestinal disorders, such as inflammatory bowel disease, including chronic abdominal pain, weight loss, malabsorption, diarrhea, and gastrointestinal bleeding. These symptoms may serve as indications for video capsule endoscopy (VCE) to evaluate for suspected Crohn's disease or small bowel bleeding. Complications of chronic RE include strictures, fistulas, bowel perforation, and obstruction.[7]

Diagnosis

Diagnosis of RE requires a thorough history to identify a prior radiation therapy, often administered years or decades before presentation with symptoms. Serologic testing for active inflammation, such as C-reactive protein (CRP), is unreliable and nonspecific for RE. Stool testing for fecal calprotectin and fecal lactoferrin is also non-diagnostic and of limited utility.[7] CT enterography (CTE) and magnetic resonance enterography (MRE) may be useful for evaluating patients with symptoms potentially related to RE. CTE and MRE are sensitive for detecting inflammation of the bowel, strictures, and fistulas. MRE offers the additional benefit of avoiding radiation exposure, making it particularly useful for younger patients or those requiring repeated imaging.[8]

Upper and lower endoscopy can assess for injury

consistent with RE and rule out alternative diagnoses. Endoscopy may reveal mucosal inflammation, ulceration, white tipped villi, and in some cases, fistulae or strictures (**Figure 1**). Histologically, acute RE is characterized by epithelial flattening, eosinophilic infiltration, and microabscess formation. Cellular atypia may also be present and can mimic dysplasia. In chronic RE, histologic features include hyalinization of the lamina propria, arteriolar intimal proliferation, and the formation of angioectasias. The presence of radiation fibroblasts within hyalinized stroma is considered a hallmark finding. These findings are analogous to those observed in cases of intestinal ischemia. This correlation makes sense as microvascular disease resulting in ischemia is a defining feature of chronic RE.[9,10]

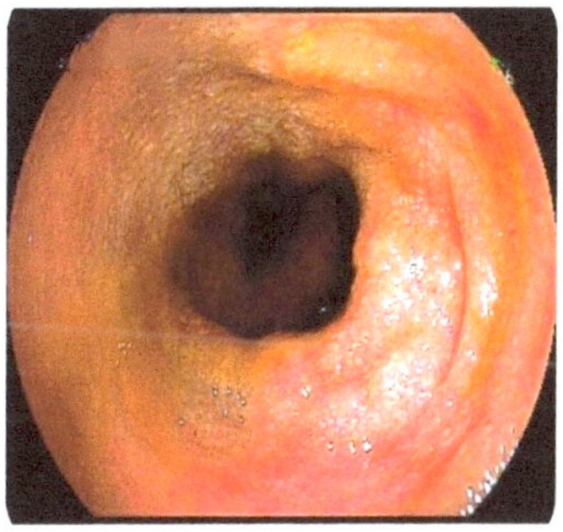

Figure 1. Small bowel erythema, villous atrophy and white tipped villi in chronic RE

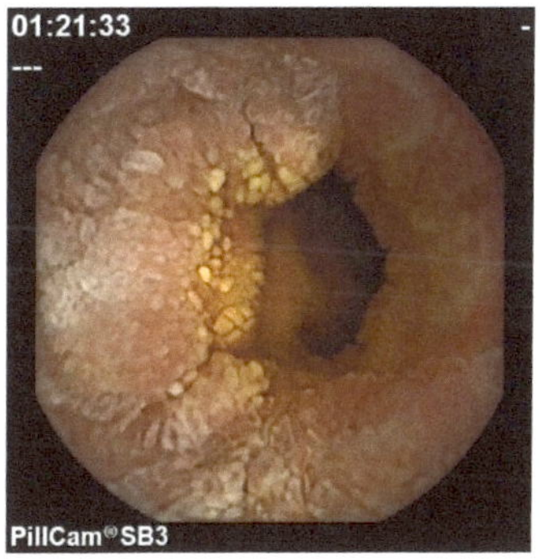

Figure 2. Inflammatory stenosis of the jejunum in chronic RE (observed by VCE).

VCE is a non-invasive method for visualizing the small intestine and can reveal features of RE such as villous atrophy, erosions, edema, stricture formation, ulceration, and bleeding angioectasias (**Figure 2**). However, the risk of capsule retention is high in this patient population. To minimize this risk, a capsule patency test should be performed before VCE in any patient with a history of abdominopelvic XRT to predict the safe passage of the capsule.[11]

Management

Prevention of radiation enteritis

Management of injury related to radiation therapy begins with prevention. Preventive measures that may decrease the risk of RE include alterations in body positioning during treatment, shielding of abdominal/pelvic segments outside of the target area, and maintaining a full bladder. Excess adipose tissue (BMI >30) may also be protective.[7] HMG-CoA reductase antagonists (ie: statin agents) and angiotensin-converting enzyme inhibitors (ACE-I) have been identified as therapies that may prevent or limit radiation injury in XRT.[12-14] In one retrospective cohort study of 308 patients undergoing pelvic XRT, patients actively treated with a statin agent or ACE-I were observed to experience significantly fewer gastrointestinal symptoms related to acute RE.[15] The glucagon-like peptide-2 analogue, teduglutide, has been shown to increase intestinal crypt stem cell survival in mice undergoing whole-body irradiation, suggesting it may have protective capabilities.[16] There have been multiple trials on the use of probiotics to prevent microbiota dysbiosis, which have shown to decrease diarrheal illness, but none have been been powered adequately to warrant endoresement.[17-21]

Acute radiation enteritis

Management of acute RE is largely supportive, including symptomatic treatment of nausea and/or diarrhea. Octreotide was studied in a randomized controlled trial versus diphenoxylate hydrochloride plus atropine sulphate, and patients with acute radiation-induced small bowel disease had faster resolution of diarrheal illness, and fewer patients required interruption of XRT.[22] In patients with severe diarrhea related to malabsorption, consultation with a dietitian may be beneficial. A diet that is low in fat and lactose-free is commonly recommended.

Chronic radiation enteritis

Options for therapy in chronic RE are limited. Cholestyramine, which impairs bile acid reabsorption in the ileum, showed up to 71% improvement in patients with radiation-induced secretory diarrhea by decreasing the incidence and severity of diarrhea.[23,24] A small retrospective 28-week study compared the combined treatment of tocopherol and pentoxifylline with supportive care, and 71% of patients saw symptomatic

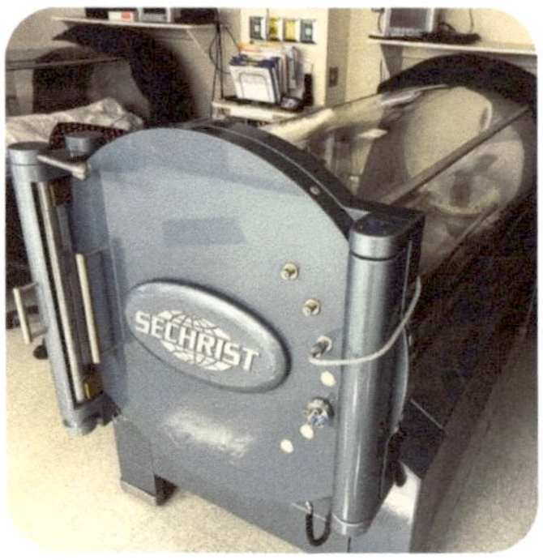

Figure 3. Standard hyperbaric chamber

improvement. It's proposed that the combination may alter the pathogenesis of radiation-induced fibrosis through antioxidant effects and inhibition of TGF-B1/Smad signaling cascade.[25,26] Case studies suggest that fecal transplantation improves diarrhea, abdominal pain, and rectal bleeding in chronic RE by promoting beneficial microbiota and reducing strains thought to be pathogenic.[27,28] The potential benefit of 5-aminosalicyclic acid derivatives in the treatment of chronic RE is unclear and requires further study. These medications decrease free radicals and inhibit prostaglandin biosynthesis to limit inflammation in patients with inflammatory bowel disease.[29]

Hyperbaric oxygen therapy (HBOT) is a well-established treatment for chronic radiation proctitis and shows promise in the management of radiation enteritis. HBOT increases tissue oxygenation within hypoxic tissues to stimulate angiogenesis, limit inflammation, and improve healing. This treatment is widely available due to its multiple applications in different disease processes. (**Figure 3**) A typical regimen includes daily sessions (100% oxygen at 2.0-2.5 atmospheres absolute) for 60-90 minutes, 5 days a week for 30-40 sessions. The typical number of sessions varies depending on the severity of symptomology and the clinical response.[31] Minimal adverse events are associated with HBOT other than otic barotrauma.

Surgical intervention is typically reserved for severe and refractory cases due to the high risk of morbidity and mortality. Frequent complications arise from poor wound healing, recurrence of obstructions, or leakage of anastomosis sites.[32] Current data suggests that ileocecal resection does not improve morbidity in patients with chronic RE.[33,34] However, surgery is eventually required in almost 30% of patients with chronic radiation enteritis to treat small bowel obstruction, strictures, or fistulae.[33]

Conclusion

Radiation enteritis is a known complication of radiation therapy for malignancies of the abdomen and pelvis. Patients with a history of prior XRT are at risk for development of chronic radiation enteritis, which may present with symptoms of chronic diarrhea, abdominal pain, and/or chronic gastrointestinal blood loss. VCE is indicated for evaluation of these symptoms, but the risk of capsule retention is increased in this patient population. The management of RE is primarily symptomatic. However, therapies which may promote healing of chronic RE, such as hyperbaric oxygen therapy, are currently being studied with promising results.

References

1. Shadad AK, Sullivan FJ, Martin JD, Egan LJ. Gastrointestinal radiation injury: prevention and treatment. World J Gastroenterol. 2013; 14;19(2):199-208.

2. Stacey R, Green JT. Radiation-induced small bowel disease: latest developments and clinical guidance. Ther Adv Chronic Dis. 2014;5(1):15-29.

3. Bismar MM, Sinicrope FA. Radiation enteritis. Curr Gastroenterol Rep. 2002;4(5):361-5.

4. Board of the Faculty of Clinical Oncology of the Royal College of Radiologists Royal. Radiotherapy Dose Fractionation. London, UK: Royal College of Radiologists; 2006.

5. Gao D, Zhang H, Sun W, Wang H, Wang H. Radiation-Induced Intestinal Injury: Molecular Mechanisms and Therapeutic Status. DNA Cell Biol. 2024;43(11):537-548.

6. Waselenko JK, MacVittie TJ, Blakely WF, et al. Medical management of the acute radiation syndrome: recommendations of the Strategic National Stockpile Radiation Working Group. Ann Intern Med. 2004;140(12):1037-51.

7. Hale MF. Radiation enteritis: from diagnosis to management. Curr Opin Gastroenterol. 2020;36(3):208-214.

8. Algin O, Turkbey B, Ozmen E, Algin E. Magnetic resonance enterography findings of chronic radiation enteritis. Cancer Imaging. 2011;11(1):189-94.

9. Khor TS, Fujita H, Nagata K, Shimizu M, Lauwers GY. Biopsy interpretation of colonic biopsies when inflammatory bowel disease is excluded. J

Gastroenterol. 2012;47(3):226-48.

10. Woodman I, Schofield JB, Haboubi N. The histopathological mimics of inflammatory bowel disease: a critical appraisal. Tech Coloproctol. 2015;19(12):717-27.

11. Assadsangabi A, Blakeborough A, Drew K, Lobo AJ, Sidhu R, McAlindon ME. Small bowel patency assessment using the patency device and a novel targeted (limited radiation) computed tomography-based protocol. J Gastroenterol Hepatol. 2015;30(6):984-9.

12. Gaugler MH, Vereycken-Holler V, Squiban C, Vandamme M, Vozenin-Brotons MC, Benderitter M. Pravastatin limits endothelial activation after irradiation and decreases the resulting inflammatory and thrombotic responses. Radiat Res. 2005;163(5):479-87.

13. Haydont V, Mathé D, Bourgier C, et al. Induction of CTGF by TGF-beta1 in normal and radiation enteritis human smooth muscle cells: Smad/Rho balance and therapeutic perspectives. Radiother Oncol. 2005;76(2):219-25.

14. Ostrau C, Hülsenbeck J, Herzog M, et al. Lovastatin attenuates ionizing radiation-induced normal tissue damage in vivo. Radiother Oncol. 2009;92(3):492-9.

15. Wedlake LJ, Silia F, Benton B, et al. Evaluating the efficacy of statins and ACE-inhibitors in reducing gastrointestinal toxicity in patients receiving radiotherapy for pelvic malignancies. Eur J Cancer. 2012;48(14):2117-24.

16. Booth C, Booth D, Williamson S, Demchyshyn LL, Potten CS. Teduglutide ([Gly2]GLP-2) protects small intestinal stem cells from radiation damage. Cell Prolif. 2004;37(6):385-400.

17. Salminen E, Elomaa I, Minkkinen J, Vapaatalo H, Salminen S. Preservation of intestinal integrity during radiotherapy using live *Lactobacillus acidophilus* cultures. Clin Radiol. 1988;39(4):435-7.

18. Delia P, Sansotta G, Donato V, et al. Use of probiotics for prevention of radiation-induced diarrhea. World J Gastroenterol. 2007;13(6):912-5.

19. Giralt J, Regadera JP, Verges R, et al. Effects of probiotic Lactobacillus casei DN-114 001 in prevention of radiation-induced diarrhea: results from multicenter, randomized, placebo-controlled nutritional trial. Int J Radiat Oncol Biol Phys. 2008;71(4):1213-9.

20. Chitapanarux I, Chitapanarux T, Traisathit P, Kudumpee S, Tharavichitkul E, Lorvidhaya V. Randomized controlled trial of live *Lactobacillus acidophilus* plus *Bifidobacterium bifidum* in prophylaxis of diarrhea during radiotherapy in cervical cancer patients. Radiat Oncol. 2010;5:31.

21. Urbancsek H, Kazar T, Mezes I, Neumann K. Results of a double-blind, randomized study to evaluate the efficacy and safety of Antibiophilus in patients with radiation-induced diarrhoea. Eur J Gastroenterol Hepatol. 2001;13(4):391-6.

22. Yavuz MN, Yavuz AA, Aydin F, Can G, Kavgaci H. The efficacy of octreotide in the therapy of acute radiation-induced diarrhea: a randomized controlled study. Int J Radiat Oncol Biol Phys. 2002;54(1):195-202.

23. Wang L, Zhou Y, Wang X, et al. Mechanism of Asbt (Slc10a2)-related bile acid malabsorption in diarrhea after pelvic radiation. Int J Radiat Biol. 2020;96(4):510-519.

24. Kurien M, Thurgar E, Davies A, Akehurst R, Andreyev J. Challenging current views on bile acid diarrhoea and malabsorption. Frontline Gastroenterol. 2018;9(2):92-97.

25. Hille A, Christiansen H, Pradier O, et al. Effect of pentoxifylline and tocopherol on radiation proctitis/enteritis. Strahlenther Onkol. 2005;181(9):606-14.

26. Hamama S, Gilbert-Sirieix M, Vozenin MC, Delanian S. Radiation-induced enteropathy: Molecular basis of pentoxifylline-vitamin E anti-fibrotic effect involved TGF-β1 cascade inhibition. Radiother Oncol. 2012;105(3):305-12.

27. Wang L, Li Y, Zhang YJ, Peng LH. Intestinal microecological transplantation for a patient with chronic radiation enteritis: A case report. World J Gastroenterol. 2024;30(19):2603-2611.

28. Ding X, Li Q, Li P, et al. Fecal microbiota transplantation: A promising treatment for radiation enteritis? Radiother Oncol. 2020;143:12-18.

29. Goldstein F, Khoury J, Thornton JJ. Treatment of chronic radiation enteritis and colitis with salicylazosulfapyridine and systemic corticosteroids. A pilot study. Am J Gastroenterol. 1976;65(3):201-8.

30. Wu C, Guan L, Yao L, Huang J. Mesalazine suppository for the treatment of refractory ulcerative chronic radiation proctitis. Exp Ther Med. 2018;16(3):2319-2324.

31. Paquette IM, Vogel JD, Abbas MA, Feingold DL, Steele SR; Clinical Practice Guidelines Committee of The American Society of Colon and Rectal Surgeons. The American Society of Colon and Rectal Surgeons

clinical practice guidelines for the treatment of chronic radiation proctitis. Dis Colon Rectum. 2018;61(10):1135-1140.

32. Galland RB, Spencer J. Surgical management of radiation enteritis. Surgery. 1986;99(2):133-9.

33. Huang Y, Guo F, Yao D, Li Y, Li J. Surgery for chronic radiation enteritis: outcome and risk factors. J Surg Res. 2016;204(2):335-343.

34. Perrakis N, Athanassiou E, Vamvakopoulou D, Kyriazi M, Kappos H, Vamvakopoulos NC, Nomikos I. Practical approaches to effective management of intestinal radiation injury: Benefit of resectional surgery. World J Gastroenterol. 2011;17(35):4013-6.

Case Study Number 11

Presented by Otis Stephen, MD, FACG

Pre-capsule Findings (included in capsule study)

An 89-year-old woman with a history of poorly controlled hypertension, stage III chronic kidney disease, and dilated cardiomyopathy (left ventricular ejection fraction = 25%) presents for further evaluation of recurrent severe anemia requiring repeated packed red blood cell (PRBC) transfusions. She has a history of mild chronic anemia over 10 years in duration attributed to anemia of chronic disease (baseline Hb = 10 g/dL). Over the past 4 months, she has been hospitalized on 3 occasions for symptomatic anemia necessitating PRBC transfusion. Her evaluation to date has included 2 upper endoscopies, 2 colonoscopies, and a push enteroscopy. Video capsule endoscopy has not been performed due to lack of availability at her local hospital.

On interview, the patient is pleasant and appropriately responsive. She denies observing bloody or tarry stool, but admits that she "never looks". Her bowel movements have been more frequent over the past few months with an unusually foul smell. She denies abdominal pain, nausea, vomiting, or weight loss. On physical examination, her lungs are clear, and she has a regular cardiac rhythm. She ambulates independently and demonstrates good functional status

A capsule endoscopy study is performed to evaluate for small bowel bleeding. Review the capsule endoscopy study and report your findings, including: gastric passage time, small bowel passage time, and observed abnormalities. Be prepared to discuss your findings and management plan with your staff prior to reviewing the diagnosis and case discussion.

Minor mucosal erythema is observed in the duodenal bulb, followed by a few tiny, red spots (**Figure 1**: 0hr 48min 48sec). Capsule hold-up is encountered in the deep small bowel beginning at 1hr 30 min and extending for almost 4 hours (until 5hrs 11min). Within this segment of hold-up, multiple views are obtained of a mass lesion characterized by abnormal mucosa, white-tipped villi, and a central depression (**Figure 2**: 1hr 45min 00sec; **Figure 3:** 1hr 47min 39sec; **Figure 4**: 3hr 43min 41sec).

Figure 1

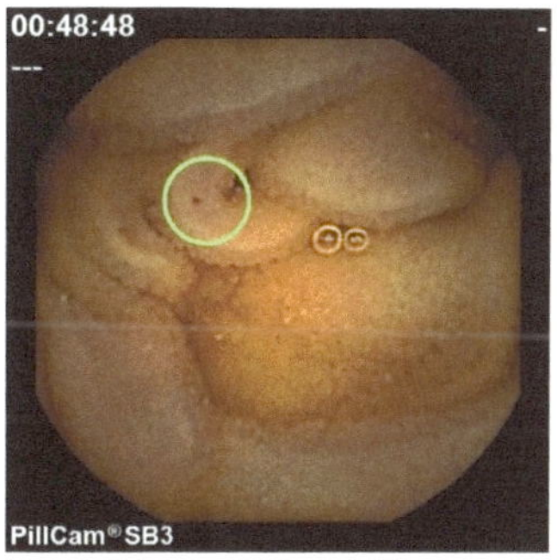

Figure 2

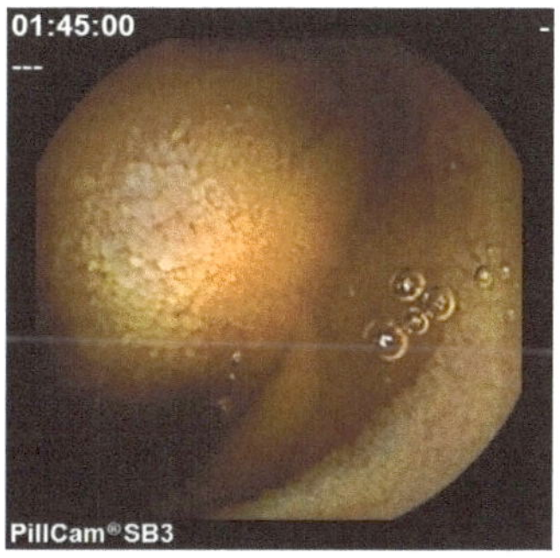

Figure 3

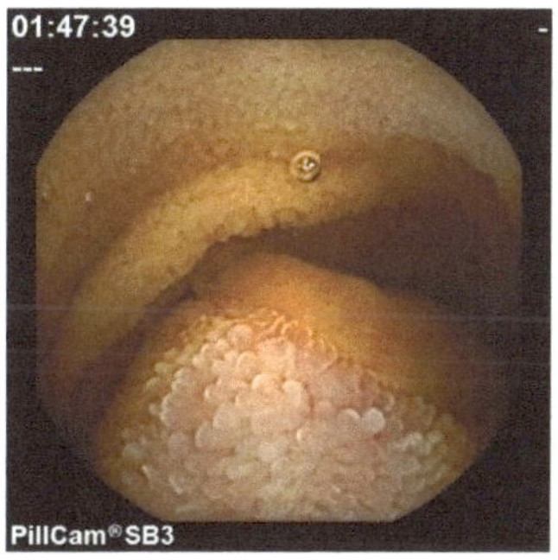

Figure 4

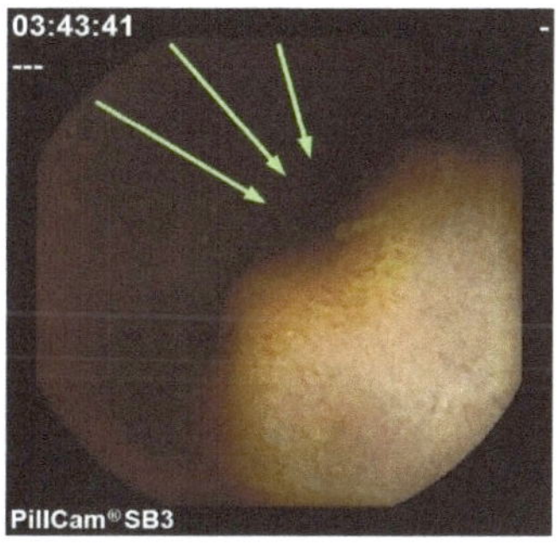

Capsule Endoscopy Findings
First Gastric Image = 0hr 0min 16sec
First Duodenal Image = 0hr 32min 09sec
Gastric passage time = 0hr 32min
First Cecal Image = 6hr 25min 54sec
Small bowel passage time = 5hr 53min

Follow-up

An anterograde double-balloon enteroscopy was performed which identified the tumor in the distal jejunum associated with central ulcer (**Figure 5**). This lesion was marked with a submucosal ink tattoo in preparation for surgical resection the following day. A small bowel resection was successful in removing the segment containing the tumor. Pathologic examination confirmed a gastrointestinal stromal tumor (GIST), measuring 3 cm with a mitotic index of fewer than 5 per high-power field.

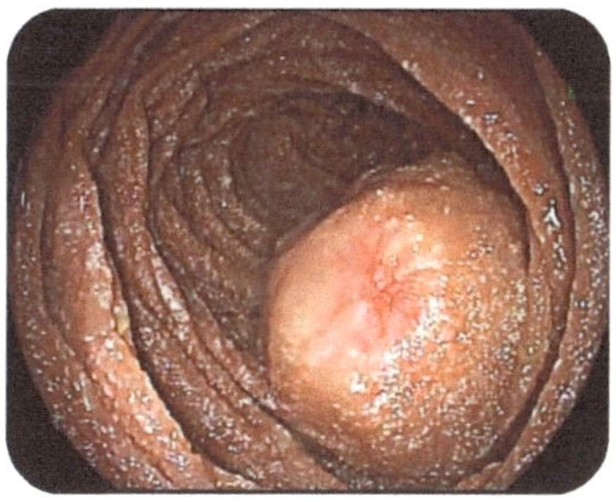

Figure 5

Chapter 11: Gastrointestinal Stromal Tumor

Catherine Loehr, MD and Daniel Raines, MD, FACG

Introduction

Gastrointestinal stromal tumors (GISTs) are mesenchymal neoplasms arising from Interstitial Cells of Cajal (ICC) or ICC precursors. GISTs represent 1 of the 4 primary small bowel tumors, alongside adenocarcinoma, lymphoma, and neuroendocrine tumors.[1-3] Gastroenterologists often become familiar with GISTs by encountering gastric tumors during upper endoscopy.[4] Small bowel GISTs are associated with a higher malignant potential compared to gastric tumors while management depends upon unique molecular features, including activating mutations in *KIT* (CD117) or *PDGFRA*.[1-2,5] Diagnosis of small bowel GISTs requires familiarity with the clinical behavior and endoscopic appearance of these tumors.

Epidemiology

GISTs are the most common mesenchymal neoplasms of the gastrointestinal tract, with an estimated 4,000 to 6,000 new diagnoses in the U.S. each year. They predominantly arise in older adults aged 60 to 65. GISTs most frequently originate in the stomach (60%–70%) and small intestine (20%–30%), with rare occurrences in the colon, rectum, and esophagus. The majority of GISTs are sporadic and driven by activating mutations in *KIT* or *PDGFRA*. While familial cases with germline mutations have been described, they are rare with only 49 *KIT* and 6 *PDGFRA* germline mutation kindreds reported. These cases are usually inherited in an autosomal dominant pattern and may present with features such as skin hyperpigmentation or dysphagia, depending on the gene mutation.[2-3,5-9]

Small bowel GISTs most commonly occur in the jejunum. These tumors are large, with mean tumor sizes ranging from 5 to 10 cm and may become exophytic, growing into the peritoneal cavity rather than intraluminaly.[10-13] Approximately 10%–30% of small bowel GISTs are discovered incidentally during imaging or surgical procedures performed for unrelated reasons.

Clinical Features

When symptomatic, most cases of small bowel GIST present with gastrointestinal bleeding. The pattern of bleeding may be overt or occult, with iron deficiency. Other presenting symptoms include abdominal pain or palpable abdominal mass, often directly related to tumor size.[6,10-11,13,14] GISTs which grow into the small bowel lumen may lead to intestinal obstruction. Exophytic tumors extending into the peritoneal cavity may be complicated by tumor rupture or peritoneal invasion.

Highly malignant small bowel GISTs are characterized by large size, high mitotic activity, irregular/invasive borders, ulceration, necrosis and exophytic growth. The liver and peritoneum are the most common sites for metastasis. Advanced disease may manifest with malignant ascites or palpable masses due to peritoneal implants. Tumor rupture, either spontaneous or iatrogenic, is associated with a high risk of peritoneal dissemination and worse prognosis.[2,11,15]

Diagnosis

Symptomatic small bowel GISTs are typically diagnosed by endoscopy and/or imaging. Video capsule endoscopy (VCE) allows for non-invasive inspection of the entire small bowel lumen. VCE may identify small bowel GISTs as submucosal lesions protruding into the lumen and associated with central ulceration and/or bleeding (**Figure 1**). Exophytic tumors may be characterized by luminal bleeding associated with abnormal vascular growth surrounding the tumor base[16-25] (**Figure 2**).

CT enterography (CTE) and MR enterography (MRE) are effective studies to detect or confirm small bowel GISTs. These hypervascular tumors enhance

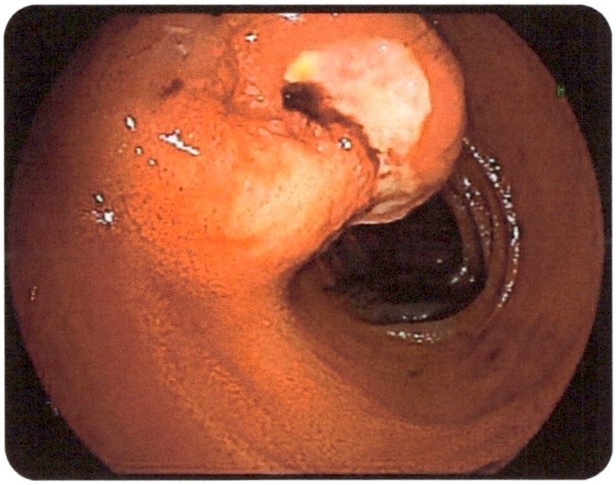

Figure 1. GIST with central ulceration protruding into the lumen.

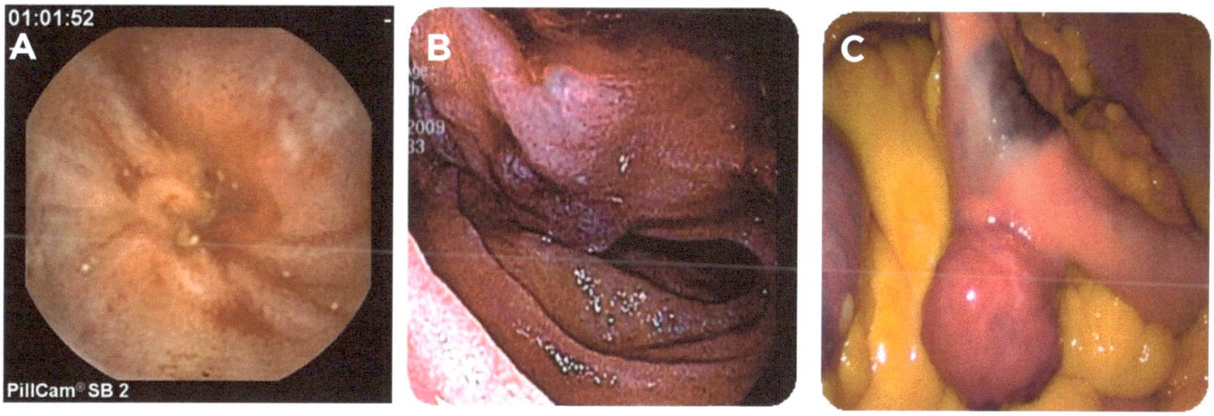

Figure 2. Exophytic GIST detected by video capsule endoscopy (a) then localized by upper device-assisted enteroscopy (b) then surgically removed (c).

conspicuously with intravenous contrast (**Figure 3**). CTE is reported as highly sensitive (up to 93%) and specific (up to 83%) for small bowel tumors in research settings.[26-33] MRE offers similar diagnostic accuracy and is preferred in younger patients to avoid radiation.[32-35] Both modalities allow assessment of tumor size and metastatic spread.[36]

Research protocols using CTE or MRE to detect small bowel tumors differ significantly from the imaging protocols used in clinical practice. A research protocol CTE may use 4 contrast phases with thin (2 mm) slices and multiplanar reconstructions (axial, coronal, sagittal) to produce nearly 3,000 images.[27,31,34-35] Reimbursement for CTE does not correlate with the number of images obtained or interpreted. Clinical CTE protocols often call for 1 phase of IV contrast with only axial images at an interval of 5 mm, generating around 80 images. If a clinical CTE protocol generates only a fraction (3%) of the images acquired in research setting, the results of CTE in a research setting may not be reproducible in practice.

Staging

Staging of small bowel GISTs is primarily based upon tumor size and mitotic index, the primary predictors of malignant potential and risk of recurrence. The majority of small bowel GISTs are relatively benign and indolent, but the risk of aggressive behavior increases with larger tumor size and higher mitotic activity. Tumors < 5 cm with ≤ 5 mitoses per 50 high-power fields (HPF) have a low risk of metastasis (< 3%), while those > 10 cm and/or with > 5 mitoses per 50 HPF have a high risk (> 50%).[1,37-38]

Imaging studies are essential for detecting metastatic or advanced disease. CT imaging of the abdomen/pelvis is standard for initial staging of small bowel

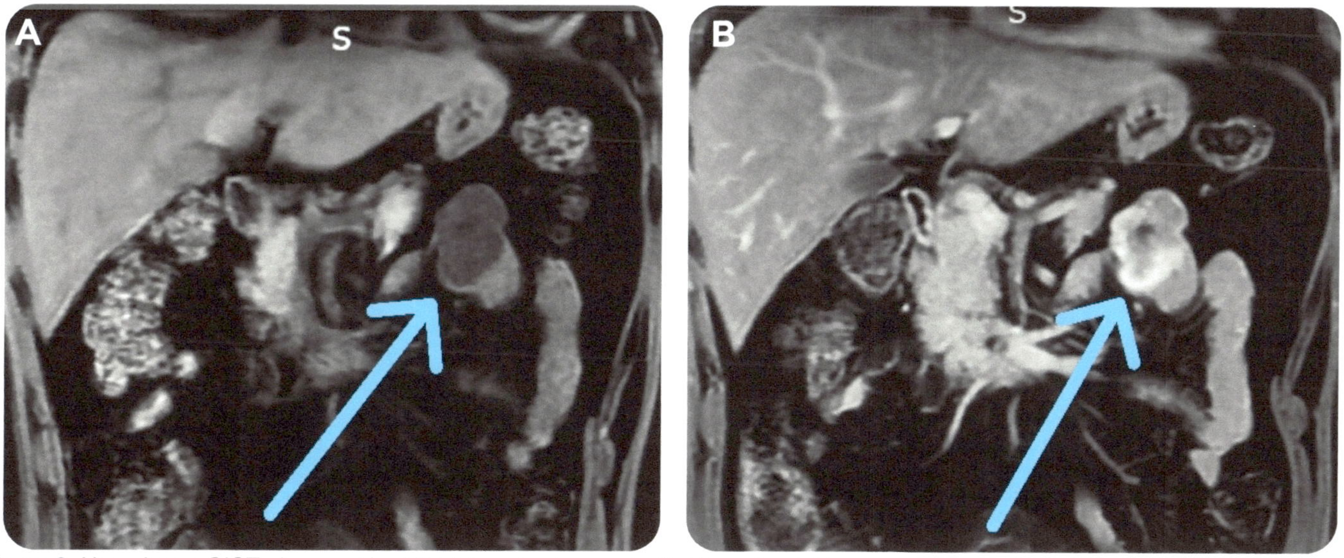

Figure 3. Hypodense GIST observed by MRI (a) and enhanced with IV contract (b).

Tumor size (cm)	Mitotic Index (per 50 HPF)	Location	Estimated risk of metastasis at 10 years
≤ 2	≤ 5	Duodenum	< 2%
≤ 2	≤ 5	Jejunum/ileum	3%-4%
> 2-5	≤ 5	Duodenum	5%-10%
> 2-5	≤ 5	Jejunum/ileum	10%-15%
> 5-10	≤ 5	Duodenum	15%-20%
> 5-10	≤ 5	Jejunum/ileum	25%-30%
Any size	> 5	Any	40%-85%
> 10	Any	Any	60%-90%

Table 1. Risk stratification for small bowel GIST based on tumor size, mitotic rate, and anatomic location. Risk estimates are based on long-term follow-up data and reflect likelihood of metastasis or disease progression at 10 years.[40-41]

GISTs, providing information related to tumor size, local invasion, and/or metastases of the liver or peritoneum. MRI is an alternative to CT imaging, particularly for liver metastases or in patients requiring reduced radiation exposure. Positron emission tomography may be used in select cases for further evaluation of metastatic disease or for treatment response.[6,39] Pathologic staging and risk stratification should be performed after surgical resection, as preoperative biopsy often cannot reliably assess mitotic index[4] (**Table 1**).

Management

Surgical resection is recommended for all small bowel GISTs, regardless of size. The recommended surgical approach involves complete en bloc resection with negative microscopic margins. Care must be taken to avoid tumor rupture. Routine lymph node dissection is not indicated, as nodal metastases are rare. Segmental small bowel resection is often curative.[38,42-43]

Imatinib (Gleevec) is the standard medical therapy following resection of high-risk tumors as well as for palliative treatment of unresectable or metastatic GIST. Imatinib is a cytostatic tyrosine kinase inhibitor that suppresses tumor growth but does not induce cell death. For high-risk patients, adjuvant imatinib at 400 mg daily for at least 3 years is recommended, as this duration improves recurrence-free and overall survival compared to shorter courses. Imatinib is also used in the neoadjuvant setting to downstage tumors and facilitate less morbid resections.[44-47]

Postoperative relapse of disease is highest within the first 2 to 3 years but can occur up to 10 years post-resection. Most recurrences are intra-abdominal, particularly within the liver and peritoneum. For high-risk patients, recommended monitoring includes imaging of the abdomen/pelvis every 4 months for a duration of 3 years, then every 6 months until year 5, then annually thereafter. Low-risk patients may be monitored with less frequent imaging.[38,48]

Conclusion

Small bowel GISTs are the most common primary tumor of the jejunum and commonly present with signs or symptoms of gastrointestinal bleeding. VCE is the diagnostic procedure of choice to evaluate for small bowel bleeding sources, such as GIST, following negative upper endoscopy/colonoscopy. Cross section imaging of the abdomen/pelvis by CTE or MRE are useful in the diagnosis and staging of small bowel GISTs. Surgical resection is the mainstay for localized disease, while tyrosine kinase inhibitors are used for advanced or high-risk cases. The risk of recurrent disease primarily correlates with 2 factors, tumor size and mitotic index.

References

1. Miettinen M, Makhlouf H, Sobin LH, Lasota J. Gastrointestinal stromal tumors of the jejunum and ileum: a clinicopathologic, immunohistochemical, and molecular genetic study of 906 cases before imatinib with long-term follow-up. Am J Surg Pathol. 2006;30(4):477-489.
2. Joensuu H, Hohenberger P, Corless CL. Gastrointestinal stromal tumour. Lancet. 2013;382(9896):973-983.

3. Khan J, Ullah A, Waheed A, et al. Gastrointestinal stromal tumors (GIST): A population-based study using the SEER database, including management and recent advances in targeted therapy. Cancers (Basel). 2022;14(15):3689.
4. Faulx AL, Kothari S, Acosta RD, et al. The role of endoscopy in subepithelial lesions of the GI tract. Gastrointest Endosc. 2017;85(6):1117–1132.
5. Kim Y, Lee SH. Pathologic diagnosis and molecular features of gastrointestinal stromal tumors: a mini-review. Front Oncol. 2024;14:1487467.
6. Wang MX, Devine C, Segaran N, Ganeshan D. Current update on molecular cytogenetics, diagnosis and management of gastrointestinal stromal tumors. World J Gastroenterol. 2021;27(41):7125-7133.
7. Alvarez CS, Piazuelo MB, Fleitas-Kanonnikoff T, Ruhl J, Pérez-Fidalgo JA, Camargo MC. Incidence and survival outcomes of gastrointestinal stromal tumors. JAMA Netw Open. 2024;7(8):e2428828.
8. Yan M, Lin J, Shu M, et al. Diagnosis, treatment, and prognosis of patients with primary familial gastrointestinal stromal tumor: A case report and literature review. Oncologist. 2023;28(12):e1134-e1141.
9. Brodey A, Kounnis V, Hawkes L, Jones RL, McVeigh TP, Cojocaru E. KIT-associated familial GIST Syndrome: Response to tyrosine kinase inhibitors and implications for risk management. Oncologist. 2022;27(8):615-620.
10. Wang Q, Li M, Bai X, et al. Unraveling the site-specific features in small intestinal stromal tumors: a retrospective study. BMC Gastroenterol. 2025;25(1):337.
11. Zhou L, Liao Y, Wu J, et al. Small bowel gastrointestinal stromal tumor: a retrospective study of 32 cases at a single center and review of the literature. Ther Clin Risk Manag. 2018;14:1467-1481.
12. Xing GS, Wang S, Sun YM, Yuan Z, Zhao XM, Zhou CW. Small bowel stromal tumors: different clinicopathologic and computed tomography features in various anatomic sites. PLoS One. 2015;10(12):e0144277.
13. Baheti AD, Shinagare AB, O'Neill AC, et al. MDCT and clinicopathological features of small bowel gastrointestinal stromal tumours in 102 patients: a single institute experience. Br J Radiol. 2015;88(1053):20150085.
14. Yang Z, Wang F, Liu S, Guan W. Comparative clinical features and short-term outcomes of gastric and small intestinal gastrointestinal stromal tumours: A retrospective study. Sci Rep. 2019;9(1):10033.
15. Fan X, Han H, Sun Z, et al. Prognostic value of bleeding in gastrointestinal stromal tumors: A meta-analysis. Technol Cancer Res Treat. 2021;20:15330338211034259.
16. Sharzehi K, Sethi A, Savides T. AGA clinical practice update on management of subepithelial lesions encountered during routine endoscopy: Expert review. Clin Gastroenterol Hepatol. 2022;20(11):2435-2443.e4.
17. Akahoshi K, Oya M, Koga T, Shiratsuchi Y. Current clinical management of gastrointestinal stromal tumor. World J Gastroenterol. 2018;24(26):2806-2817.
18. Nakano A, Nakamura M, Watanabe O, et al. Endoscopic characteristics, risk grade, and prognostic prediction in gastrointestinal stromal tumors of the small bowel. Digestion. 2017;95(2):122-131.
19. Honda W, Ohmiya N, Hirooka Y, et al. Enteroscopic and radiologic diagnoses, treatment, and prognoses of small-bowel tumors. Gastrointest Endosc. 2012;76(2):344-354.
20. Yano T, Yamamoto H. Endoscopic Diagnosis of Small Bowel Tumor. Cancers (Basel). 2024;16(9):1704.
21. Nakatani M, Fujiwara Y, Nagami Y, et al. The usefulness of double-balloon enteroscopy in gastrointestinal stromal tumors of the small bowel with obscure gastrointestinal bleeding. Intern Med. 2012;51(19):2675-2682.
22. Rondonotti E, Koulaouzidis A, Georgiou J, Pennazio M. Small bowel tumours: Update in diagnosis and management. Curr Opin Gastroenterol. 2018;34(3):159-164.
23. Zagorowicz ES, Pietrzak AM, Wronska E, et al. Small bowel tumors detected and missed during capsule endoscopy: Single center experience. World J Gastroenterol. 2013;19(47):9043-9048.
24. Rondonotti E, Pennazio M, Toth E, et al. Small-bowel neoplasms in patients undergoing video capsule endoscopy: a multicenter European study. Endoscopy. 2008;40(6):488-495.
25. Spada C, Riccioni ME, Familiari P, et al. Video capsule endoscopy in small-bowel tumours: a single centre experience. Scand J Gastroenterol. 2008;43(4):497-505.
26. Gerson LB, Fidler JL, Cave DR, Leighton JA. ACG Clinical Guideline: Diagnosis and management of small bowel bleeding. Am J Gastroenterol. 2015;110(9):1265-87.
27. Li R, Ye S, Zhou C, Liu F, Li X. A systematic review and meta-analysis of magnetic resonance and computed tomography enterography in the diagnosis of small intestinal tumors. PeerJ. 2023;11:e16687.
28. Gurudu SR, Bruining DH, Acosta RD, et al. The role of endoscopy in the management of suspected small-bowel bleeding. Gastrointest Endosc. 2017;85(1):22-31.
29. Yaghoobi M, Tan J, Alshammari YTATA, Scandrett K, Mofrad K, Takwoingi Y. Video capsule endoscopy versus computed tomography enterography in assessing suspected small bowel bleeding: A systematic review and diagnostic test accuracy meta-analysis. Eur J Gastroenterol Hepatol. 2023;35(11):1253-1262.
30. Hakim FA, Alexander JA, Huprich JE, Grover M, Enders FT. CT-enterography may identify small bowel tumors not detected by capsule endoscopy: Eight years experience at Mayo Clinic Rochester. Dig Dis Sci. 2011;56(10):2914-2919.

31. Masselli G, Di Tola M, Casciani E, et al. Diagnosis of small-bowel diseases: prospective comparison of multi-detector row CT enterography with MR enterography. Radiology. 2016;279(2):420-431.
32. Tu H, Chen Q, Tu J, et al. Small bowel gastrointestinal stromal tumors: The value of CT enterography in assessing pathological aggressiveness. J Comput Assist Tomogr. 2024;48(5):713-718.
33. Vasconcelos RN, Dolan SG, Barlow JM, et al. Impact of CT enterography on the diagnosis of small bowel gastrointestinal stromal tumors. Abdom Radiol (NY). 2017;42(5):1365-1373.
34. Amzallag-Bellenger E, Soyer P, Barbe C, et al. Prospective evaluation of magnetic resonance enterography for the detection of mesenteric small bowel tumours. Eur Radiol. 2013;23(7):1901-1910.
35. Amzallag-Bellenger E, Soyer P, Barbe C, et al. Diffusion-weighted imaging for the detection of mesenteric small bowel tumours with magnetic resonance–Enterography. Eur Radiol. 2014;24(11):2916-2926.
36. Sengupta N, Kastenberg DM, Bruining DH, et al. The role of imaging for gastrointestinal bleeding: Consensus recommendations from the American College of Gastroenterology and Society of Abdominal Radiology. Am J Gastroenterol. 2024;119(3):438-449.
37. Sander B, Cameron S, Gunawan B, Füzesi L. Optimal thresholds of risk parameters for gastrointestinal stromal tumors. Eur J Surg Oncol. 2020;46(1):180-188.
38. Koo DH, Ryu MH, Kim KM, et al. Asian consensus guidelines for the diagnosis and management of gastrointestinal stromal tumor. Cancer Res Treat. 2016;48(4):1155-1166.
39. Vernuccio F, Taibbi A, Picone D, et al. Imaging of gastrointestinal stromal tumors: From diagnosis to evaluation of therapeutic response. Anticancer Res. 2016;36(6):2639-2648.
40. Trinh VQ, Dashti NK, Cates JMM. A proposed risk assessment score for gastrointestinal stromal tumors based on evaluation of 19,030 cases from the National Cancer Database. J Gastroenterol. 2021;56(11):964-975.
41. Zhang H, Liu Q. Prognostic indicators for gastrointestinal stromal tumors: A review. Transl Oncol. 2020;13(10):100812.
42. Everett M, Gutman H. Surgical management of gastrointestinal stromal tumors: Analysis of outcome with respect to surgical margins and technique. J Surg Oncol. 2008;98(8):588-593.
43. Nishida T, Goto O, Raut CP, Yahagi N. Diagnostic and treatment strategy for small gastrointestinal stromal tumors. Cancer. 2016;122(20):3110-3118.
44. Croom KF, Perry CM. Imatinib mesylate: In the treatment of gastrointestinal stromal tumours. Drugs. 2003;63(5):513-522.
45. Sanford M, Scott LJ. Imatinib: As adjuvant therapy for gastrointestinal stromal tumour. Drugs. 2010;70(15):1963-1972.
46. Penel N, Le Cesne A, Blay JY. Adjuvant treatment of gastrointestinal stromal tumor: State of the art in 2025. Eur J Cancer. 2025;222:115473.
47. von Mehren M, Joensuu H. Gastrointestinal stromal tumors. J Clin Oncol. 2018;36(2):136-143.
48. Joensuu H, Martin-Broto J, Nishida T, et al. Follow-up strategies for patients with gastrointestinal stromal tumour treated with or without adjuvant imatinib after surgery. Eur J Cancer. 2015;51(12):1611-1617.

CAPSULE ENDOSCOPY BY CASE STUDY
Case Study Number 12

Presented by by Matthew G. Bell, MD and Shabana F. Pasha, MD, FACG

Pre-capsule Findings (included in capsule study)

A 70-year-old woman with a history of hypertension, type 2 diabetes, coronary artery disease, and chronic kidney disease presents for further evaluation of anemia (hemoglobin of 8gm/dl). She was diagnosed with iron deficiency anemia 1 year prior to this visit. Initial evaluation of her anemia 10 months ago, including upper endoscopy and colonoscopy, did not identify a source of chronic gastointestinal blood loss. Her anemia has progressed over the past 6 months resulting in the need for transfusion of 2 units of packed red blood cells.

The patient currently denies any symptoms of melena, hematochezia, diarrhea, abdominal pain, weight loss, or epistaxis. She takes aspirin 81 mg day but denies any other NSAID use. Her medication list includes clopidogrel for coronary artery disease with a history of coronary stent placed over 10 years ago. Physical exam is unremarkable including evaluation for mucocutaneous telangiectasias.

A capsule endoscopy study is performed to evaluate for small bowel bleeding. Review the capsule endoscopy study and report your findings, including: gastric passage time, small bowel passage time, and observed abnormalities. Be prepared to discuss your findings and management plan with your staff prior to reviewing the diagnosis and case discussion.

Multiple angioectasias are observed in the proximal small bowel, including at least 3 classic lesions in the proximal jejunum (**Figure 1**: 0hr 53min 35sec; **Figure 2**: 0hr 53min 42sec; **Figure 3**: 0hr 53min 50sec). Examination of the remaining small bowel is unremarkable.

Capsule Endoscopy Findings
First Gastric Image = 0hr 7min 39sec
First Duodenal Image = 0hr 51min 48sec
Gastric passage time = 0hr 44min
First Cecal Image = 3hr 38min 15sec
Small bowel passage time = 2hr 54min

Figure 1

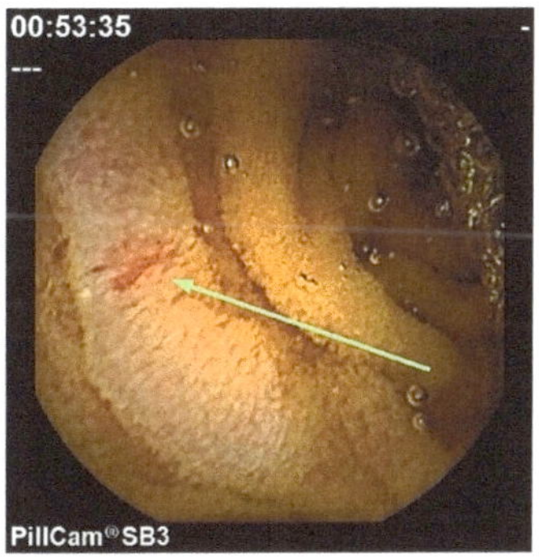

Figure 2

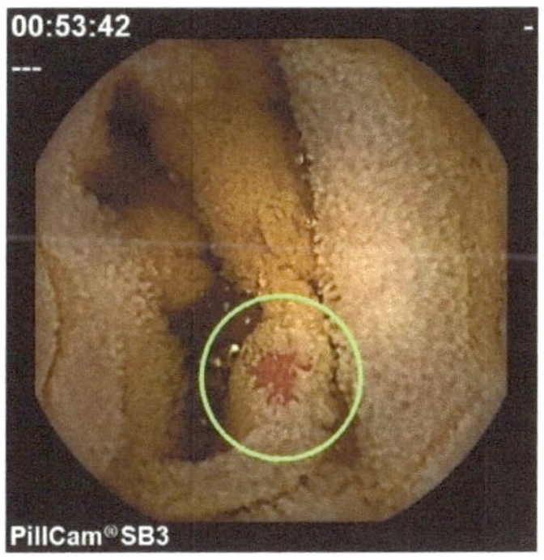

Figure 3

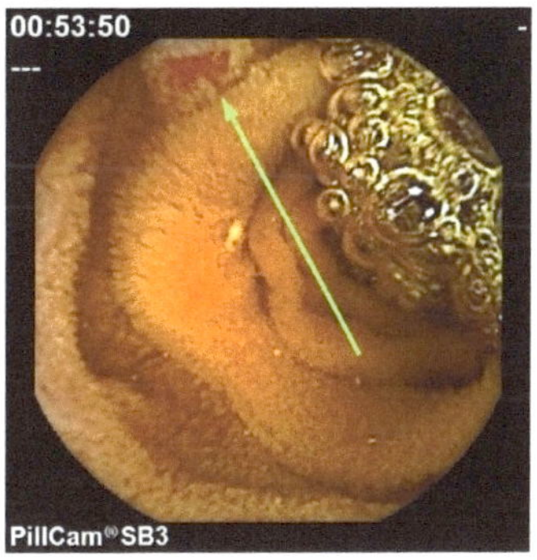

Follow-up

An anterograde enteroscopy was performed with ablation of multiple (5) angioectasias in the proximal and mid jejunum (**Figure 4**) In addition, a course of parenteral iron therapy was prescribed and clopidogrel was discontinued following consultation with cardiology. Reassessment of the patient's anemia 6 months later demonstrated an improvement in serum hemoglobin to 12mg/dl.

Figure 4

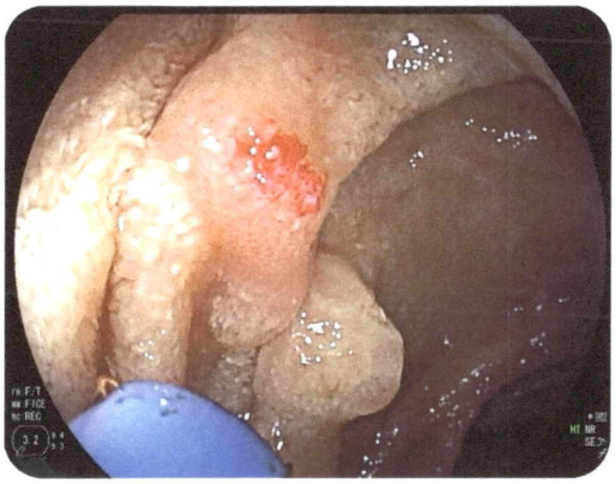

Chapter 12: Non-Hereditary Angioectasias

Matthew G. Bell, MD and Shabana F. Pasha, MD, FACG

Introduction

Non-hereditary gastrointestinal (GI) angioectasias are common vascular lesions of the GI tract and are the most common small bowel (SB) bleeding source in patients older than 50. "Angioectasia" refers to abnormal dilation of submucosal veins accompanied by ectasia of the overlying mucosal capillaries.[1] Although the terms angioectasia, angiodysplasia, and arteriovenous malformation (AVM) are used interchangeably in clinical practice, AVM refers to a larger subtype of angioectasia characterized by loss of precapillary sphincter function and a direct communication between an artery and a vein, bypassing the capillary bed.[2]

The Yano-Yamamoto endoscopic classification of small bowel vascular lesions has provided a framework to standardize endoscopic findings and terminology (**Figure 1**).[3] SB AE's are classified as type 1 lesions, which may be subclassified as type 1a when characterized by punctate erythema (<1 mm) and type 1b when characterized by patchy erythema (2-3 mm). In addition, the Saurin criteria offer a validated system for grading the bleeding potential of vascular and other lesions identified on capsule endoscopy, and thereby aid in the selection of patients who might benefit from endoscopic treatment (**Table 1**).[4, 5]

Pathophysiology

Historically, GI angioectasias were considered to be degenerative vascular lesions.[6] The understanding of their underlying etiopathogenesis has evolved, and is now considered to be multifactorial. It has been proposed that chronic, low-grade obstruction of submucosal veins may play a major role in the pathogenesis of angioectasias.[7] Intermittent venous obstruction results in local hypoxia, which stimulates the upregulation of angiogenic factors such as vascular endothelial growth factor (VEGF), promoting the formation of fragile, ectatic vessels that are prone to bleeding.[8]

Certain populations have shown a higher propensity for angioectasia formation. GIAEs are more commonly found in patients above the age of 50 years, and especially those with cardiovascular disease. Patients with aortic stenosis (AS) or ventricular assist device (LVAD) support and resultant acquired von Willebrand factor (vWF) deficiency are at increased risk for GIAEs.[9] High shear stress in AS and LVAD may result in degradation of vWF multimers, thus impairing hemostasis and contributing to dysregulated angiogenesis.[10] This mechanism serves as the proposed basis for the long-observed association between AS and GI angioectasia—Heyde's syndrome.[11, 12] Chronic kidney disease contributes to angioectasia development through a combination of chronic mucosal hypoxia and increased angiogenic signaling. Conditions such as occlusive arterial disease, chronic obstructive pulmonary disease, and pulmonary hypertension may result in inadequate

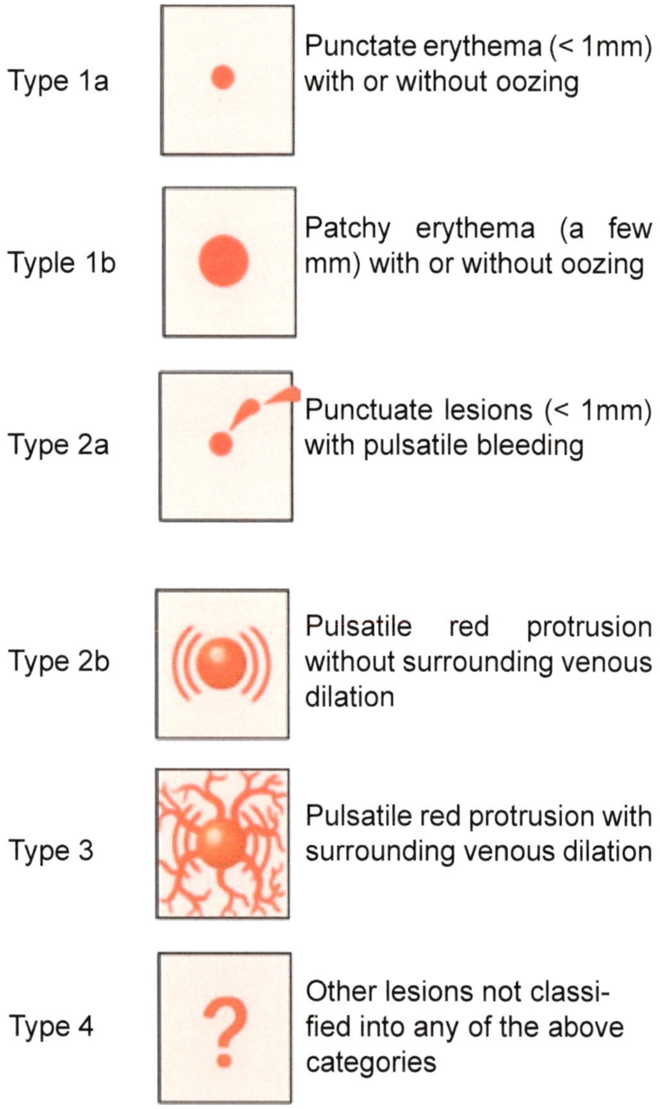

Figure 1. Yano Yamamoto classification of small bowel vascular lesions.

Lesion Type	Bleeding Potential	Example
P0	None	Visible submucosal veins Diverticula without the presence of blood Nodules without mucosal break
P1	Uncertain	Red spots in the intestinal mucosa Small or isolated erosions
P2	High	Typical angiomas Large ulcerations Tumors Varices

Table 1. Saurin classification of small bowel lesions.

delivery of oxygen to the intestinal mucosa resulting in stimulation of angiogenesis. Ultimately, GIAEs likely arise from the interplay of degenerative, mechanical, and hematologic alterations all of which contribute to aberrant vessel formation and impaired hemostasis.[9]

Clinical Presentation

The true prevalence of nonhereditary GIAEs in the general population is unknown. They can be present throughout the gastrointestinal tract and are incidentally found in 1%-2% of patients undergoing endoscopic evaluation.[1,13] The majority of GIAEs are asymptomatic and commonly found incidentally in the right colon and/or cecum.[1,14,15] In patients with GIAEs complicated by bleeding, these lesions are most prevalent in the jejunum (80%) followed by the duodenum (51%), stomach (22.8%), and right colon (11.4%). Up to 60% of patients with bleeding GIAEs develop lesions in multiple locations, such as the duodenum and right colon.[16,17]

As previously mentioned, common comorbidities associated with angiectasia formation include valvular heart disease, end-stage renal disease and advanced age. These risk factors as well as anticoagulation/antiplatelet use are associated with increased risk of bleeding from angiectasias.[9] SB angioectasias may be the underlying source in approximately 60% of patients presenting with suspected SB bleeding.[18-20]

Angioectasias typically present with occult blood loss and iron deficiency anemia but may also result in overt bleeding, presenting with melena or hematochezia. They can be challenging to detect and treat effectively due to their small size, multiple lesions, location within and behind mucosal folds, and propensity to ooze intermittently and at a slow rate.[2,9] AVMs are often larger in size compared to other angioectasias, and present with arterial bleeding.[4]

Diagnosis

On endoscopic evaluation, angioectasias appear as flat lesions with arborizing blood vessels arising from a central red spot (**Figures 2 and 3**). This characteristic endoscopic appearance may not be as evident in the small bowel as in the colon or upper GI tract and may result in unwarranted endoscopic treatment of false positive lesions or red spots.
As the distribution of GIAEs is predominantly in the proximal small bowel and right colon, these lesions

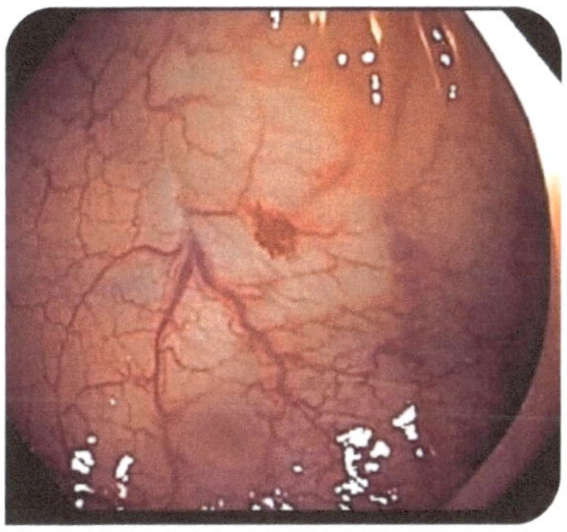

Figure 2. Angioectasia in the right colon seen on colonoscopy

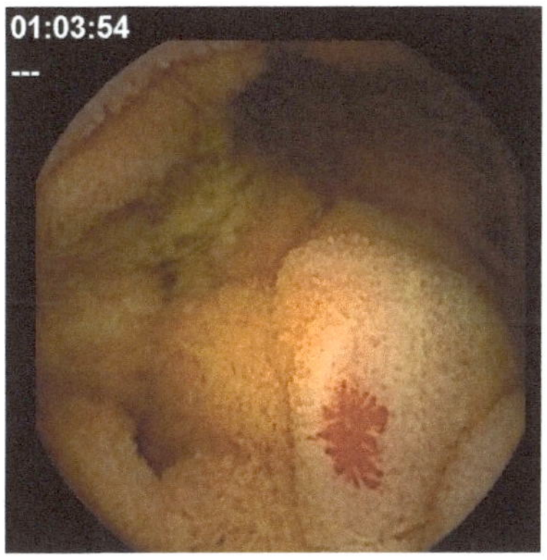

Figure 3. Small bowel angioectasia seen on capsule endoscopy

are often visualized during standard upper endoscopy and colonoscopy. During endoscopic evaluation of unexplained iron deficiency anemia or overt gastrointestinal bleeding, careful attention for mucosal lesions, including inspection behind the folds may improve detection of GIAEs. In addition, performing a push enteroscopy in high-risk patients, also allows examination of the distal duodenum and proximal jejunum for detection of additional lesions.[17]

The American College of Gastroenterology and other GI societies recommend video capsule endoscopy (VCE) as the first diagnostic test for suspected SB bleeding after negative bidirectional endoscopy.[21] VCE is easy to perform, allows noninvasive visualization of the entire SB, and detects bleeding and nonbleeding angioectasias.[21, 22] Its main limitations include lack of interventional capability, potential for missed lesions, and inaccurate localization due to variable capsule transit time. Capsule retention is reported in 1%-2% of all VCE examinations performed for suspected SB bleeding.[23]

In patients presenting with overt bleeding and hemodynamic instability, CT angiography (CTA) is preferred over endoscopic evaluation due to its availability and rapid interpretation. CTA has largely replaced technetium 99m nuclear medicine scans due to superior diagnostic capability, more accurate localization of bleeding source within the gastrointestinal tract, and faster time to mesenteric angiography.[24] CTA has a bleeding rate detection threshold of approximately 0.3 mL/min. It may therefore be unrevealing in cases of intermittent or slow bleeding.[25, 26]

Device-assisted enteroscopy (DAE) has diagnostic yield similar to capsule endoscopy in patients with suspected small bowel bleeding.[27] However, DAE is typically reserved for cases in which a small bowel bleeding sources has been identified by VCE or CTA. Antegrade DAE carries a higher diagnostic and therapeutic yield compared to retrograde DAE due to predilection of angioectasias in the proximal small bowel.[28 22]

Endoscopic Management of GIAEs

GIAEs with active bleeding or high potential for bleeding (according to the Saurin or Yano-Yamamoto criteria) can be treated with various endoscopic methods. These treatment options include argon plasma coagulation (APC), electrocautery, mechanical hemostasis (hemoclips), and injection therapy.[22, 29] The choice of endoscopic intervention is largely endoscopist and lesion dependent. Argon plasma coagulation is a safe technique due to noncontact thermal coagulation and limited depth of coagulation injury and is the preferred endoscopic treatment modality for most endoscopists.[30] Submucosal saline injection may reduce the risk of deep thermal injury in the treatment of large right colon angioectasias. In addition to conventional modalities, radiofrequency ablation and sclerotherapy for treatment of SB angioectasias has been described in case series.[31, 32]

Although endoscopic therapy is effective in reducing transfusion requirements, recurrent bleeding is reported in 30%-40% of patients with underlying GIAEs regardless of endoscopic intervention.[33] Increased risk of rebleeding is seen in patients with larger angioectasias (5 mm or greater), heart failure, and those who are actively smoking. Interestingly, studies have shown no association between rebleeding risk and chronic kidney disease.[18,34] Further research is needed to determine specific risk factors that increase risk of rebleeding as these patients may benefit from closer surveillance and more aggressive intervention.

Medical Therapy for GIAEs

Medical therapy serves as an important adjunct to endoscopic ablation in patients with symptomatic anemia due to bleeding GIAEs. Aggressive supplementation of iron, including parenteral iron therapy, is essential in patients with depleted iron stores due to chronic GI blood loss. Somatostatin analogs, such as octreotide and lanreotide, have been found to significantly reduce the need for blood transfusions in patients with GIAEs. Somatostatin analogs may downregulate VEGF, inhibit vasodilation, reduce splanchnic blood flow, and improve platelet aggregation. Octreotide and lanreotide are both available as long-acting intramuscular injections administered with a clinical response rate of 40% to 76%.[35,36] Adverse events most commonly include diarrhea, cholelithiasis and glucose intolerance.[30] Thalidomide is an oral medication with anti-angiogenic properties. In a large multicenter randomized controlled trial (n=150), treatment with thalidomide resulted in a 50% reduction in rebleeding in most patients (51%) treated with 50 mg daily and two-thirds (69%) treated with 100 mg daily, compared to 16% with placebo.[37] Side effects associated with thalidomide included somnolence, neuropathy, constipation, and elevation in liver enzymes. Bevacizumab, a monoclonal antibody against VEGF, may be effective in the treatment of GIAEs, but carries a high risk of bowel perforation and thromboembolic events.[38] Hormonal therapy and tranexamic acid have been studied in the management of GIAEs without demonstrated benefit.[39, 40]

Conclusion

Non-hereditary angioectasias are the most common source of small bowel bleeding in adults over 50. Advances in endoscopic and imaging techniques have improved detection and treatment of these lesions. When conventional upper endoscopy and colonoscopy fail to reveal a bleeding source, video capsule endoscopy serves as a valuable noninvasive diagnostic tool. The results from capsule endoscopy may be used for diagnosis as well as to direct endoscopic intervention. Medical therapy with somatostatin analogs or thalidomide may provide benefit to patients with bleeding GIAEs but the use of these agents is limited due to risk of side effects and cost. Further research is needed to determine the underlying mechanisms of GIAE formation and identify medical interventions which may benefit this patient population.

References

1. Foutch PG, Rex DK, Lieberman DA. Prevalence and natural history of colonic angiodysplasia among healthy asymptomatic people. Am J Gastroenterol. 1995;90:564-7.
2. Regula J, Wronska E, Pachlewski J. Vascular lesions of the gastrointestinal tract. Best Pract Res Clin Gastroenterol. 2008;22(2):313-28.
3. Yano T, Yamamoto H, Sunada K, et al. Endoscopic classification of vascular lesions of the small intestine (with videos). Gastrointest Endosc. 2008;67:169-72.
4. Saurin JC, Delvaux M, Gaudin JL, et al. Diagnostic value of endoscopic capsule in patients with obscure digestive bleeding: Blinded comparison with video push-enteroscopy. Endoscopy. 2003;35:576-84.
5. Saurin JC, Delvaux M, Vahedi K, et al. Clinical impact of capsule endoscopy compared to push enteroscopy: 1-year follow-up study. Endoscopy. 2005;37:318-23.
6. Boley SJ, Sammartano R, Adams A, et al. On the nature and etiology of vascular ectasias of the colon. Degenerative lesions of aging. Gastroenterology. 1977;72:650-60.
7. Committee ASoP, Pasha SF, Shergill A, et al. The role of endoscopy in the patient with lower GI bleeding. Gastrointest Endosc. 2014;79:875-85.
8. Junquera F, Saperas E, de Torres I, et al. Increased expression of angiogenic factors in human colonic angiodysplasia. Am J Gastroenterol. 1999;94:1070-6.
9. Sami SS, Al-Araji SA, Ragunath K. Review article: Gastrointestinal angiodysplasia - pathogenesis, diagnosis and management. Aliment Pharmacol Ther. 2014;39:15-34.
10. Kang J, Hennessy-Strahs S, Kwiatkowski P, et al. Continuous-flow LVAD support causes a distinct form of intestinal angiodysplasia. Circ Res 2017;121:963-969.
11. Loscalzo J. From clinical observation to mechanism—Heyde's syndrome. N Engl J Med 2012;367:1954-6.
12. Heyde E. Gastrointesinal bleeding in aortic stenosis. N Engl J Med 1958:196.
13. Bermont A, Abu-Freha N, Cohen DL, et al. Epidemiology and risk factors for angiodysplasias of the upper and lower gastrointestinal tract: A large population-based study. Dig Liver Dis. 2025;57:220-224.
14. Foutch PG. Angiodysplasia of the gastrointestinal tract. Am J Gastroenterol. 1993;88:807-18.
15. Bollinger E, Raines DL. Distribution of bleeding gastrointestinal angioectasias in a Western population. World J Gastroenterology. 2012;18(43): 6235-9.
16. Davie M, Yung DE, Douglas S, Plevris JN, Koulaouzidis A. Mapping the distribution of small bowel angioectasias. Scand J Gastroenterol. 2019;54:597-602.
17. Plotkin E, Imaeda A. Small Intestinal angioectasias are not randomly distributed in the small bowel and most may be reached by push enteroscopy. J Clin Gastroenterol. 2016;50:561-5.
18. Arieira C, Magalhaes R, Dias de Castro F, et al. Small bowel angioectasias rebleeding and the identification of higher risk patients. Dig Dis Sci. 2021;66:175-180.
19. Raju GS, Gerson L, Das A, et al. American Gastroenterological Association (AGA) Institute medical position statement on obscure gastrointestinal bleeding. Gastroenterology. 2007;133:1694-6.
20. Garcia-Compean D, Del Cueto-Aguilera AN, Jimenez-Rodriguez AR, et al. Diagnostic and therapeutic challenges of gastrointestinal angiodysplasias: A critical review and view points. World J Gastroenterol. 2019;25:2549-2564.
21. Gerson LB, Fidler JL, Cave DR, et al. ACG Clinical Guideline: Diagnosis and Management of Small Bowel Bleeding. Am J Gastroenterol 2015;110:1265-87.
22. ASGE Standards of Practice Committee, Gurudu SR, Bruining DH, et al. The role of endoscopy in the management of suspected small-bowel bleeding. Gastrointest Endosc. 2017;85:22-31.
23. Rezapour M, Amadi C, Gerson LB. Retention associated with video capsule endoscopy: systematic review and

meta-analysis. Gastrointest Endosc. 2017;85:1157-1168 e2.
24. Yaxley KL, Mulhem A, Godfrey S, et al. The accuracy of computed tomography angiography compared with technetium-99m labelled red blood cell scintigraphy for the diagnosis and localization of acute gastrointestinal bleeding: A systematic review and meta-analysis. Curr Probl Diagn Radiol 2023;52:546-559.
25. Wortman JR, Landman W, Fulwadhva UP, et al. CT angiography for acute gastrointestinal bleeding: What the radiologist needs to know. Br J Radiol. 2017;90:20170076.
26. Dobritz M, Engels HP, Schneider A, et al. Detection of intestinal bleeding with multi-detector row CT in an experimental setup. How many acquisitions are necessary? Eur Radiol 2009;19:2862-9.
27. Pasha SF, Leighton JA, Das A, et al. Double-balloon enteroscopy and capsule endoscopy have comparable diagnostic yield in small-bowel disease: A meta-analysis. Clin Gastroenterol Hepatol. 2008;6:671-6.
28. Sanaka MR, Navaneethan U, Kosuru B, et al. Antegrade is more effective than retrograde enteroscopy for evaluation and management of suspected small-bowel disease. Clin Gastroenterol Hepatol. 2012;10:910-6.
29. Nennstiel S, Machanek A, von Delius S, et al. Predictors and characteristics of angioectasias in patients with obscure gastrointestinal bleeding identified by video capsule endoscopy. United European Gastroenterol J. 2017;5:1129-1135.
30. Kwan V, Bourke MJ, Williams SJ, et al. Argon plasma coagulation in the management of symptomatic gastrointestinal vascular lesions: experience in 100 consecutive patients with long-term follow-up. Am J Gastroenterol. 2006;101:58-63.
31. Igawa A, Oka S, Tanaka S, et al. Polidocanol injection therapy for small-bowel hemangioma by using double-balloon endoscopy. Gastrointest Endosc. 2016;84:163-7.
32. Lara LF, Silva R, Thakkar S, et al. Multicenter case series of patients with small-bowel angiodysplasias treated with a small-bowel radiofrequency ablation catheter. VideoGIE. 2020;5:162-167.
33. Jackson CS, Gerson LB. Management of gastrointestinal angiodysplastic lesions (GIADs): A systematic review and meta-analysis. Am J Gastroenterol. 2014;109:474-83.
34. Kaufman D, Leslie G, Marya N, et al. Small intestinal angioectasia: Characterization, risk factors, and rebleeding. J Clin Gastroenterol. 2017;51:720-727.
35. Goltstein L, Grooteman KV, Rocco A, et al. Effectiveness and predictors of response to somatostatin analogues in patients with gastrointestinal angiodysplasias: A systematic review and individual patient data meta-analysis. Lancet Gastroenterol Hepatol. 2021;6:922-932.
36. Brown C, Subramanian V, Wilcox CM, et al. Somatostatin analogues in the treatment of recurrent bleeding from gastrointestinal vascular malformations: An overview and systematic review of prospective observational studies. Dig Dis Sci. 2010;55:2129-34.
37. Chen H, Wu S, Tang M, et al. Thalidomide for recurrent bleeding due to small-intestinal angiodysplasia. N Engl J Med. 2023;389:1649-1659.
38. Albitar HAH, Almodallal Y, Papadakis KA, et al. Intravenous bevacizumab reduces transfusion requirements and endoscopic interventions in patients with gastric antral vascular ectasia and small bowel angioectasia. Gastroenterology. 2020;158:1162-1163 e4.
39. Junquera F, Feu F, Papo M, et al. A multicenter, randomized, clinical trial of hormonal therapy in the prevention of rebleeding from gastrointestinal angiodysplasia. Gastroenterology. 2001;121:1073-9.
40. HALT-IT Trial Collaborators. Effects of a high-dose 24-h infusion of tranexamic acid on death and thromboembolic events in patients with acute gastrointestinal bleeding (HALT-IT): an international randomised, double-blind, placebo-controlled trial. Lancet. 2020;395:1927-1936.

Case Study Number 13

Presented by Daniel Wild, MD, FACG and Ryne Ramaker, MD

Pre-capsule Findings (included in capsule study)

A 47-year-old woman with a history of hypertension and generalized anxiety disorder presents as a referral from her primary physician for iron deficiency anemia. She has no prior history of anemia or iron deficiency in the past. Her last menstrual period was over 2 years ago. She admits to occasional abdominal pain recently but denies associated nausea, diarrhea, early satiety or weight loss. Family history is negative for celiac disease, inflammatory bowel disease, and colorectal cancer. An initial endoscopic evaluation, including upper endoscopy with duodenal biopsies and colonoscopy with inspection of the terminal ileum, is unrevealing. Laboratory results are notable for a hemoglobin of 9gm/dl with a serum ferritin of 11 ng/ml.

A capsule endoscopy study is performed to evaluate for small bowel bleeding. Review the capsule endoscopy study and report your findings, including: gastric passage time, small bowel passage time, and observed abnormalities. Be prepared to discuss your findings and management plan with your staff prior to reviewing the diagnosis and case discussion.

Capsule Endoscopy Findings
First Duodenal Image = 0hr 7min 14sec
First Cecal Image = 5h 47min 27sec
Small bowel passage time = 5hr 40min

Video capsule image capture starts in the duodenal bulb. The proximal small bowel is normal in appearance. Within the mid small bowel (3 hours), capsule transit is delayed. Capsule hold up is observed for approximately 1 hour prior to transit into a distal segment of bowel which contains red blood (**Figure 1**: 4hrs 5min 23sec) followed by a stenosis with ulceration (**Figure 2**: 4hrs 35min 59sec).

Follow-up

Intubation of the deep small bowel by anterograde double balloon enteroscopy identifies the area of stenosis with ulceration (**Figure 3**). Biopsies are obtained and the site is marked in a submucosal India Ink tattoo. A diagnosis of small bowel lymphoma is made by pathology.

Figure 1

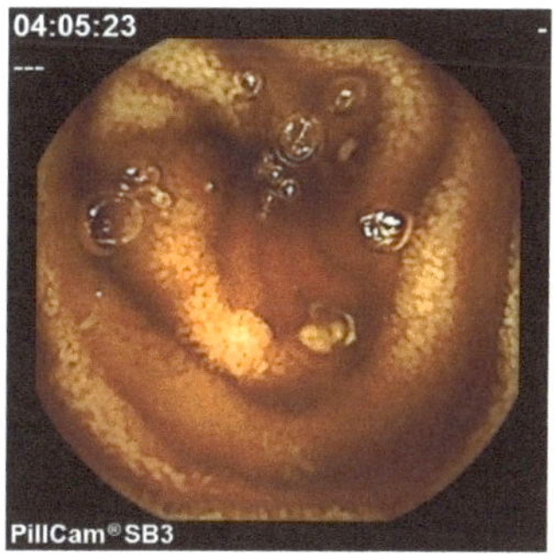

Figure 2

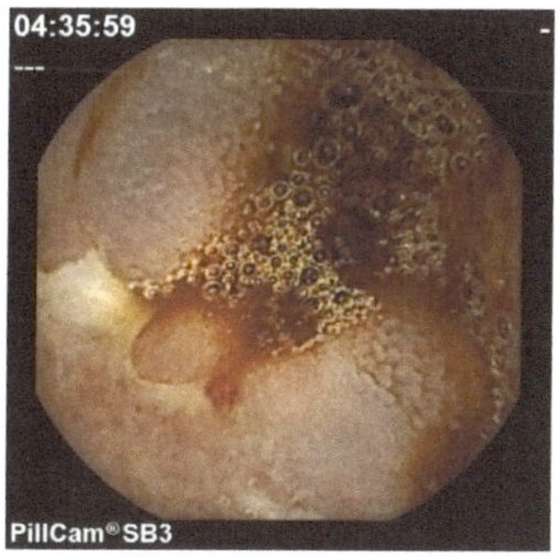

Figure 3

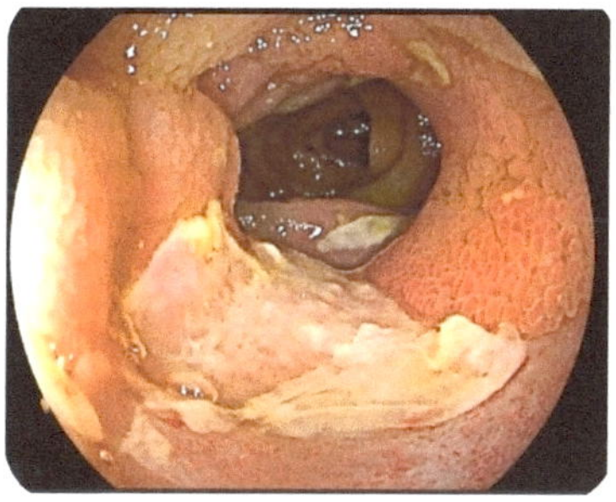

Chapter 13: Small Bowel Lymphoma

Daniel Wild, MD, FACG and Ryne Ramaker, MD

Epidemiology

The gastrointestinal (GI) tract is the most common site for extranodal non-Hodgkin's lymphoma (NHL), representing 5%-20% of all cases, but primary small bowel lymphomas are rare.[1] A German registry of 371 patients with primary GI NHL showed that only 9% of the tumors had a primary site of origin between the duodenum and terminal ileum, with another 7% arising between the terminal ileum and cecum.[2] Even compared to other small bowel tumors, primary small bowel lymphomas are uncommon. In 2 large retrospective studies, 1 from Japan featuring small bowel tumors detected with double balloon enteroscopy (DBE) and 1 from Italy featuring small bowel tumors detected on capsule endoscopy, only 22%-23% of the primary small bowel tumors were lymphomas.[3,4]

Primary small bowel lymphoma is even less common in the U.S. population. According to the National Cancer Data Base, lymphoma represented 17% of the small bowel tumors registered from 1985 to 1995, making it the third most common small bowel malignancy behind carcinoid (44%) and adenocarcinoma (33%).[5] In a recent study of 218 patients diagnosed with small bowel mass lesions by device-assisted enteroscopy across 3 major U.S. referral centers, only 2 patients (1%) were found to have lymphoma.[6]

Classification

The majority of small bowel lymphomas are of B-cell origin.[1] In studies from Germany and Austria 73%-83% of these lymphomas were of B-cell origin and 79%-83% were classified as high grade.[2,7] Small bowel lymphomas can be classified into the following 4 groups.

Enteropathy Associated T-Cell Lymphoma (EATL)

EATL comprises less than 1% of all NHL.[8] It is associated with celiac sprue, particularly in patients with type II refractory disease. EATL is derived from the monoclonal expansion of a population of intraepithelial T-lymphocytes and likely stems from chronic inflammation.

Extranodal Marginal Zone 8-Cell Lymphoma (MZL)

MZL of mucosa associated lymphoid tissue (MALT) is a low grade lymphoma arising from epithelial mucosa. Within the GI tract, MALT lymphoma occurs primarily in the stomach as a consequence of long-standing gastritis from *Helicobacter pylori* infection.[9] Small bowel involvement can occur in association with gastric MALT lymphoma but is rare.[10] In contrast to gastric MALT lymphoma, *H. pylori* infection is not associated with primary extra nodal MZL of the small bowel.[11-13] Chronic immune stimulation due to auto-immune diseases or other infections are thought to be a risk factor for the development of primary extra nodal MZL. Immune-proliferative small intestinal disease ("alpha heavy chain disease") is a variant of extranodal MZL that is essentially absent in the industrialized world. Its prevalence in developing and impoverished nations and response to antibiotics in early stage disease strongly suggest that parasitic and enteric infections of the small bowel contribute to the development of the disease.[14] The proliferative cells are IgA-secreting B-cells which produce an alpha-heavy chain paraprotein that is often detectable in the serum.[1] Extranodal MZL has an indolent growth pattern, but may transform to a more aggressive high-grade B cell lymphoma.

Primary intestinal follicular lymphoma

Primary intestinal follicular lymphoma is a rare disease entity. Overall, follicular lymphoma accounts for only 2% of all GI NHL.[15] These lesions are most commonly found in the duodenum.[16] The growth pattern of follicular lymphoma is relatively indolent.[17]

Other Lymphomas

Mantle cell lymphoma (or multiple lymphomatous polyposis), Burkitt's Lymphoma, and diffuse large B cell lymphoma can occur in the small bowel, although they often simultaneously present at other sites in the gastrointestinal tract at the time of diagnosis. In a case series of 31 consecutive patients with primary gastrointestinal tract mantle cell lymphoma, 57% of cases involved the stomach and 90% involved the colon.[18]

Presentation

Small bowel lymphomas cause a wide range of non-specific symptoms and often have an insidious presentation. In a large German registry, small bowel lymphomas most commonly presented with abdominal pain (75%) but were also associated with a decrease in appetite (41%), ileus (37.5%), weight loss (34%), emesis (31.3%), and/or gastrointestinal bleeding (6.3%). In a study from Korea, 50% of the cases of small bowel lymphoma were asymptomatic upon diagnosis.[19] Recurrent fevers greater than 104ºF degrees, drenching night sweats, and unintentional weight loss (B symptoms) were relatively rare, occurring in only 15.6% of cases.[2] Pain was the presenting feature in 79% of patients in a Chinese series with 40% of these patients reporting B symptoms.[20]

In general, small bowel lymphomas occur later in life, with a mean age of 62 at diagnosis and a male predominance that has been reported as to be as high as 2:1.2 The incidence of EATL peaks in the sixth decade and is often marked by clinical relapse in a patient with previously well-controlled celiac sprue. Presenting symptoms may also include acute bleeding, obstruction, or perforation.[21,22] Patients with extranodal MZL arising from the small bowel may present with gastric outlet obstruction, perforation, or intussuception. Patients with IPSID present earlier in life with a median age of 25 at diagnosis. These patients may also present with abdominal pain, chronic diarrhea, severe weight loss, and malabsorptive features such as growth retardation.[1] Ascites, fever, hypocalcemia, and organomegaly have also been reported.[23] An alpha-chain protein is detectable serologically in up to 70% of these patients.[24] Patients with primary intestinal follicular lymphoma may present with upper abdominal pain, weight loss, or anemia.[17]

Diagnosis

Guidelines for the diagnostic evaluation of NHL are available at www.NCCN.org, and are updated regularly. In cases in which an abnormality is identified on VCE, tissue sampling is required to confirm a diagnosis of lymphoma. Fine needle aspiration or core needle biopsies are generally inadequate for diagnosis. Sufficient tissue should be obtained for a gross morphological evaluation, as well as tissue immunohistochemistry, flow cytometry, cytogenetics, and fluorescence in situ hybridization (FISH). According to WHO criteria, formal pathological diagnosis requires morphologic, immunophenotypic, and genotypic features.

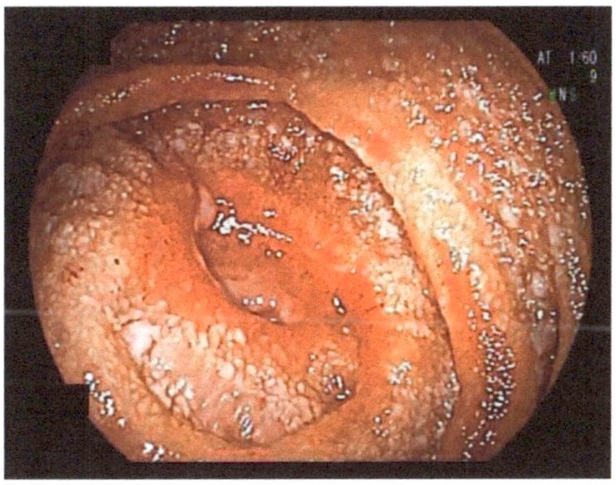

Figure 1. Small bowel lymphoma complicated by an inflammatory stricture.

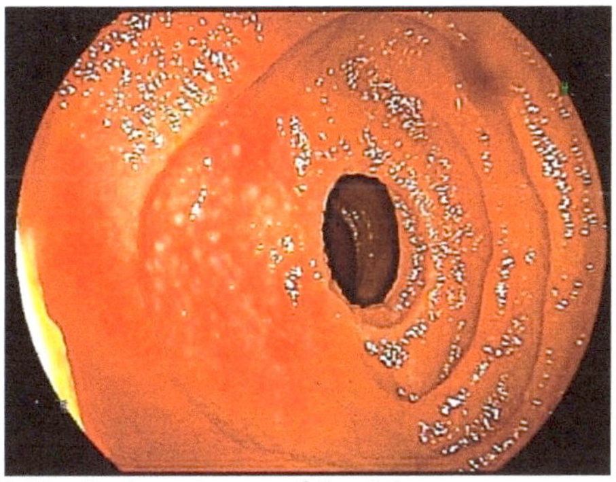

Figure 2. Follicular lymphoma of the jejunum.

The appearance of lymphoma on VCE is variable and non-specific with features that mimic those seen in other small bowel tumors as well as in celiac sprue and Crohn's disease. These features include mucosal erosions, ulcers and ulcerated strictures such as those seen in the case example as well as nodules or masses[4, 25] (**Figure 1**). In the only study of VCE in patients with known primary intestinal lymphoma, the authors observed that mucosal abnormalities develop in either an ulcerative pathway with villous atrophy followed by the formation of plaques and ulcers or a proliferative pathway resulting in the formation of polyps or nodules.[26] VCE may diagnose EATL in patients with refractory celiac sprue. In these patients, the lesion appears as ulceration and stenosis.[27] The endoscopic appearance of GI follicular lymphoma has been reported as multiple, small, whitish nodules[17] (**Figure 2**).

Staging

Staging of NHL begins with a detailed history with particular attention given to B symptoms. Physical examination includes an evaluation of enlarged lymph nodes and the size of the liver and spleen. The ring of tonsillar tissue located in the posterior oral cavity (Waldeyer's ring) is commonly enlarged in patients with lymphoma. Routine laboratory studies include a complete blood count, comprehensive metabolic panel, and lactate dehydrogenase. A bone marrow biopsy is indicated to rule out other sites of extra nodal disease. A complete staging evaluation also includes either a diagnostic CT of the chest, abdomen, and pelvis or a PET-CT.[24]

The Ann Arbor staging system is used for nodal NHL; however, this system is insufficient for prognostication of gastrointestinal lymphomas.[25] A modified form of Ann Arbor Staging is frequently used for extranodal disease. In this system, disease that is limited to a single site in the intestinal tract is considered stage IE (extranodal= E). Stage II disease refers to multiple lymph node chains on one side of the diaphragm, and stage III refers to disease on both sides of the diaphragm. If multiple extranodal sites are affected, or multiple lymph nodes are involved, the disease is classified as stage IV.[26] Alternative staging systems for small bowel lymphomas have been proposed, such as the Lugano classification system and Paris system.[27,28]

The Paris system combines depth of invasion and distant involvement using TNMB classification. In this system, the T stage separates disease confined to the mucosa (T1m), confined to the submucosa (T1sm), infiltrating the muscularis propria or subserosa (T2), penetrating the serosa without adjacent structure involvement (T3), and invasion of adjacent structures (T4). The N stage separates disease with no nodal involvement (N0), regional node involvement (N1), distant abdominal node involvement (N2), and extra-abdominal node involvement (N3). The M stage classifies disease by extent of metastatic spread as either a single site of disease (M0), non-continuous involvement of a separate gastrointestinal location (M1), or involvement of other tissues (M2). Finally, the B stage separates disease without bone marrow involvement (B0) from those with infiltration of the bone marrow (B1).[29]

Multiple retrospective analyses comparing the modified Ann Arbor, Lugano, and Paris systems have found the Paris system is the only classification capable of clinically significant prognostic stratification of intestinal lymphomas.[30,31] Newer staging systems for select patient populations, such as elderly patients, have been proposed, but have not yet been widely implemented.[32]

Treatment

Therapies for primary small bowel lymphoma are guided by the disease subtype and may range from observation alone to high-dose chemotherapy.

EATL currently has no clear standard of care treatment. Unresectable disease is most commonly treated with combination chemotherapy with regimens typically including cyclophosphamide, an anthracycline, vincristine, and prednisone; however, response rates to therapy are typically less than 50%.[32,33,34]

Extranodal MZL of MALT is often treated with radiation therapy alone in the setting of Ann Arbor stage I and II disease.[35,36,37] Alternatively, surgical resection or rituximab monotherapy can be considered.[38,39,40] For more advanced disease stages, curative surgery is not possible. Either radiation therapy or systemic therapy with chemotherapy and rituximab are treatment options.[41,42] IPSID is a unique subset for which early-stage disease can be treated with antibiotics targeting the instigating pathogen alone. More advanced disease is treated similarly to MALT lymphoma.[43,44]

Primary intestinal follicular lymphoma is an indolent disease that rarely progresses to an advanced stage, and spontaneous remissions have been observed in some patients receiving no active treatment.[45,46] The majority of patients managed with observation alone. However, treatment with radiation therapy or chemotherapy with rituximab are potential treatment options.[47]

Other lymphomas, such as mantle cell lymphoma, DLBCL, and Burkitt's lymphoma generally present with advanced disease, and are treated with systemic therapy according to disease-specific algorithms.[48]

Prognosis

The prognosis for patients with primary small bowel lymphoma varies based on their disease subtype and stage at diagnosis. The prognosis for patients with EATL is exceptionally poor. Cohort studies of patients treated with combination chemotherapy found most patients survive less than a year. Retrospective studies have found improved outcomes for patients who undergo autologous stem cell transplantation in first remission.[49]

The prognosis for patients with primary extranodal MZL of the small bowel presenting with localized disease (Ann Arbor stages I or II) is excellent, mainly due to its responsiveness to local therapy and the indolent growth of the disease. Cohort studies that include small bowel disease have found 5-year overall survival rates of 100% for early-stage disease patients treated with radiation therapy.[50,51]

IPSID is fatal in the absence of therapy, but prognosis improves with treatment. A case series of 23 consecutive patients treated in Turkey reported a 5-year overall survival of 70%, and almost half of all patients receiving a tetracycline alone were disease free at 5 years.[52,53,54]

The prognosis for patients with localized primary intestinal follicular lymphoma is favorable. A retrospective analysis of 73 cases of primary intestinal follicular lymphoma managed by observation alone reported an 87.1% overall survival at 10 years.[55] In a recent study of VCE enhanced by a deep convolutional neural network, interpretive algorithms could assess whether follicular lymphomas in the small bowel progressed, regressed or remained unchanged during a surveillance interval.[56]

Conclusion

Primary small bowel lymphomas are a rare and diverse group of malignancies that present significant diagnostic and therapeutic challenges due to their variable clinical manifestations, histologic subtypes, and disease behaviors. Accurate diagnosis requires a high index of suspicion, especially in patients with nonspecific gastrointestinal symptoms or known risk factors such as celiac disease, and should be supported by adequate tissue sampling for histopathologic and molecular evaluation. Capsule endoscopy and device-assisted enteroscopy play important roles in the initial identification of lesions, though cross-sectional imaging and systemic staging remain essential for treatment planning. Management strategies must be tailored to the lymphoma subtype and extent of disease, ranging from observation in indolent cases to aggressive multimodal therapies for high-grade or disseminated disease. Prognosis is likewise heterogeneous, with favorable outcomes seen in early-stage MZL and follicular lymphoma, and poor survival in cases of EATL and advanced-stage disease. Continued advancements in diagnostic modalities, classification systems, and targeted therapies are essential to improving outcomes for patients with these uncommon but clinically significant malignancies.

References

1. Gill SS, Heuman DM, Mihas AA. Small intestinal neoplasms. J Clin Gastroenterol 2001, 33:267-282.
2. Koch P, del Valle F, Berdel WE, et al. Primary gastrointestinal non-Hodgkin's lymphoma: Anatomic and histologic distribution, clinical features, and survival data of 371 patients registered in the German Multicenter Study GIT NHL 01/92. J Clin Oncol. 2001; 19:3861-3873.
3. Mitsui K, Tanaka S, Yamamoto H, et al. Role of double-balloon endoscopy in the diagnosis of small-bowel tumors: the first Japanese multicenter study. Gastrointest Endosc. 2009; 70:498-504.
4. Spada C, Riccioni ME, Familiari P, Marchese M, Bizzotto A, Costamagna G. Video capsule endoscopy in small-bowel tumours: A single centre experience. Scand J Gastroenterol. 2008; 43:497-505.
5. Howe JR, Karnell LH, Menck HR, Scott-Conner C. The American College of Surgeons Commission on Cancer and the American Cancer Society. Adenocarcinoma of the small bowel: Review of the National Cancer Data Base, 1985-1995. Cancer. 1999; 86:2693-2706.
6. Noujaim MG, Dorsey C, Parish A, et al. Clinical features and management of small bowel masses detected during device-assisted enteroscopy: A multi-center experience. Gastroenterology Res. 2022;15(6):353-363.
7. Radaszkiewicz T, Dragosics B, Bauer P. Gastrointestinal malignant lymphomas of the mucosa-associated lymphoid tissue: Factors relevant to prognosis. Gastroenterology. 1992; 102:1628-1638.
8. Zettl A, deLeeuw R, Haralambieva E, Mueller-Hermelink HK. Enteropathy-type T-cell lymphoma. Am J Clin Pathol. 2007; 127:701-706.
9. Hussell T, Isaacson PG, Crabtree JE, Spencer J. The response of cells from low-grade B-cell gastric lymphomas of mucosaassociated lymphoid tissue to *Helicobacter pylori*. Lancet. 1993; 342:571-574.
10. Dolak W, Raderer M, Maresch J, et al. Detection of gastric MALT lymphoma spreading to the small bowel by enteroscopy. Endoscopy. 2011; 43:731-733.
11. Tadmor T, Rainis T, Bejar J, Attias D, Lavy A. Primary duodenal mucosa-associated lymphoid tissue (MALT) lymphoma—A rare presentation of gastric outlet obstruction. Can J Gastroenterol. 2007;21:393-395.

12. Jang WC, Kim VS, Hong SW, Kang YK. [Small intestinal perforation caused by primary jejunal MALT lymphoma]. Korean J Gastroenterol. 2008;51:215-218.
13. Erol MF, Karakayali AS, Ozer S, Yildiz M, Celepli S, Kaptanoğlu B. Mucosa-associated lymphoid tissue lymphoma of the ileum as the cause of an intestinal invagination. J Pediatr Surg. 2008;43(8):e13-5.
14. Khojasteh A, Haghshenass M, Haghighi P. Current concepts immunoproliferative small intestinal disease. A "Third-World lesion". N Engl J Med. 1983;308:1401-1405.
15. Anderson JR, Armitage JO, Weisenburger DD. Epidemiology of the non-Hodgkin's lymphomas: Distributions of the major subtypes differ by geographic locations. Non-Hodgkin's Lymphoma Classification Project. Ann Oncol. 1998;9:717-720.
16. Takata K, Okada H, Ohmiya N, et al. Primary gastrointestinal follicular lymphoma involving the duodenal second portion is a distinct entity: A multicenter, retrospective analysis in Japan. Cancer Sci. 2011;102:1532-1536.
17. Schmatz AI, Streubel B, Kretschmer-Chott E, et al. Primary follicular lymphoma of the duodenum is a distinct mucosal/submucosal variant of follicular lymphoma: A retrospective study of 63 cases. J Clin Oncol. 2011; 29:1445-1451.
18. Ruskone-Fourmestraux A, Delmer A, Lavergne A, et al. Multiple lymphomatous polyposis of the gastrointestinal tract: Prospective clinicopathologic study of 31 cases. Groupe D'etude des Lymphomes Digestifs. Gastroenterology. 1997;112:7-16.
19. Yoo AY, Lee BJ, Kim WS, et al. Clinicopathological features of small bowel tumors diagnosed by video capsule endoscopy and balloon-assisted enteroscopy: A single center experience. Clin Endosc. 2021;54(1):85-91.
20. 20. Li B, Shi YK, He XH, et al. Primary non-Hodgkin lymphomas in the small and large intestine: clinicopathological characteristics and management of 40 patients. Int J Hematol. 2008;87:375-381.
21. Green PH, Cellier C. Celiac disease. N Engl J Med. 2007;357:1731-1743.
22. Swinson CM, Slavin G, Coles EC, Booth CC. Coeliac disease and malignancy. Lancet. 1983;1:111-115.
23. Nassar VH, Salem PA, Shahid MJ, et al. "Mediterranean abdominal lymphoma" or immunoproliferative small intestinal disease. Part II: Pathological aspects. Cancer. 1978;41(4):1340-1354.
24. Rambaud JC, Modigliani R, Phuoc BK, et al. Non-secretory alpha-chain disease in intestinal lymphoma. N Engl J Med. 1980; 303(1):53.
25. Boot H. Diagnosis and staging in gastrointestinal lymphoma. Best Pract Res Clin Gastroenterol. 2010;24(1):3-12.
26. Musshoff K. [Clinical staging classification of non-Hodgkin's lymphomas (author's transl)]. Strahlentherapie. 1977;153(4):218-221.
27. Rohatiner A, d'Amore F, Coiffier B, et al. Report on a workshop convened to discuss the pathological and staging classifications of gastrointestinal tract lymphoma. Ann Oncol. 1994;5(5):397-400.
28. Ruskoné-Fourmestraux A, Dragosics B, Morgner A, Wotherspoon A, De Jong D. Paris staging system for primary gastrointestinal lymphomas. Gut. 2003;52(6):912-913.
29. Hwang HS, Yoon DH, Suh C, Park CS, Huh J. Intestinal diffuse large B-cell lymphoma: an evaluation of different staging systems. J Korean Med Sci. 2014;29(1):53-60.
30. Chang S, Shi X, Xu Z, Liu Q. TNM staging system may be superior to Lugano and Ann Arbor systems in predicting the overall survival of patients with primary gastrointestinal lymphoma. J BUON. 2015;20(3):812-819.
31. Wang J, Ren W, Zhang C, Wang X. A New staging system based on the dynamic prognostic nomogram for elderly patients with primary gastrointestinal diffuse large B-cell lymphoma. Front Med (Lausanne). 2022;9:860993.
32. Delabie J, Holte H, Vose JM, et al. Enteropathy-associated T-cell lymphoma: Clinical and histological findings from the international peripheral T-cell lymphoma project. Blood. 2011;118(1):148-155.
33. Babel N, Paragi P, Chamberlain RS. Management of enteropathy-associated T-cell lymphoma: An algorithmic approach. Case Rep Oncol. 2009;2(1):36-43.
34. Wöhrer S, Chott A, Drach J, et al. Chemotherapy with cyclophosphamide, doxorubicin, etoposide, vincristine and prednisone (CHOEP) is not effective in patients with enteropathy-type intestinal T-cell lymphoma. Ann Oncol. 2004;15(11):1680-1683.
35. Teckie S, Qi S, Chelius M, et al. Long-term outcome of 487 patients with early-stage extra-nodal marginal zone lymphoma. Ann Oncol. 2017;28(5):1064-1069.
36. Fang P, Gunther JR, Pinnix CC, et al. A prospective trial of radiation therapy efficacy and toxicity for localized mucosa-associated lymphoid tissue (MALT) lymphoma. Int J Radiat Oncol Biol Phys. 2021;109(5):1414-1420.
37. MacManus MP, Roos D, O'Brien P, et al. Prospective Phase II trial of radiation therapy in localised non-gastric marginal zone lymphoma with prospective evaluation of autoimmunity and Helicobacter pylori status: TROG 05.02/ALLG NHL15. Eur J Cancer. 2021;152:129-138.
38. Conconi A, Martinelli G, Thiéblemont C, et al. Clinical activity of rituximab in extranodal marginal zone B-cell lymphoma of MALT type. Blood. 2003;102(8):2741-2745.
39. Okamura I, Imai H, Mori K, et al. Rituximab monotherapy as a first-line treatment for pulmonary mucosa-associated lymphoid tissue lymphoma. Int J Hematol. 2015;101(1):46-51.

40. Zucca E, Conconi A, Pedrinis E, et al. Nongastric marginal zone B-cell lymphoma of mucosa-associated lymphoid tissue. Blood. 2003;101(7):2489-2495.
41. Rummel MJ, Niederle N, Maschmeyer G, et al. Bendamustine plus rituximab versus CHOP plus rituximab as first-line treatment for patients with indolent and mantle-cell lymphomas: An open-label, multicentre, randomised, phase 3 non-inferiority trial. Lancet. 2013;381(9873):1203-1210.
42. Flinn IW, van der Jagt R, Kahl BS, et al. Randomized trial of bendamustine-rituximab or R-CHOP/R-CVP in first-line treatment of indolent NHL or MCL: The BRIGHT study. Blood. 2014;123(19):2944-2952.
43. Al-Saleem T, Al-Mondhiry H. Immunoproliferative small intestinal disease (IPSID): A model for mature B-cell neoplasms. Blood. 2005;105(6):2274-2280.
44. AlYamany R, Kharfan-Dabaja MA, Hamadani M, Alshaibani A, Aljurf M. The evolution of our understanding of immunoproliferative small intestinal disease (IPSID) over time. Current Oncology. 2022;29(5):3759-3769.
45. Weindorf SC, Smith LB, Owens SR. Update on gastrointestinal lymphomas. Arch Pathol Lab Med. 2018;142(11):1347-1351.
46. Tari A, Asaoku H, Takata K, et al. The role of "watch and wait" in intestinal follicular lymphoma in rituximab era. Scand J Gastroenterol. 2016;51(3):321-328.
47. Marks E, Shi Y. Duodenal-Type Follicular Lymphoma: A Clinicopathologic Review. Arch Pathol Lab Med. 2018;142(4):542-547.
48. Olszewska-Szopa M, Wróbel T. Gastrointestinal non-Hodgkin lymphomas. Adv Clin Exp Med. 2019;28(8):1119-1124.
49. Jantunen E, Boumendil A, Finel H, et al. Autologous stem cell transplantation for enteropathy-associated T-cell lymphoma: A retrospective study by the EBMT. Blood. 2013;121(13):2529-2532.
50. Ito E, Ogino I, Sugiura M, et al. Long-term outcomes of early-stage non-stomach gastrointestinal mucosa-associated lymphoid tissue lymphoma treated with radiation therapy. Anticancer Res. 2023;43(6):2851-2857.
51. Ishikawa E, Nakamura M, Satou A, Shimada K, Nakamura S. Mucosa-associated lymphoid tissue (MALT) lymphoma in the gastrointestinal tract in the modern era. Cancers (Basel). 2022;14(2):446.
52. Akbulut H, Soykan I, Yakaryilmaz F, et al. Five-year results of the treatment of 23 patients with immunoproliferative small intestinal disease: a Turkish experience. Cancer. 1997;80(1):8-14.
53. Salimi M, Spinelli JJ. Chemotherapy of Mediterranean abdominal lymphoma. Retrospective comparison of chemotherapy protocols in Iranian patients. Am J Clin Oncol. 1996;19(1):18-22.
54. Afroza S, Zabin M, Uddin M, Ahmed S. Immunoproliferative small intestinal disease – A case report. Bangladesh Oncology Journal. 2009;4(2):90-92.
55. Iwamuro M, Tanaka T, Ennishi D, et al. Long-term outcomes of patients with primary intestinal follicular lymphoma managed with watch-and-wait strategy. Sci Rep. 2023;13(1):5858.
56. Sumioka A, Tsuboi A, Oka S. Disease surveillance evaluation of primary small-bowel follicular lymphoma using capsule endoscopy images based on a deep convolutional neural network. Gastrointest Endosc. 2023;98(6):968-976.e3.

Case Study Number 14

Presented by Christian S. Jackson, MD, FACG and Daniel Raines, MD, FACG

Pre-capsule Findings (included in capsule study)

A 66-year-old man with a past medical history significant for prostate cancer, coronary artery disease with myocardial infarction, hypertension, hyperlipidemia, hypothyroidism was admitted to the hospital for symptomatic iron deficiency anemia. He complained of fatigue and dyspnea on exertion but denied any history of melena, hematochezia, nausea/vomiting, abdominal pain, or weight loss. Inpatient evaluation by EGD and colonoscopy were unremarkable for a cause of iron deficiency anemia. He was discharged from the hospital following transfusion of packed red blood cells. An outpatient video capsule endoscopy (VCE) is ordered to evaluate for small bowel bleeding.

A capsule endoscopy study is performed to evaluate for small bowel bleeding. Review the capsule endoscopy study and report your findings, including: gastric passage time, small bowel passage time, and observed abnormalities. Be prepared to discuss your findings and management plan with your staff prior to reviewing the diagnosis and case discussion.

A friable mass is observed in the mid-small bowel (26%-41% of small bowel transit time). The mass is associated with active bleeding and lymphagiectasia (**Figure 1**: 1hr 47min 48sec; **Figure 2**: 1hr 47min 55sec; **Figure 3**: 1hr 48min 7sec).

Capsule Endoscopy Findings
First Gastric Image = 0hr 1min 12sec
First Duodenal Image = 1hr 0min 15sec
Gastric passage time = 0hr 59min
First Cecal Image = 3hr 22min 52sec
Small bowel passage time = 2hr 22min

Figure 1

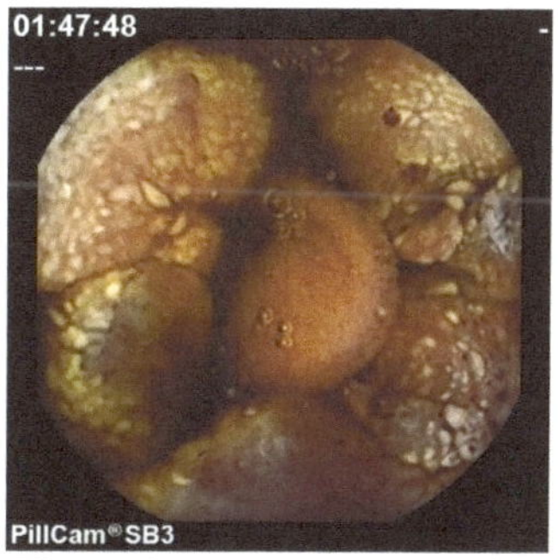

Figure 2

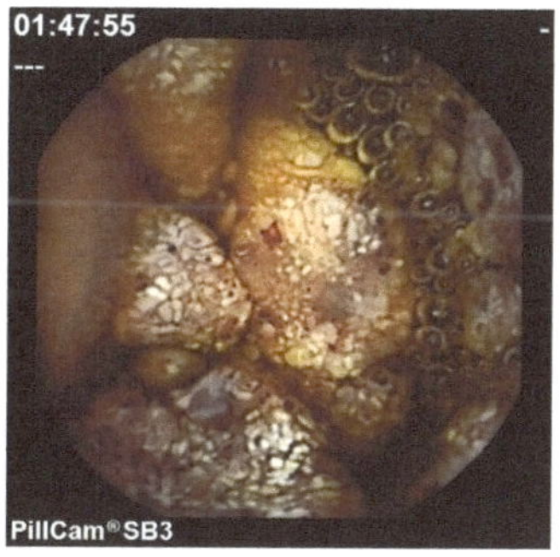

Figure 3

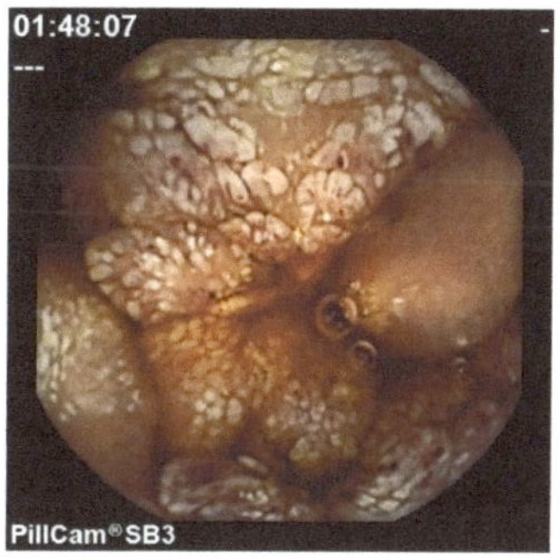

Follow-up

An anterograde single balloon enteroscopy was performed to further evaluate the abnormality observed by VCE. This exam was revealing for a friable mass lesion in the mid-jejunum (**Figure 4**). The mass was 4 cm in length and occupied 75% of the small bowel lumen. Biopsies of the mass revealed prominent lymphangiectasia. Subsequent evaluation by CT enterography demonstrated a jejunal mass with multiple grape-like filling defects. The patient was elected for laparotomy with small bowel resection due to concern for a potential malignancy. Pathologic analysis of the mass revealed a benign small bowel lymphangioma.

Figure 4

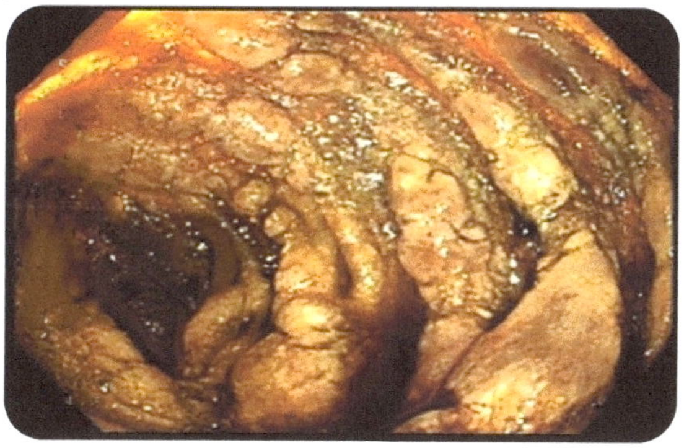

Chapter 14: Benign Small Bowel Lesions

Christian S. Jackson, MD, FACG and Daniel Raines, MD, FACG

Introduction

The incidence of small bowel lesions has increased dramatically with the widespread adoption of VCE, CT/MR enterography, and device-assisted enteroscopy (DAE). To effectively manage small bowel lesions identified by capsule endoscopy, readers should be equipped with a differential diagnosis for these lesions which includes benign small bowel pathologies in addition to malignant tumors. In this chapter, benign submucosal lesions commonly observed by VCE are discussed while a complete list of lesions can be found in **Table 1**. Small bowel lesions associated with polyposis syndromes (familial adenomatous polyposis, Peutz-Jeghers syndrome, juvenile polyposis, Cowden's syndrome) or premalignant conditions, such as celiac disease or Crohn's disease, are discussed in other chapters.

Benign Mesenchymal Tumors	**Focal Lymphangiectasia**
Lipoma	**Sporadic epithelial polyps**
Leiomyoma	Hamartoma
Hemangioma	Adenoma
Lymphangioma	Hyperplastic
Neuroma/schwannoma	**Granuloma**
Inflammatory fibroid polyp	

Table 1. Benign small bowel lesions.

Lymphangioma

Lymphangiomas are generally asymptomatic or responsible for nonspecific symptoms, including abdominal pain, diarrhea, and bleeding. In this case, the patient presented with iron deficiency anemia and was subsequently diagnosed with jejunal cavernous lymphangioma, an uncommon presentation. Cavernous lymphangiomas are usually identified in infants and children with most lesions found around the head and neck, trunk or extremities. Lymphangiomas account for 22% of small bowel tumors seen in children but are a smaller percentage (~28%) in adults.[1,2] The histological features of cavernous lymphangioma were first described by Gaudier and Gorse in 1913.[3] This tumor consists of single-layer endothelial-lined lymphatic spaces containing chylous or serous material. Lymphangiomas of the small bowel can be subtyped into cavernous or cystic presentation. For symptomatic cystic lesions or tumors larger than 37 mm, surgical resection is the treatment of choice.[4] In selected patients, endoscopic resection is a feasible option.

Focal Lymphangiectasia

Lymphangiectasias consist of dilated lymphatic vessels of the mucosa and submucosa which appear as white or yellowish foci as they are lipid-filled. Superficial lesions or "microcystic lymphangiectasias" are characterized by a cluster of tiny, white dots which represent dilated lacteals. Cystic dilation of larger lymphatic vessels in the submucosa produces a uniform, yellow blot under the mucosa which has been termed cystic lymphangiectasia, chylous cyst or xanthoma.[5]

Focal lymphangiectasias are commonly observed in the small bowel during capsule endoscopy but are rarely of any clinical significance. These lesions may appear as submucosal masses if they are raised (**Figures 1 and 2**). In rare cases, cystic lymphangiectasias may be associated with bleeding or abdominal pain when ulcerated or unusually large.[6,7] Focal lymphangiectasias should be managed

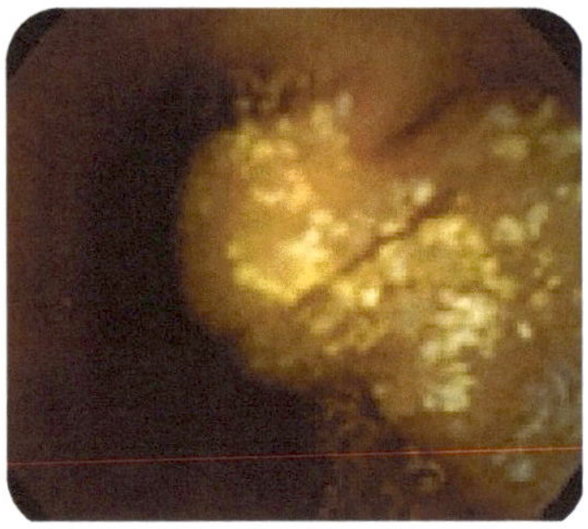

Figure 1. Polypoid lesion observed in the ileum on capsule endoscopy.

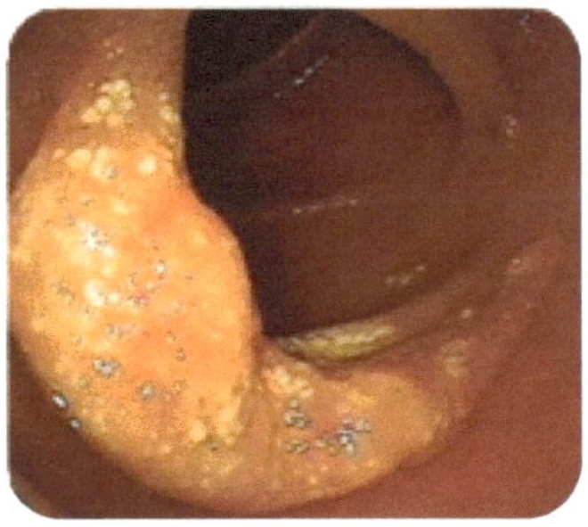

Figure 2. Retrograde double balloon enteroscopy image of the same lesion. Biopsy of the lesion confirmed a benign cystic lymphangiectasia.

conservatively. A secondary or expert review of VCE images with this finding is typically conclusive.

Small Bowel Lipoma

Gastrointestinal lipomas are benign, submucosal tumors which commonly occur in the colon (65%) but can also be found in the small bowel and stomach. Esophageal lipomas are very rare.[8] The vast majority of gastrointestinal lipomas are asymptomatic and discovered incidentally during routine endoscopy. During standard endoscopy, lipomas appear as discrete, soft masses associated with a yellowish mucosa! discoloration. These lesions can be commonly diagnosed by their characteristic appearance combined with their pliability upon manipulation with the biopsy forceps or "pillow sign."

The diagnosis of lipomas observed in the small bowel by VCE is more challenging. Small bowel lipomas may mimic malignant submucosal lesions such as gastrointestinal stromal tumor or carcinoid tumor (**Figure 3**). In cases in which concern malignancy persists or a small bowel lipoma is suspected to be symptomatic, additional evaluation by CT/MR enterography or DAE may be required (**Figure 4**). Small bowel lipomas exhibit a characteristic adipose density on CT, ranging between -80 and -120 Hounsfield units (HU), which can be diagnostic (**Figure 5**).[9,10]

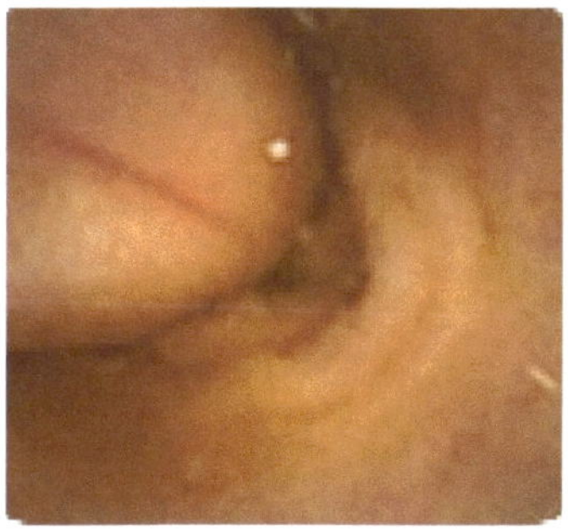

Figure 3. Lipoma of the ileum observed on capsule endoscopy.

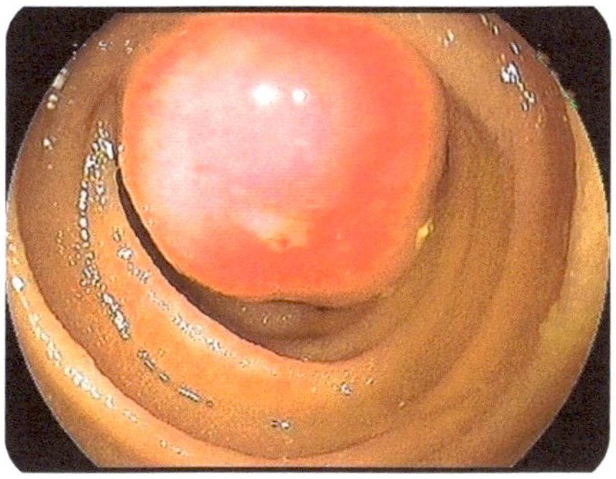

Figure 4. Jejunal lipoma with central ulceration observed by upper DBE

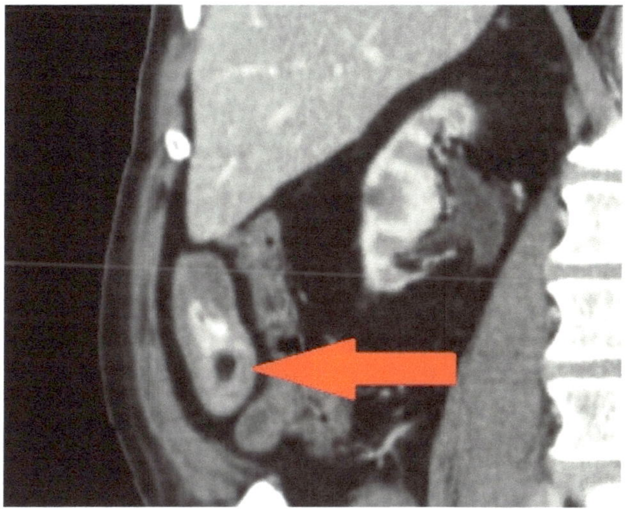

Figure 5. Coronal CT image of a bleeding lipoma (focus of fat density with extravasation of IV contrast superiorly).

Symptomatic gastrointestinal lipomas are generally greater than 2 cm in size and may present with bleeding, intestinal obstruction or intussusception.[11-13] Surgical resection is the mainstay of therapy for symptomatic lesions as endoscopic resection is associated with a high risk of perforation, especially with lesions > 2 cm in size. Pedunculated lesions which seem amenable to snare polypectomy may include invaginated layers of the muscularis propria and serosa in the stalk. Endoscopic treatment is possible by rupturing the capsule of lipoma using a forceps or cautery. However, the use of this technique must be more widely studied before it may be considered as a standard therapy.[14-16]

Inflammatory Fibroid Polyp

Inflammatory fibroid polyps (IFPs) are rare, benign, submucosal lesions of the gastrointestinal tract. They were first described by Vanek in 1949 as "gastric submucosal granulomas with eosinophilic infiltration" although the term IFP was proposed later by Helwig and Ranier.[17,18] IFPs have historically been considered as derived from benign reactive process similar to granulomas.[19-21] However, recent evidence supports a neoplastic process. IFP tissue samples stain positive for CD34 as observed with other stromal tumors. Genetic analysis of IFPs consistently reveals specific genetic mutations including PDGFRA tyrosine kinase mutation.[22,23]

IFPs most commonly occur in the stomach (37%), small bowel (37%), and rectosigmoid colon (36%).[24] Theses solitary lesions range 0.4 cm to 3 cm in size although IFPs up to 20 cm have been reported.[24,25] Most IFPs are discovered incidentally during routine endoscopy. Symptomatic IFP's of the small bowel often present with intussusception. Small bowel IFPs may also present with gastrointestinal bleeding due to extension of lesion from the submucosa into the mucosa with ulceration[24,26] (**Figure 6**). Endoscopic confirmation of a diagnosis of IFP is difficult as standard endoscopic biopsies are inadequate and malignant lesions such as GISTs cannot be excluded. On endoscopic ultrasound, IFP appears as a homogenenous, hypo-echogenic lesion located in the second or third sonographic layer with indistinct margins.[27] Surgical resection is the treatment of choice for IFP although resection by endoscopic snare technique is possible.[28,29] Complete resection is required for cure as well as to dispel concern for malignancy.

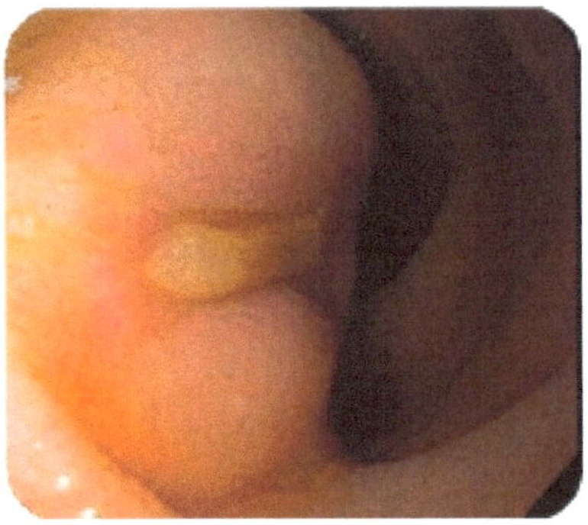

Figure 6. Jejunal inflammatory fibroid polyp.

Histology of IFPs demonstrates a proliferation of fibroid connective tissue with spindle cells and inflammatory cell infiltration. Prominent eosinophilia is common but is not required for diagnosis. Perivascular onion concentric fibroblastic proliferation (onion skinning) may be found in the majority of cases.[22-24] IFPs generally stain positive for CD34 and negative for CD117/kit antigen.[22,23]

Sporadic Epithelial Polyps

Subcentimeter adenomas are typically found in the duodenum but can develop in the deep small bowel. Analogous to adenomatous polyps of the colon, small bowel adenomas may evolve into adenocarcinoma. Adenomas greater than 26 mm in size have an increased risk of progression to malignancy.[30,31] Non-ampullary duodenal adenomas are subclassified as intestinal-type and gastric-type according to their histologic phenotype. While little is known regarding the molecular features of jejunal or ileal adenomas, the most frequent genetic alterations of intestinal-type NADAs involve *APC* and *KRAS* genes, as observed with colorectal adenomas.[32] Small bowel adenomas may be endoscopically removable by endoscopic mucosal resection or may require surgery.[30]

Hyperplastic polyps may occasionally be found by VCE and are often associated with ectopic gastric tissue (**Figure 7**). Sporadic hamartomas may occur in the small bowel as solitary lesions rather than related to a polyposis syndrome. Hyperplastic polyps and hamartomas of the small bowel may be removed endoscopically, precluding the need for surgery.[30-32] Lastly, granulomas may extend through the small bowel mucosa to mimic epithelial polyps (**Figure 8**). Polypoid granulomas may also be removed

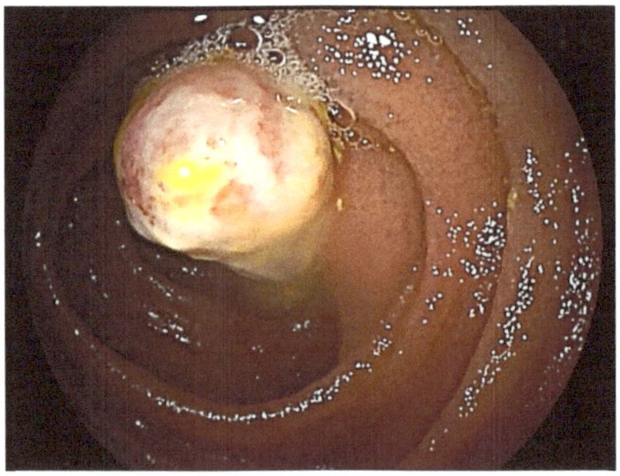

Figure 7. Hyperplastic polyp with ulceration.

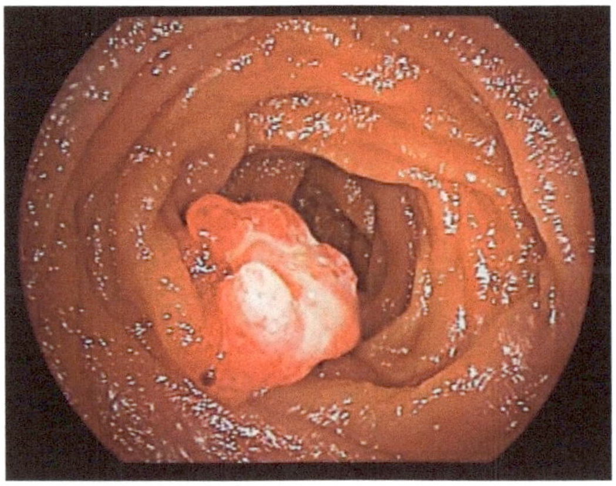

Figure 8. Granuloma.

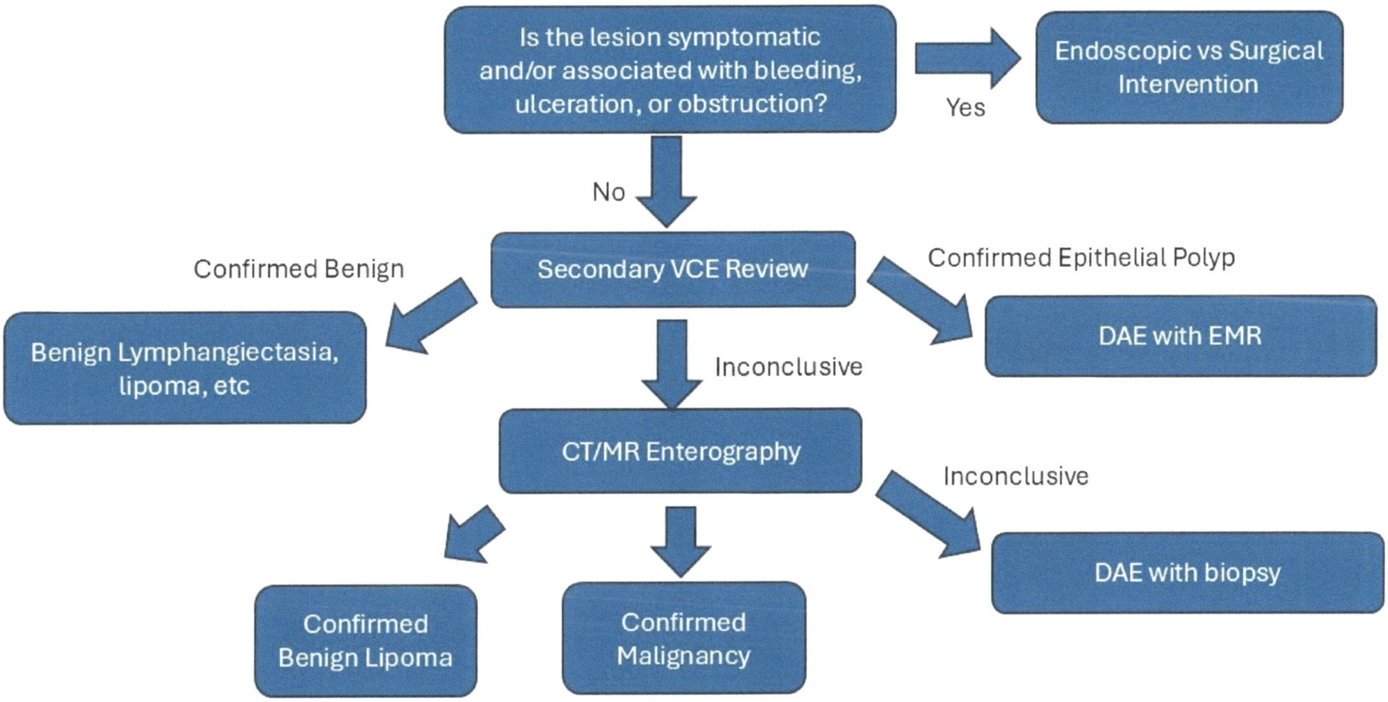

Figure 9. Management of Indeterminate SB Lesions. CT, computed tomography; DAE, device-assisted enteroscopy EMR, endoscopic mucosal resection; MR, magnetic resonance; VCE, video capsule endoscopy.

endoscopically but are likely to recur unless the underlying inflammatory condition is resolved.

Management of Benign Lesions

Small bowel lesions found by VCE may be managed conservatively if asymptomatic and confidently diagnosed as benign. Lesions complicated by ulceration or bleeding should be treated through surgery or DAE. Benign lesions may be diagnosed through consultation with a second capsule reader. If this review is inconclusive, CT/MR enterography is capable of confidently diagnosing small bowel lipomas as well as malignancy. Lesions which cannot be diagnosed may require direct inspection by DAE with biopsy and/or surgical resection to exclude a malignant process (**Figure 9**).

References

1. Alqahtani A, Nguyen LT, Flageole H, Shaw K, Laberge JM. 25 years' experience with lymphangiomas in children. J Pediatr Surg. 1999;34(7):1164-8.
2. Hanagiri T, Baba M, Shimabukuro T, et al. Lymphangioma in the small intestine: Report of a case and review of the Japanese literature. Surg Today. 1992;22(4):363-7.
3. Gaudier H, Gorse P. [Abdomino-scrotal retroperitoneal cystic lymphangioma]. Presse Méd 1913;22:458-89.
4. Khan K, Kleess L, Ganga R, DePaz H, Santopietro R. Small bowel lymphangioma causing ileo-ileal intussusception in adults. Int J Surg Case Rep. 2017;41:469–72.
5. Bellutti M, Mönkemüller K, Fry LC, Dombrowski F, Malfertheiner P. Characterization of yellow plaques found in the small bowel during double-balloon enteroscopy. Endoscopy. 2007;39(12):1059-63.
6. Chen CP, Chao Y, Li CP, Lo WC, Wu CW, Tsay SH, Lee RC, Chang FY. Surgical resection of duodenal lymphangiectasia: a case report. World J Gastroenterol. 2003;9(12):2880-2.
7. Mishkin D. Normal variants. In: de Rranchis R, Lewis BS, Mishkin DS, eds. Capsule Endoscopy Simplified. Thorofare, NJ: Slack Inc; 2010:43-59.
8. Taylor AJ, Stewart ET, Dodds WJ. Gastrointestinal lipomas: a radiologic and pathologic review. AJR Am J Roentgenol. 1990;155(6):1205-10.
9. Kakitsubata Y, Kakitsubata S, Nagatomo H, Mitsuo H, Yamada H, Watanabe K. CT manifestations of lipomas of the small intestine and colon. Clin Imaging. 1993;17(3):179-82.
10. Thompson WM. Imaging and findings of lipomas of the gastrointestinal tract. AJR Am J Roentgenol. 2005;184(4):1163-71.
11. Paksoy M, Böler DE, Baca B, et al. Laparoscopic transgastric resection of a gastric lipoma presenting as acute gastrointestinal hemorrhage. Surg Laparosc

Endosc Percutan Tech. 2005;15(3):163-5.
12. Slavin JD Jr, Islam QT, Spencer RP, Martinez H. Jejunal lipoma as a source of gastrointestinal bleeding. Clin Nucl Med. 2000;25(11):946.
13. Zissin R. Enteroenteric intussusception secondary to a lipoma: CT diagnosis. Emerg Radiol. 2004;11(2):107-9.
14. Aydin HN, Bertin P, Singh K, Arregui M. Safe techniques for endoscopic resection of gastrointestinal lipomas. Surg Laparosc Endosc Percutan Tech. 2011;21(4):218-22.
15. Shinsaku F, Ryo Y, Tatsuya M, et al. Gastric lipoma successfully treated by endoscopic unroofing. Digestive Endoscopy. 2003; 1527:228-231.
16. Hizawa K, Kawasaki M, Kouzuki T, Aoyagi K, Fujishima M. Unroofing technique for the endoscopic resection of a large duodenal lipoma. Gastrointest Endosc. 1999;49:391-2.
17. Vanek J. Gastrointestinal submucosal granuloma with eosinophilic infiltration. Am J Pathol. 1949; 33:397-411.
18. Helwig EB, Ranier A. Inflammatory fibroid polyps of the stomach. Surg Gynecol Obstet. 1953; 96:355-367.
19. Johnstone JM, Morson BC. Inflammatory fibroid polyp of the gastrointestinal tract. Histopathology. 1978; 34:349-361.
20. Wille P, Borchard F. Fibroid polyps of intestinal tract are inflammatory-reactive proliferations of CD34-positive perivascular cells. Histopathology. 1998 Jun;32(6):498-502.
21. Daum 0, Hes 0, Vanecek T et al. Vanek's tumor (inflammatory fibroid polyp). Report of 36 cases and comparison with three cases of the original Vanek's series. Ann Diagn Pathol. 2003;15:337-347.
22. Lasota J, Wang ZF, Sobin LH, et al. Mutations, earlier reported in gastrointestinal stromal tumors, are common in small intestinal inflammatory fibroid polyps. A study of 60 cases. Mod Pathol. 2009;28:1049–1056.
23. Huss S, Wardelmann E, Goltz D, et al. Activating PDGFRA mutations in inflammatory fibroid polyps occur in exons 25, 37 and 36and are associated with tumour localization. Histopathology. 2012;61:59-68.
24. Liu TC, Lin MT, Montgomery EA, Singhi AD. Inflammatory fibroid polyps of the gastrointestinal tract: spectrum of clinical, morphologic, and immunohistochemistry features. Am J Surg Pathol. 2013;37(4):586-92.
25. Mohamud SO, Motorwala SA, Daniel AR, Tworek JA, Shehab TM. Giant ileal inflammatory fibroid polyp causing small bowel obstruction: a case report and review of the literature. Cases J. 2008;1(1):341.
26. O'Kane AM, O'Donnell ME, McCavert M, Taylor K, Lee J, Wilkinson AJ. Inflammatory fibroid polyp of the ileum causing recurrent intussusception and chronic ischaemia: a case report. Cases J. 2008;1(1):244.
27. Matsushita M, Hajiro K, Okazaki K, Takakuwa H. Gastric inflammatory fibroid polyps: endoscopic ultrasonographic analysis in comparison with the histology. Gastrointest Endosc. 1997;46(1):53-7.
28. Wolff JH, Twaddell WS, Darwin PE. Endoscopic resection of an ileal inflammatory fibroid polyp using retrograde single-balloon enteroscopy. Clin Gastroenterol Hepatol. 2009;7(11):e66-7.
29. Kim SG, Choi KD, Kim JS, Jung HC, Song IS. Ileal inflammatory fibroid polyp: a rare cause of obscure gastrointestinal bleeding diagnosed by wireless capsule endoscopy. Dig Dis Sci. 2006;51(5):906-8.
30. de Latour RA, Kilaru SM, Gross SA. Management of small bowel polyps: A literature review. Best Pract Res Clin Gastroenterol. 2017;31(4):401-408.
31. Saurin JC, Benech N, Pioche M. Management of small bowel polyps: from small to big. Curr Opin Gastroenterol. 2019;35(3):250-256.
32. Vanoli A, Grillo F, Furlan D, Arpa G, Grami O, Guerini C, Riboni R, Mastracci L, Di Sabatino A. Small Bowel Epithelial Precursor Lesions: A Focus on Molecular Alterations. Int J Mol Sci. 2021;22(9):4388.

Case Study Number 15

Presented by Stephany Nguyen, MD and Daniel Raines, MD, FACG

Pre-capsule Findings (included in capsule study)

A 51-year-old man with a past medical history significant for hypertension, type II diabetes, coronary artery disease, and renal cell carcinoma is referred by his oncologist for further evaluation of an abnormal imaging finding within the small bowel. The patient has been routinely surveilled by oncology for evidence of disease activity following radical nephrectomy for clear cell renal cell carcinoma 4 years ago.

On most recent imaging, a focal area of abnormal metabolic activity was identified in the distal ileum by fused positron emission tomography-computed tomography (PET-CT) scan. The patient currently denies gastrointestinal symptoms, including abdominal pain, altered bowel habits, or unintentional weight loss. A screening colonoscopy performed 6 months ago was normal. On physical examination, the only notable finding is a posterior surgical scar consistent with prior nephrectomy.

A capsule endoscopy study is performed for further evaluation of an abnormality of the distal ileum observed by PET-CT . Review the capsule endoscopy study and report your findings, including: gastric passage time, small bowel passage time, and observed abnormalities. Be prepared to discuss your findings and management plan with your staff prior to reviewing the diagnosis and case discussion.

Capsule Endoscopy Findings
First Gastric Image = 0hr 0min 54sec
First Duodenal Image = 0hr 11min 39sec
Gastric passage time = 11min
First Cecal Image = 2hr 11min 32sec
Small bowel passage time = 2hr 0mm

Figure 1

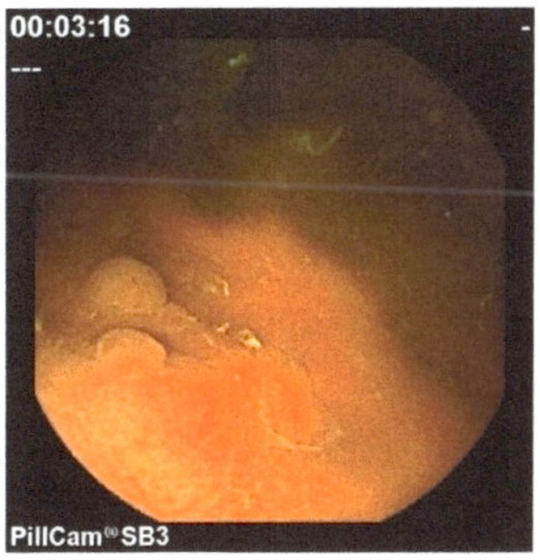

Figure 2

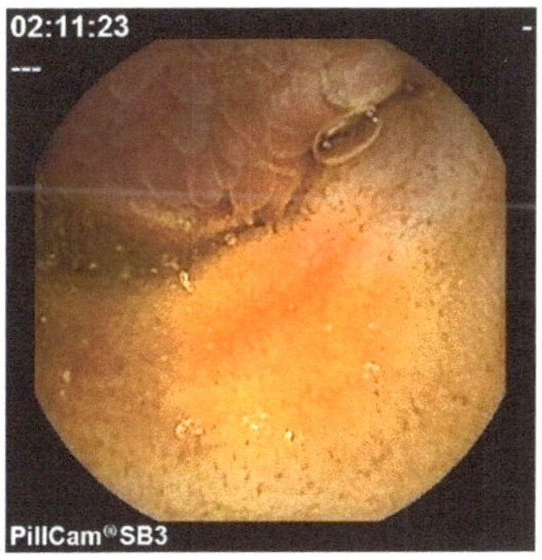

Figure 3

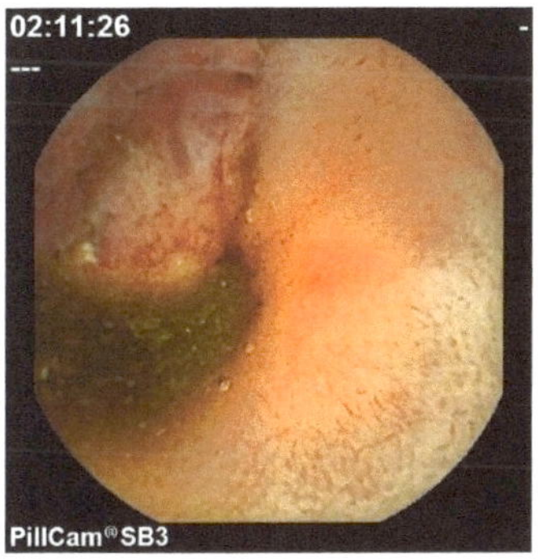

Several small (<1 cm) polyps are observed in the gastric body and are consistent with benign fundic gland polyps (**Figure 1:** 0hr 3min 16sec). Capsule transit through the stomach, duodenum, and jejunum is otherwise unremarkable. Prior to capsule entry into the cecum, a polypoid lesion of the terminal ileum is observed. This lesion is associated with surface ulceration and a frond-like villous architecture (**Figure 2**: 2hr 11min 23sec ; **Figure 3:** 2hr 11min 26sec).

Follow-up

A retrograde double balloon endoscopy was performed to further evaluate the abnormalities identified on PET-CT (**Figure 4**) and VCE. This examination confirmed the presence of an ulcerated polypoid lesion in the terminal ileum with bleeding (**Figure 5**). To achieve hemostasis and obtain tissue for histologic evaluation, this lesion was partially resected by hot snare after submucosal injection with saline. Pathology of the resected specimen was consistent with metastatic clear cell renal cell carcinoma.

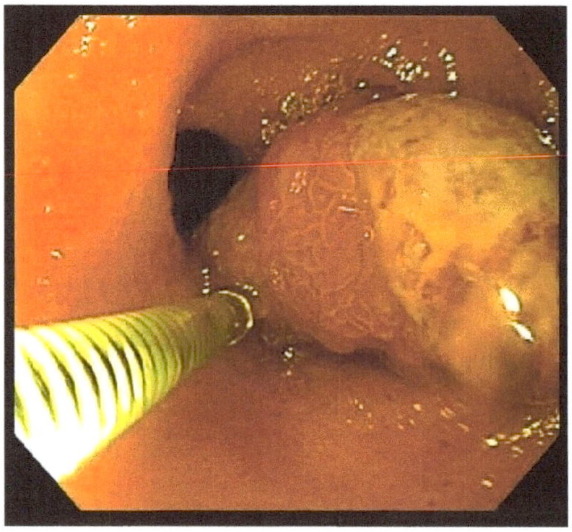

Figure 4

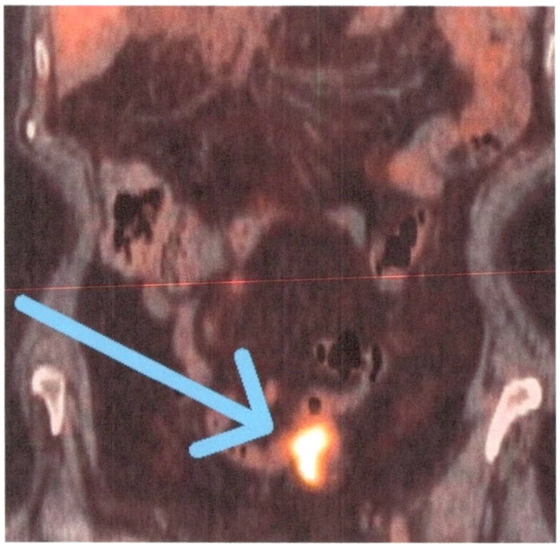

Figure 5

Chapter 15: Metastatic Small Bowel Malignancy

Stephany Nguyen, MD and Daniel Raines, MD, FACG

Introduction

Metastatic small bowel malignancy is more common than the 4 primary small bowel tumors, adenocarcinoma, gastrointestinal stromal tumor, neuroendocrine tumor, and lymphoma.[1] Routes of metastasis to the small bowel include hematogenous spread, intraperitoneal seeding, direct extension, and lymphogenous spread.[2,3] Metastatic disease of the small bowel commonly presents with overt or occult gastrointestinal bleeding as an indication for video capsule endoscopy (VCE). Evaluation by VCE or device assisted endoscopy (DAE) may also be indicated for evaluation of suspected small bowel metastases identified by imaging.

Epidemiology

Melanoma accounts for the majority (50%-70%) of cases of metastatic small bowel malignancy.[1] This malignancy has a predilection for metastasis to the gastrointestinal tract as melanoma expresses chemokine receptor CCR9. This receptor promotes migration to CCR9 ligands, which are highly expressed in the small bowel.[4,5] Up to 60% of patients diagnosed with advanced melanoma have small bowel metastasis on autopsy although only 10% are diagnosed premortem[1] (**Figure 1**).

Hematogenous spread to the small bowel occurs in other common malignancies, including breast cancer, lung cancer, and renal cell cancer. Breast cancer is the most common malignancy and second highest cause of cancer-related death amongst women in the United States. It is estimated that 28% to 50% of breast cancers metastasize to the small bowel (**Figure 2**).[6] Lung cancer is the second most common cancer amongst men and women in the United States and is the leading cause of cancer-related deaths. The reported incidence of small bowel metastasis from lung cancer is approximately 0.2% to 2% (**Figure 3**).[7] Renal cell carcinoma is the third most common genitourinary cancer with a rate of small bowel metastasis ranging from 1% to 15%.[8,9]

Other mechanisms of small bowel metastasis are intraperitoneal seeding, direct extension, and lymphogenous spread.[2,3] Colon and ovarian cancers are the most common types of cancer to spread to the small bowel via intraperitoneal seeding.[2] Metastasis by direct extension can occur from pancreatic, biliary, or colon cancers.[2] Testicular cancer can metastasize to the small bowel via the lymphatic system in rare (1.4%) of cases.[3] Esophageal cancer has been reported to metastasize to the small bowel; however, it is unknown whether the mechanism is due to hematogenous or lymphogenous spread.[10]

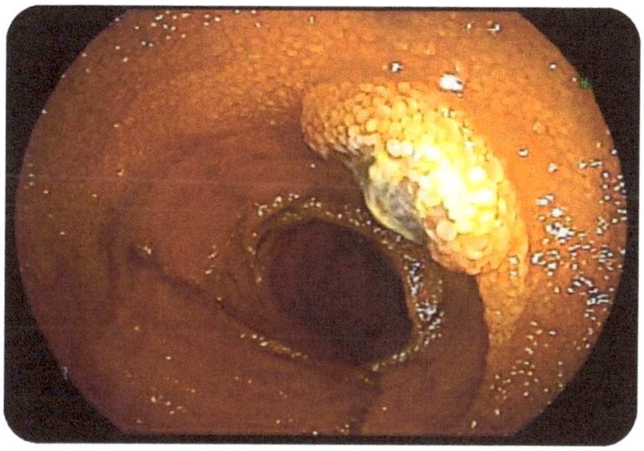

Figure 1. Metastatic melanoma of the jejunum.

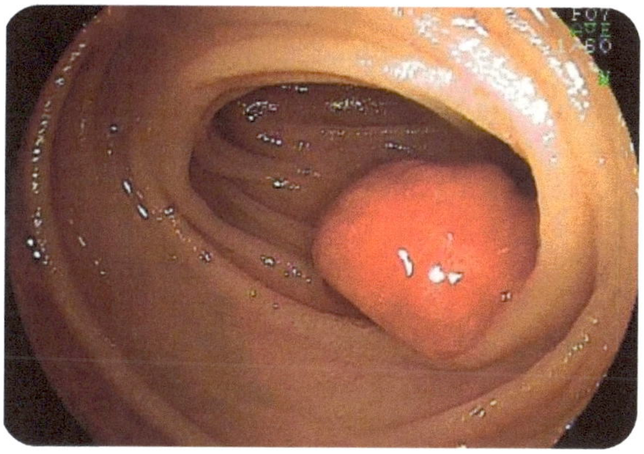

Figure 2. Breast cancer metastasis to the ileum.

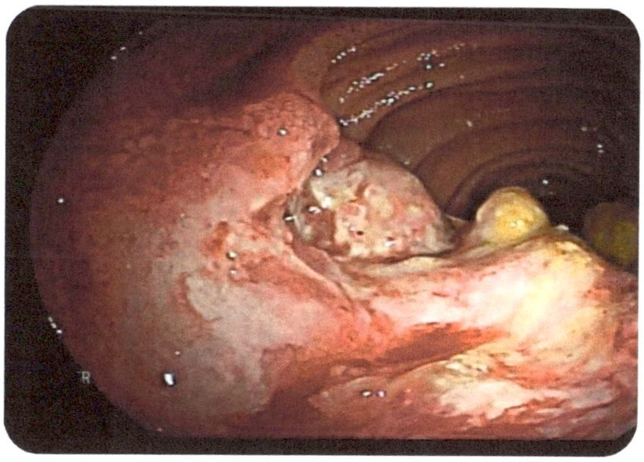

Figure 3. Jejunal metastatic adenocarcinoma of the lung.

Chapter 15: Metastatic Small Bowel Malignancy

Clinical Features

Metastatic disease of the small bowel may remain asymptomatic or present with a variety of complications, such as gastrointestinal bleeding, obstruction, intussusception, or perforation. The most common presenting symptom is chronic gastrointestinal blood loss.[1,3,9,11] The pattern of bleeding in these cases is commonly occult with slow or intermittent bleeding resulting in progressive anemia with iron deficiency. In rare cases, small bowel metastases may result in acute presentation with bowel perforation. Asymptomatic tumors are often detected by surveillance imaging performed by oncology. Endoscopic examination of the small bowel may be requested in these cases to confirm or exclude malignancy.

Diagnosis

VCE is recommended as a primary means to evaluate for suspected small bowel bleeding, including gastrointestinal bleeding due to malignant disease.[12] Small bowel metastases observed by VCE may be characterized as exophytic mass lesions associated with ulceration and/or bleeding.[13,14] Metastatic melanoma which invades the small bowel mucosa may be distinctive in color as "coal-black", often with a peripheral ring of white-tipped villi (**Figure 4**).[15]

Cross sectional imaging by computed tomography enterography and magnetic resonance enterography may identify metastatic lesions of the small bowel as single or multiple polypoid masses.[16] Focal wall thickening of the small bowel may also be present.[16] Fused PET-CT is highly sensitive for metastatic malignancy, including metastatic small bowel disease. However, this imaging study cannot always differentiate hypermetabolic activity related to malignancy, inflammation, or artifact. Abnormalities observed by imaging often require subsequent endoscopic evaluation by VCE and/or DAE.

Management

Management options of small bowel metastases include resection, chemotherapy, radiation therapy, and/or palliative care. The choice of management depends on cancer type and extent of metastasis. Surgical resection can be performed for focal metastatic lesions.[17] Endoscopic resection of hemorrhagic lesions by DAE has also been reported as a palliative measure (**Figure 5a, b**).[12] Chemotherapy and radiation therapy are effective for treatment of metastatic disease due breast cancer, lung cancer, renal cell cancer, and testicular cancer.[6,11,17,18,19,20] Immunotherapy may be considered in patients with metastatic melanoma, breast cancer, and renal cell cancer.[6,17,19,21]

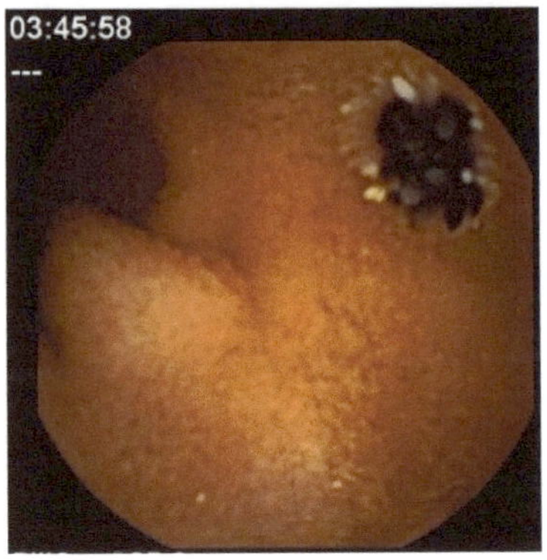

Figure 4. Metastatic melanoma identified by video capsule endoscopy.

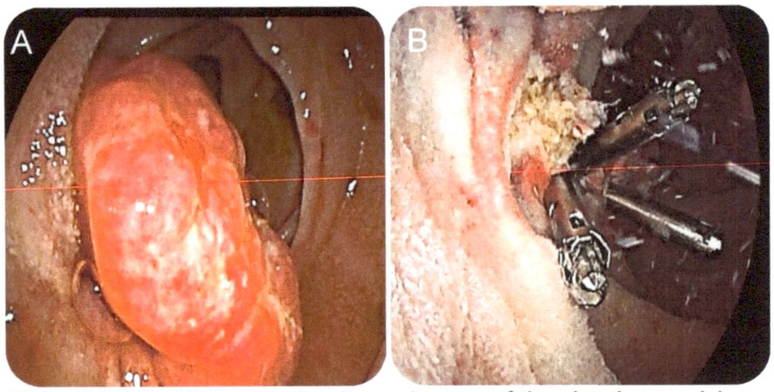

Figure 5. Metastatic renal cell carcinoma of the duodenum (a) treated by endoscopic mucosal resection (b) .

Conclusion

Malignancies which are prevalent in the U.S. often metastasize to the small bowel, including melanoma, breast cancer, lung cancer, and renal cell cancer. Colonic and ovarian malignancies may also metastasize to the small bowel through direct extension, intraperitoneal seeding, or lymphogenous spread.[2,3] Symptomatic metastases of the small bowel typically present with gastrointestinal bleeding, while asymptomatic lesions may be identified by cross sectional imaging. Endoscopic evaluation of the small bowel by VCE and/or DAE may be diagnostic in these cases. Focal lesions may be considered for surgical or endoscopic resection. Chemotherapy, immunotherapy, and/or radiation therapy may be effective in suppressing tumor growth.

References

1. Zoumpos A, Ho NAH, Loeschhorn-Becker R, Schuppert F. Haemorrhagic small bowel melanoma metastasis: a clinical rarity. BMJ Case Rep. 2019 11;12(9):e230454.
2. Sailer J, Zacherl J, Schima W. MDCT of small bowel tumours. Cancer Imaging. 2007;7(1):224-33.
3. Dassouli C, El Manjra C, Errami AA, Oubaha S, Samlani Z, Krati K. Small bowel metastases from a testicular choriocarcinoma revealed by gastrointestinal bleeding: a case report. Pan Afr Med J. 2021;39:259.
4. Chipuc S, Bacalbasa N, Rodica A, Toma L, Iliescu L, Baciu C, Zgura A. Beyond the surface: A Case report of a patient with small bowel metastasis and melanoma history. Diagnosis and Management. Chirurgia (Bucur). 2024;119(eCollection):1.
5. Serrao EM, Costa AM, Ferreira S, et al. The different faces of metastatic melanoma in the gastrointestinal tract. Insights Imaging. 2022;13(1):161.
6. Saied A, Bhati C, Sharma R, Garrean S, Salti G. Small bowel obstruction from breast cancer metastasis: a case report and review of the literature. Breast Dis. 2011;33(4):183-8.
7. Alhusari L, Abdallah M, Al-Madani A, Nwanwene K, Lawrence LM, Pacioles T. A rare presentation of small bowel perforation secondary to microscopic metastasis of non-small cell lung cancer (NSCLC): A Case Report. Cureus. 2023;15(12):e50383.
8. Bellio G, Cipolat Mis T, Kaso G, Dattola R, Casagranda B, Bortul M. Small bowel intussusception from renal cell carcinoma metastasis: a case report and review of the literature. J Med Case Rep. 2016;10(1):222.
9. Vashi PG, Abboud E, Gupta D. Renal cell carcinoma with unusual metastasis to the small intestine manifesting as extensive polyposis: successful management with intraoperative therapeutic endoscopy. Case Rep Gastroenterol. 2011;5(2):471-8.
10. Ono R, Ogino H, Kawachi J, et al. Small intestinal metastases from esophageal carcinoma presenting as a perforation: A case report and review of the literature. Int J Surg Case Rep. 2018;48:104-108.
11. Gonzalez JJ, Wahab A, Gonzalez E, Udager AM, Reichert ZR. Upper gastrointestinal bleeding due to a duodenal metastasis from primary testicular squamous cell carcinoma. Am J Case Rep. 2020;21:e922007.
12. Vlachou E, Koffas A, Toumpanakis C, Keuchel M. Updates in the diagnosis and management of small-bowel tumors. Best Pract Res Clin Gastroenterol. 2023;64-65:101860.
13. Zhong Y, Tang X, Deng B. Capsule endoscopy-based diagnosis of lung squamous cell carcinoma associated with abdominal pain and metastasis to small intestine: A case report. Case Rep Oncol. 2023;16(1):102-108.
14. Cohen DL. Small bowel metastasis from renal cell carcinoma identified on capsule endoscopy. ACG Case Rep J. 2013;1(1):3.
15. Todeschini A, Loconte I, Contaldo A, Ierardi E, Di Leo A, Principi M. Small bowel metastatic melanoma: an emblematic “coal-black” appearance at videocapsule endoscopy. Medicina (Kaunas). 2021;57(12):1313.
16. Jasti R, Carucci LR. Small bowel neoplasms: A pictorial review. Radiographics. 2020;40(4):1020-1038.
17. Huang D, Lynch C, Serra LM, et al. Primary site stereotactic ablative body radiotherapy in localized, recurrent, and metastatic renal cell carcinoma. Clin Transl Radiat Oncol. 2024;49:100879.
18. Kosciuszek ND, Noel P, Takabe K, et al. Intraluminal small bowel metastasis from primary lung cancer. World J Oncol. 2022;13(6):409-416.
19. Todorovic Đ, Stojanovic B, Filip M, et al. Small bowel perforation due to renal carcinoma metastasis: A comprehensive case study and literature review. Diagnostics (Basel). 2024;14(7):761.
20. Muhanna A, Nimri F, Almomani ZA, Al Momani L, Likhitsup A, Hamid F. Small bowel metastasis as a presentation of testicular seminoma. Cureus. 2021;13(9):e17962.
21. Larkin J, Chiarion-Sileni V, Gonzalez R, et al. Five-year survival with combined nivolumab and ipilimumab in advanced melanoma. N Engl J Med. 2019;381(16):1535-1546.

Case Study Number 16

Presented by Autumn Collins, MD and John J. Hutchings, MD, FACG

Pre-capsule Findings (included in capsule study)

A 26-year-old woman with a history of recurrent, acute pancreatitis is admitted for observation due to symptoms of intractable nausea, vomiting, and abdominal pain. Her symptoms developed over a course of several hours and have persisted for 2 days. She describes her pain as constant in nature and localized to the epigastric region. Her abdomen is somewhat tender to palpation without rebound or involuntary guarding. Initial lab results are remarkable for a serum lipase level of 467 u/L (normal = 10 - 63 u/L). During routine CT imaging of the abdomen, an abnormal segment of small bowel with circumferential thickening is identified. The radiologist interprets this abnormality is concerning for a new diagnosis of small bowel adenocarcinoma.

A capsule endoscopy study is performed for further evaluation of this imaging abnormality. Review the capsule endoscopy study and report your findings, including: gastric passage time, small bowel passage time, and observed abnormalities. Be prepared to discuss your findings and management plan with your staff prior to reviewing the diagnosis and case discussion.

An area of capsule hold up is observed in the jejunum (likely mid-jejunum). Capsule transit is delayed within a segment of small bowel characterized by gross mucosal edema associated with discoloration. Several folds appear as potential submucosal vascular structures or "venous blebs" (**Figure 1:** 1hr 53min 31sec; **Figure 2:** 1hr 53min 36sec).

Follow-up

Capsule Endoscopy Findings
First Gastric Image = 0h 0min 20sec
First Duodenal Image = 1h 27min 25sec
Gastric passage time = 1h 27min
First Cecal Image = 4h 47min 2sec
Small bowel passage time = 3hr 20min

Figure 1

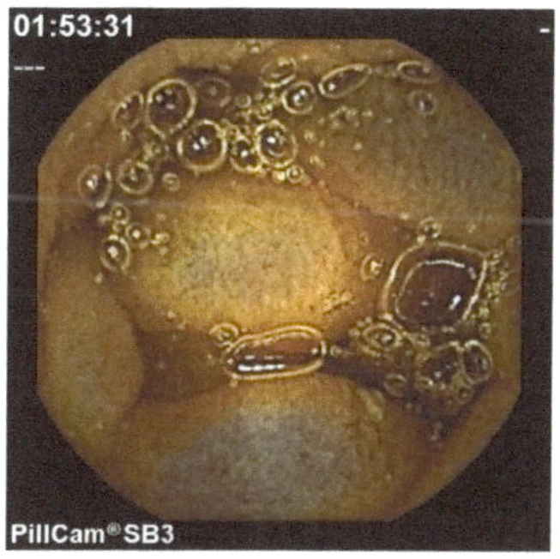

Figure 2

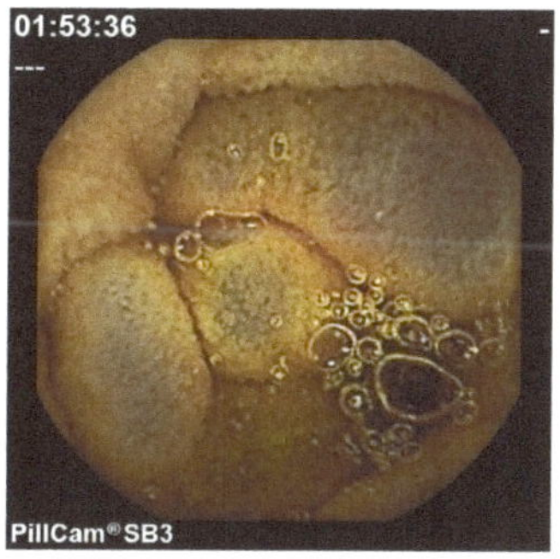

Review of the patient's CT images with radiology highlighted a focal area of bowel wall thickening accompanied by adjacent inflammatory change (**Figure 3**). An anterograde single-balloon enteroscopy identified a short (5 cm) segment of marked edema in the mid-jejunum (**Figure 4**). The proximal and distal margins of the abnormal segment were tattooed with India Ink. Mucosal biopsies are obtained but fail to reveal a specific pathology. Due to concern for an intramural malignancy and lack of improvement in the patient's ability to tolerate oral intake, laparoscopic resection of the abnormal segment of bowel is performed. A diagnosis of heterotopic pancreas complicated by inflammation (heterotopic pancreatitis) is made by pathology (**Figure 5**).

Figure 3

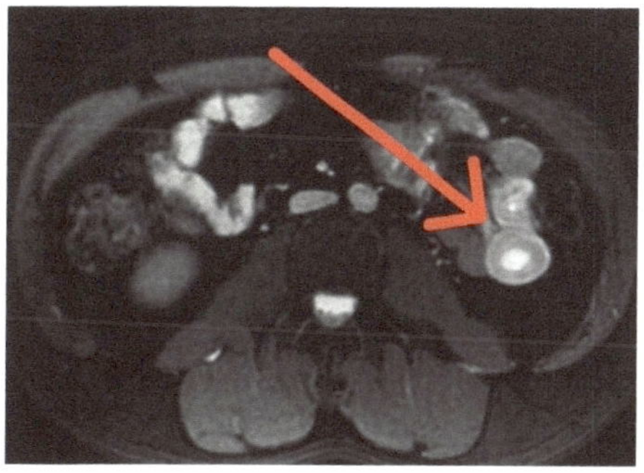

Figure 4

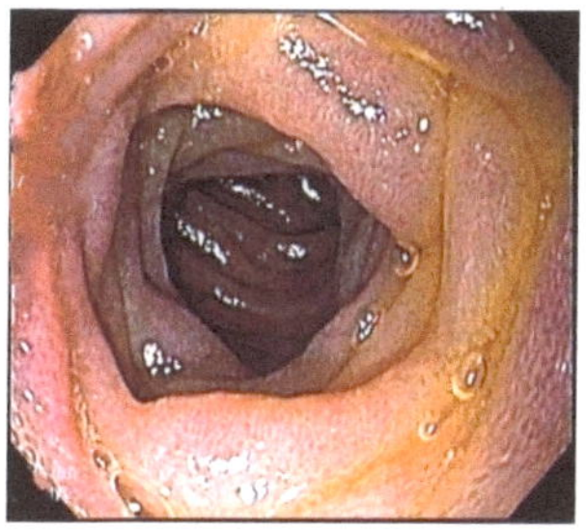

Figure 5

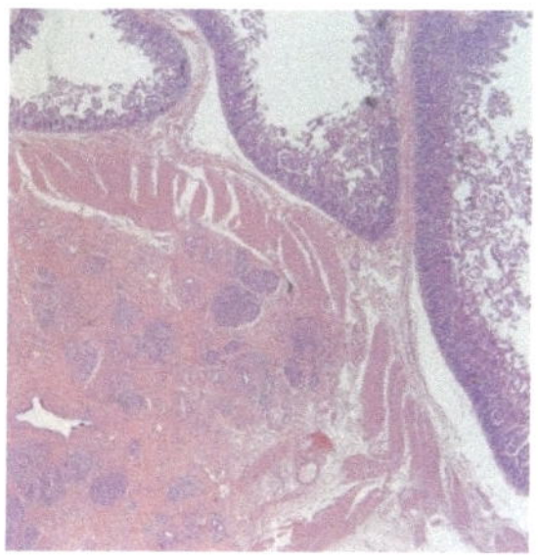

Chapter 16: Heterotopic Pancreas

Autumn Collins, MD and John J. Hutchings, MD, FACG

Introduction

Heterotopic pancreas (HP) is a congenital anomaly in which pancreatic tissue exists outside its normal anatomical location and lacks continuity with the main pancreatic gland. The true incidence is unknown as most cases are asymptomatic, but autopsy results indicate a prevalence of 0.5% to 13.7%.[1] HP is twice as common in males and typically is not discovered until the fifth or sixth decade of life.[2] It most frequently occurs in the submucosa of the gastric antrum (30%) and proximal portion of the duodenum (30%) in close proximity to the main pancreas.[3] HP has been reported in other locations such as the esophagus, gallbladder, Meckel's diverticulum, biliary tree, mesentery, and spleen.[1]

HP is an entity not uncommonly encountered in gastroenterology practice. Awareness of this condition should prevent overtreatment of asymptomatic cases and allow for consideration of HP in the differential diagnosis of recurrent pancreatitis, focal small bowel inflammation, or small bowel mass. This chapter will discuss the pathogenesis, clinical manifestations, diagnosis, and management of HP.

Pathophysiology

Two main theories have been proposed to explain the embryologic development of HP: the migration theory and the metaplasia theory.[4] The migration theory posits that during embryogenesis, as dorsal and ventral pancreatic buds arise from the foregut endoderm and undergo rotation and fusion, small clusters of pancreatic progenitor cells may fail to integrate with the main pancreatic gland. These displaced cells are embedded in the developing wall of the stomach, duodenum, or other foregut-derived structures as ectopic pancreatic tissue.[1] The end result is differentiation of local endodermal cells into pancreatic tissue at ectopic sites (**Figure 1**).[4,5,6]

The metaplasia theory suggests that endodermal cells in the gastrointestinal tract retain the potential to differentiate into pancreatic tissue under certain molecular conditions. Experimental data has shown that the loss of regulatory factors such as Hes1 and GATA4 can reprogram local endodermal progenitors toward a pancreatic fate, leading to the formation of pancreatic tissue in abnormal locations.[4,5]

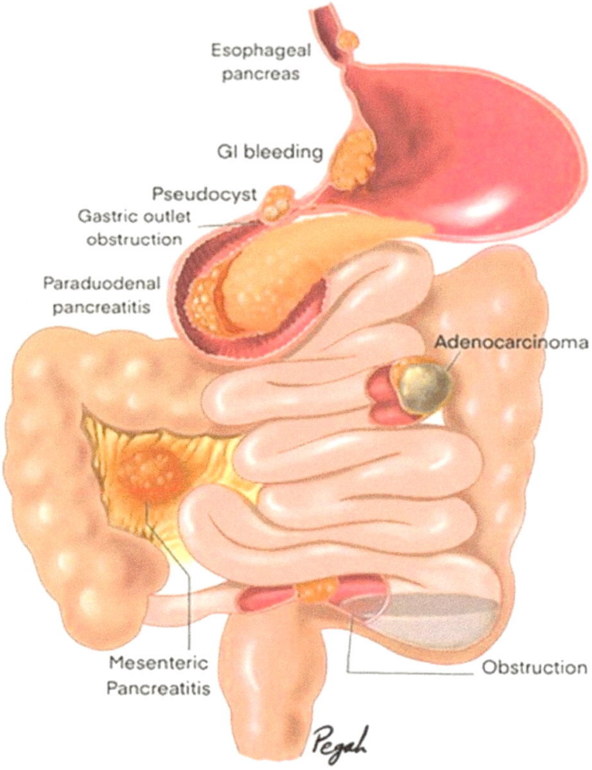

Figure 1. Complications of HP by anatomic location: esophageal pancreatitis, gastric hemorrhage, pseudocyst, gastric outlet obstruction, paraduodenal pancreatitis, adenocarcinoma, mesenteric pancreatitis, and large bowel obstruction. *Adapted from Soheyla.*[7]

Clinical Features

The clinical presentation of HP is highly variable and depends largely on the size and anatomical location of the ectopic tissue. Most cases of HP are asymptomatic and discovered incidentally during imaging, endoscopy, or surgery. However, when symptoms do occur, they typically reflect the local effects of the ectopic tissue.

Pancreatic Rest (Gastric Heterotopic Pancreas)

Pancreatic rest most commonly occurs in the gastric antrum or prepyloric region, typically within the submucosal layer (**Figure 2**). When symptomatic, patients may present with non-specific symptoms such as chronic epigastric pain or dyspepsia while larger lesions can result in gastric outlet obstruction.[8]

Duodenal Heterotopic Pancreas

The duodenum is the second most common site of

HP, with lesions typically located in the submucosa or muscularis propria of the duodenal wall. Symptomatic cases of duodenal HP commonly present with non-specific abdominal pain but may also be complicated by gastrointestinal bleeding or duodenal obstruction. Paraduodenal pancreatitis, characterized by chronic inflammation and cystic changes within the duodenal wall, is a unique complication of duodenal HP (**Figure 3**).[8-10]

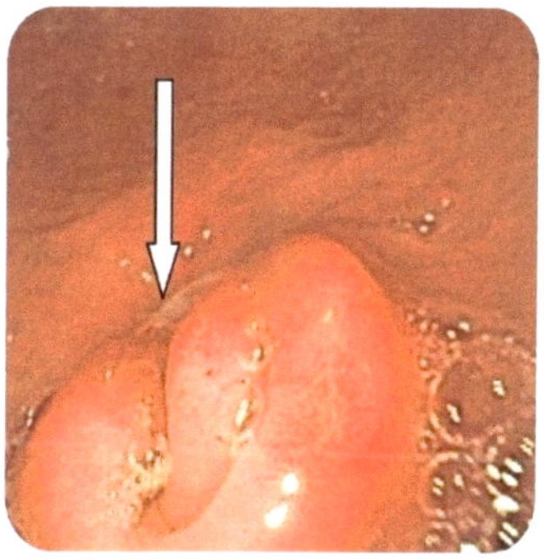

Figure 2: Characteristic appearance of gastric HP (pancreatic rest) of the antrum with central umbilication on upper endoscopy.

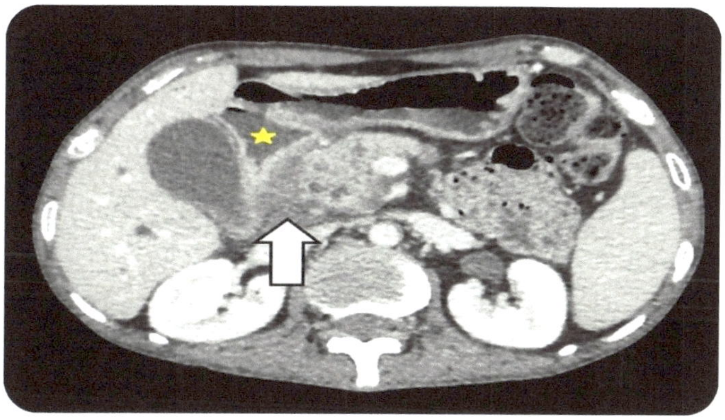

Figure 3. CT image with hypoenhancing soft tissue within the pancreaticoduodenal groove (white arrow) resulting in obstruction of the duodenum with upstream dilatation of the duodenal cap (yellow star). Reprinted from Clinical Radiology, 2014; 69(3), Arora A, et al with permission from Elsevier.[9]

Jejunal Heterotopic Pancreas

Jejunal HP is less common than gastric or duodenal HP, but is more likely to become symptomatic. Symptomatic cases of jejunal HP may be characterized by abdominal pain, vomiting, and abdominal distension due to functional obstruction of the jejunal lumen. Unlike HP in the stomach or duodenum, jejunal lesions are more likely to result in acute complications such as intussusception or perforation.[1,11]

Other Locations of Heterotopic Pancreas

HP has been reported to occur in other foregut-derived structures such as the esophagus, gallbladder, Meckel's diverticulum, biliary tree, mesentery, and spleen. When symptoms do occur, they tend to correlate with the location of the ectopic tissue. However, these symptoms rarely lead directly to a diagnosis; in many cases, HP is discovered incidentally during evaluation for other conditions. Case reports have described esophageal HP presenting with dyspepsia, nausea, and abdominal bloating, while gallbladder HP has been identified following cholecystectomy for presumed biliary colic.[2,12] Pancreatic tissue has been identified in around 6% of all patients with Meckel's diverticulum, often presenting as recurrent hematochezia.[13]

Diagnosis

Diagnosis of HP is based upon clinical presentation, endoscopic findings, imaging studies, and, in certain cases, tissue sampling.[14] Gastric HP, or pancreatic rest, is commonly observed by routine upper endoscopy as a rounded, subepithelial lesion with central umbilication in the gastric antrum (Figure 2). Pancreatic rest may be diagnosed by typical endoscopic features alone, precluding the need for additional studies such as cross sectional imaging or endoscopic ultrasound (EUS).[15] In atypical cases, EUS with fine-needle aspiration (FNA) or endoscopic mucosal resection (EMR) can be used to confirm a diagnosis of HP.[15-17] Surgical intervention is reserved cases in which evaluation by EUS with FNA or EMR are inconclusive or suggestive of malignancy.[1,16]

The role of endoscopy is limited if HP presents in other locations, such as within a Meckel's diverticulum or the biliary tree. Diagnosis of HP in these locations is typically made incidentally during surgery, imaging, or autopsy.[1,18] If HP tissue becomes inflammed (ie heterotopic pancreatitis), elevations in serum amylase and/or lipase may be observed.[19,20] Imaging studies useful in the diagnosis of HP including standard cross sectional imaging (CT/MRI) and/or nuclear medicine studies. Deposits of HP may be identifiable by standard cross sectional imaging, especially if associated with inflammatory changes or fluid collections.[21,22] Actively inflamed heterotopic pancreatic tissue may also be identifiable by 18F-FDG PET/CT.[21]

Histologically, HP differs from the main pancreatic gland by often exhibiting an incomplete or unbalanced representation of ducts, acinar cells, and islet cells. The Gaspar-Fuentes classification categorizes HP into 4 types based on cellular components. Type I consists of typical pancreatic tissue containing acini, ducts, and islets. Type II is composed of pancreatic ducts alone, while Type III contains only acinar cells. Type IV is made up solely of islet cells. While this system is useful for histopathologic confirmation of HP, it does not influence clinical management.[1, 23]

Management

Heterotopic pancreas is most commonly an asymptomatic, incidental finding. Conservative management is appropriate for asymptomatic patients when the diagnosis is established and in the absence of concerning features. It is important to educate patients that HP is a benign condition with a very low risk of malignant transformation or other complications. No specific medical therapy or routine surveillance is required for these patients.[1,16,18]

Surgical or endoscopic resection is indicated in symptomatic cases of HP as well as lesions which are large (>2 cm) or growing rapidly. The choice between endoscopic surgical approaches depends on factors such as lesion size, location, and depth. For small, superficial, and accessible lesions, EMR is preferred, as it is minimally invasive and has a high rate of symptom resolution. In cases of HP associated with complications such as intestinal obstruction, bleeding, or perforation, surgical resection is typically required. Conservative management is not appropriate for symptomatic cases, as symptoms rarely resolve without intervention.[7,24]

Conclusion

Heterotopic pancreas is routinely encountered in gastroenterology practice. Though typically an incidental finding, HP can present with a range of symptoms depending on its location. Diagnosis relies on a combination of clinical suspicion, endoscopy, imaging, and, when needed, histopathology. While the majority of cases require no intervention, symptomatic or suspicious lesions should be resected. Awareness of this entity is important for recognition of benign HP of the gastric antrum (pancreatic rest) and consideration of symptomatic HP as an uncommon cause of complications such as heterotopic pancreatitis, intestinal obstruction, or gastrointestinal bleeding.

References

1. Rezvani M, Menias C, Sandrasegaran K, Olpin JD, Elsayes KM, Shaaban AM. Heterotopic pancreas: Histopathologic features, imaging findings, and complications. Radiographics. 2017 Mar-Apr;37(2):484-499.
2. Shamoon D, Sostre V, Patel V, Volfson A. A Case of Heterotopic Pancreatic Tissue Discovered in the Distal Esophagus. Case Rep Gastrointest Med. 2020;2020:4695184.
3. Borghei P, Sokhandon F, Shirkhoda A, Morgan DE. Anomalies, anatomic variants, and sources of diagnostic pitfalls in pancreatic imaging. Radiology. 2013;266(1):28-36.
4. Fukuda A, Kawaguchi Y, Furuyama K, et al. Ectopic pancreas formation in Hes1 -knockout mice reveals plasticity of endodermal progenitors of the gut, bile duct, and pancreas. J Clin Invest. 2006;116(6):1484-93.
5. Rodríguez-Seguel E, Villamayor L, Arroyo N, De Andrés MP, Real FX, Martín F, Cano DA, Rojas A. Loss of GATA4 causes ectopic pancreas in the stomach. J Pathol. 2020;250(4):362-373.
6. Jørgensen MC, de Lichtenberg KH, Collin CA, et al. Neurog3-dependent pancreas dysgenesis causes ectopic pancreas in Hes1 mutant mice. Development. 2018;145(17):dev163568.
7. Soheyla F. Heterotopic Pancreas [Internet]. Acute and Chronic Pancreatitis [Working Title]. IntechOpen; 2025. Available from: http://dx.doi.org/10.5772/intechopen.1008706
8. LeCompte MT, Mason B, Robbins KJ, et al. Clinical classification of symptomatic heterotopic pancreas of the stomach and duodenum: A case series and systematic literature review. World J Gastroenterol. 2022;28(14):1455-1478.
9. Arora A, Dev A, Mukund A, Patidar Y, Bhatia V, Sarin SK. Paraduodenal pancreatitis. Clin Radiol. 2014;69(3):299-306.
10. Adsay NV, Zamboni G. Paraduodenal pancreatitis: a clinico-pathologically distinct entity unifying "cystic dystrophy of heterotopic pancreas", "para-duodenal wall cyst", and "groove pancreatitis". Semin Diagn Pathol. 2004;21(4):247-54.
11. Chin NH, Wu JM, Chen KC, Lee TH, Lin CK, Chung CS. pancreatic heterotopia in the small bowel: A case report and literature review. Pancreas. 2022;51(6):700-704.
12. Chen N, Gu J. Heterotopic pancreas of the gallbladder: A case report of a rare and commonly incidental finding. Ann Hepatobiliary Pancreat Surg. 2025;29(2):205-208.
13. Chen S, Zhang H, Yu X, Chen Y. Heterotopic pancreas in Meckel's diverticulum in an adult man with lower gastrointestinal bleeding: a case report and literature review. AME Case Rep. 2023;7:19.
14. Kim JY, Lee JM, Kim KW, et al. Ectopic pancreas: CT findings with emphasis on differentiation from

small gastrointestinal stromal tumor and leiomyoma. Radiology. 2009;252(1):92-100.
15. Standards of Practice Committee; Faulx AL, Kothari S, Acosta RD, et al. The role of endoscopy in subepithelial lesions of the GI tract. Gastrointest Endosc. 2017;85(6):1117-1132.
16. Zhang X, Peng L, Wang Z, et al. Extensive heterotopic pancreas in a rare site: A case report and a review of literature. Medicine (Baltimore). 2023;102(9):e32241.
17. Khashab MA, Cummings OW, DeWitt JM. Ligation-assisted endoscopic mucosal resection of gastric heterotopic pancreas. World J Gastroenterol. 2009;15(22):2805-8.
18. Zhang Y, Sun X, Gold JS, Sun Q, Lv Y, Li Q, Huang Q. Heterotopic pancreas: a clinicopathological study of 184 cases from a single high-volume medical center in China. Hum Pathol. 2016;55:135-42.
19. Bush N, Akshintala VS. Interpretation of serum pancreatic enzymes in pancreatic and nonpancreatic conditions. Curr Opin Gastroenterol. 2023;39(5):403-410.
20. Hameed AM, Lam VW, Pleass HC. Significant elevations of serum lipase not caused by pancreatitis: a systematic review. HPB (Oxford). 2015;17(2):99-112.
21. Ruan M, Liu M, Cheng L, Xie W, Chen L. Increased 18F-FDG uptake of heterotopic pancreatitis in the small intestine: A CARE-compliant case report. Medicine (Baltimore). 2016;95(36):e4465.
22. Jacquet-Francillon N, Passot G, Galan A, Tordo J, Dhomps A. Diagnosis of Ectopic Pancreas in Small Intestine With 18F-DOPA PET/CT. Clin Nucl Med. 2021;46(12):e589-e591.
23. hin KM, Tan DMY, Chan NHL, Goh BKP. Successful preoperative diagnosis of heterotopic pancreas in the duodenum. Int J Surg Case Rep. 2019;55:125-128.
24. Rimal D, Thapa SR, Munasinghe N, Chitre VV. Symptomatic gastric heterotopic pancreas: clinical presentation and review of the literature. Int J Surg. 2008;6(6):e52-4.

Case Study Number 17

Presented by Pegah Carroll, MD and Nisha Loganantharaj, MD

Pre-capsule Findings (included in capsule study)

A 28-year-old woman with an established diagnosis of Crohn's disease (CD) presents for monitoring of response to medical therapy. She was initially diagnosed with isolated small bowel CD 6 months ago by video capsule endoscopy (VCE) indicated for symptoms of abdominal pain, chronic diarrhea, and iron deficiency anemia. Following evaluation by standard upper endoscopy and colonoscopy, video capsule endoscopy findings were diagnostic for multiple (3) segments of small bowel disease activity characterized by deep mucosal ulcers and stenosis. These segments of disease activity were localized within the mid small bowel (distal jejunum) and distal small bowel (mid ileum and distal/terminal ileum). A definitive diagnosis of CD was confirmed by tissue biopsy obtained by retrograde device-assisted enteroscopy. This patient reports that her symptoms of abdominal pain and diarrhea have improved by 60% over the past 6 months on infliximab although she remains iron deficient. A repeat VCE study is ordered to evaluate for mucosal healing on infliximab. Prior to VCE, a patency capsule is administered in clinic then identified in the rectum by abdominal X-ray 30hrs after ingestion.

A capsule endoscopy study is performed for surveillance of CD. Review the capsule endoscopy study and report your findings, including: gastric passage time, small bowel passage time, and observed abnormalities. Be prepared to discuss your findings and management plan with your staff prior to reviewing the diagnosis and case discussion.

Capsule Endoscopy Findings
First Gastric Image = 0h 0min 30sec
First Duodenal Image = 0h 8min 54sec
Gastric passage time = 0h 8min
First Cecal Image = 3h 43min 0sec
Small bowel passage time = 3hr 35min

Following entry into the duodenal bulb, several small (<3 mm) apthous ulcers are observed (**Figure 1:** 10min 45sec). Capsule transit through the ileum appears to be delayed with capsule hold up beginning ~2 hours into the study. In the distal ileum, 1 deep ulcer <5 mm in size is encountered (**Figure 2:** 3hr 17min 49sec) within a solitary area of stenosis (**Figure 3:** 3hrs 23min 32sec). The video capsule traverses the stenosis immediately prior to entry into the cecum.

Follow-up

Small bowel disease activity identified by VCE prior to and following treatment with infliximab are compared. These findings provide evidence of a response to medical therapy with only 1 remaining stenosis with ulcer within the terminal ileum. A clinic visit is scheduled to discuss adjustment of medical therapy versus continued monitoring for complete mucosal healing.

Figure 1

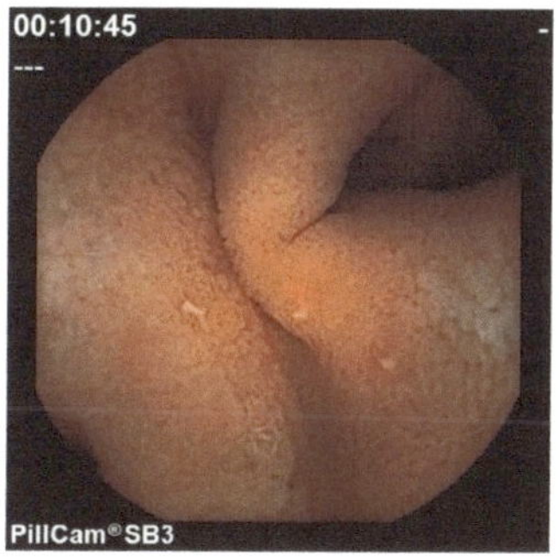

Figure 2

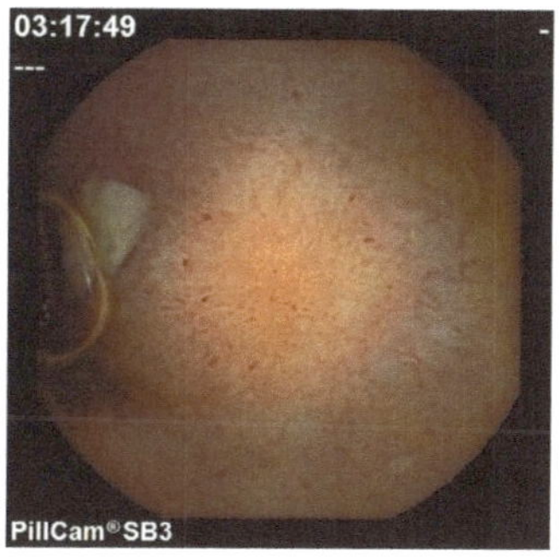

Figure 3

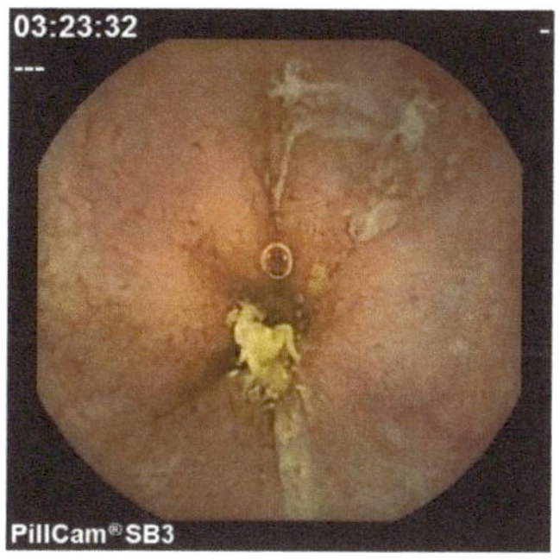

CASE STUDY DISCUSSIONS — CASE NUMBER 17

Chapter 17: Staging & Surveillance of Crohn's Disease

Pegah Carroll, MD and Nisha Loganantharaj, MD

Introduction

Crohn's disease (CD) is a complex and challenging chronic inflammatory disease of the upper and lower gastrointestinal tract with an often-progressive course. Controlling inflammation in Crohn's disease can help prevent progression to complications. It is estimated that over half of all patients with CD will develop penetrating disease complicated by fistulas or strictures.[1] Recent studies have emphasized the importance of staging of CD, including evaluation for small bowel involvement, as well as surveillance to confirm response to therapy with mucosal healing. Current medical evidence supports the use of objective testing in staging and surveillance of CD, including serum C-reactive protein (CRP), fecal calprotectin (FCP), video capsule endoscopy (VCE), CT/MR enterography, and intestinal ultrasound.

The STRIDE II initiative provides management direction for inflammatory bowel disease in the clinical practice setting.[2] The STRIDE II target pathway for active inflammatory bowel disease begins with identifying appropriate therapy based on the patient's individual risk profile. Of foremost importance to patients and clinicians alike is symptomatic response, a short-term target. However, symptomatic response in Crohn's disease doesn't necessarily correlate with healing of mucosal inflammation.[3] The long-term goals of therapy for inflammatory bowel disease, such as improved quality of life and absence of disability, correlate closely with mucosal healing (**Figure 1**).

Staging of Crohn's Disease

Endoscopy is considered the gold standard for the diagnosis of CD and determining disease extent. Ileocolonoscopy is diagnostic for CD in 74%-100% of cases.[5] However, small bowel involvement may remain undetected by standard ileocolonoscopy and upper endoscopy. Video capsule endoscopy is highly sensitive (up to 90%) for small bowel CD with a negative predictive value approaching 100%.[6,7,8,9] The capability of VCE to identify and characterize small bowel disease activity in Crohn's supports the use of capsule endoscopy in staging and surveillance of CD.[10]

Two standardized scoring systems, including the Lewis Score and Capsule Endoscopy Crohn's Disease Activity Index (CECDAI), have been validated for use in quantifying small bowel inflammation observed by VCE.[10] These systems include parameters which predict the likelihood of small bowel CD based upon degree of inflammation. There is data to support that CD is unlikely with a Lewis score <135.[11-13] A Lewis score between 135 and 790 corresponds to mild inflammation while a score >790 corresponds to severe inflammation.[9] For the CECDAI, a score of <3.8 suggests that CD is unlikely while a score of

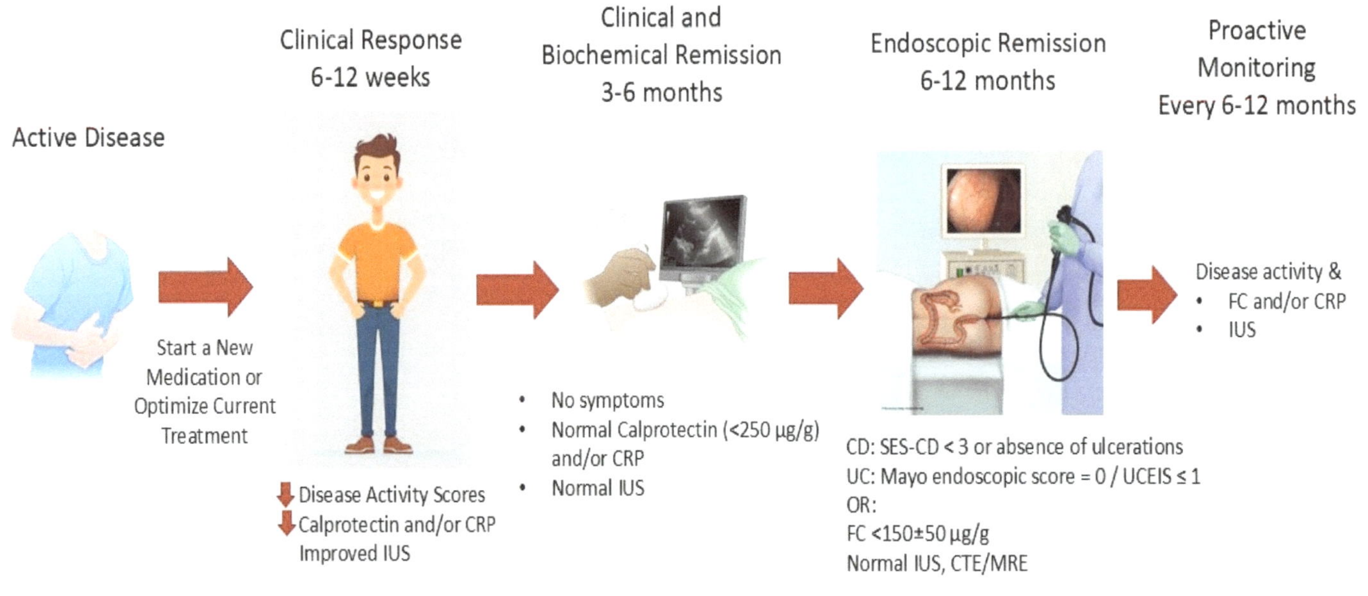

Figure 1. Disease activity monitoring for inflammatory bowel disease. Reprinted from Gaidos et al.[4]

>5.8 indicates severe inflammation.[14] These scoring systems may also be useful for prognosis as well as diagnosis of small bowel CD. Recent research suggests that a Lewis score >350 or a CECDAI score >4 are predictive of an increased risk of disease relapse and/or requirement for therapeutic intervention.[10, 15]

Pillcam™ software provides a convenient means for calculating Lewis score. This calculation divides the small bowel into 3 equal parts, or tertiles, based on time from duodenal image to the first cecal image. Tertile scores are determined based on number, size, and distribution of ulcers, as well as extent of villous edema. These parameters are multiplied to produce a score for each tertile.[16] Stenoses are evaluated independently. The Lewis score is derived by the sum of the worst tertile score and the stenosis score.[9] FCP is considered an accurate reflection of intestinal inflammation and has been shown to correlate more closely to Lewis score as compared to the CECDAI score.[14]

The CECDAI scoring system is similar to the Lewis score. Using this system, the small bowel is divided into 2 segments (proximal and distal). Each segment is assigned a score based upon degree of inflammation, extent of disease, and presence of strictures. The total score for each segment is calculated by multiplying the inflammation score (A) by the extent of disease score (B) followed by the addition of the stricture score (C). The sum of the proximal and distal segment scores equals the total CECDAI score.[16]

Small Bowel CD Surveillance

Symptoms correlate poorly with inflammatory activity in CD. Objective testing is therefore required for effective management.[17] The use of biomarkers allows for serial objective surveillance of Crohn's disease. CALM was the first study to utilize information from biomarker testing in adjusting management of CD to improve outcomes.[18] CRP and FCP are the main inflammatory biomarkers used for monitoring in CD. Improvement in CRP is one of the early treatment targets recommended by the International Organization for the Study of Inflammatory Bowel Disease.[2] Although CRP testing is widely available, it is a marker of systemic inflammation, therefore, not specific for intestinal inflammation.[19] CRP may fail to correlate with intestinal inflammation in some

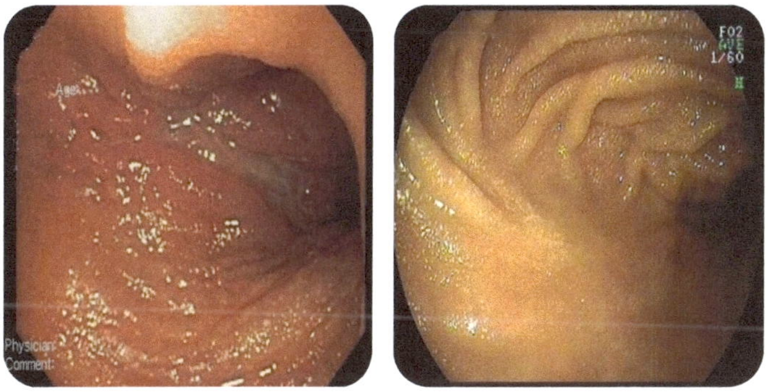

Figure 2. Active Crohn's disease of the jejunum (a) and mucosal healing on infliximab (b).

patients. This is particularly true in patients with small bowel CD.[20,21] One study found that a lower number of patients with ileal disease (43.2%) mounted a CRP as compared to patients with colonic (70%) or ileocolonic disease (72.6%).[22] FCP is a well-established biomarker of inflammation and an intermediate treatment target based on STRIDE II recommendations.[2] Although 2 small studies have shown that FCP can correlate well with capsule endoscopy findings, it should be noted that in one of the studies capsule endoscopy correlation was observed only in those patients with FCP < 100 ug/g and not in those with higher FCP levels.[23,24] Kopylov et al did not find a significant correlation between both CRP and FCP to significant inflammation on capsule endoscopy.[25] The cumulative findings of this research imply that the use of biomarkers alone may be inadequate for monitoring small bowel CD activity.

Imaging studies may be used for luminal evaluation, assessment of disease activity, and response to treatment. Cross sectional imaging is particularly useful for evaluation of stenoses and fistulizing disease. The sensitivity of CTE for Crohn's disease ranges from 74% to 93% with a specificity of 64%-100%. The sensitivity and specificity of MRE for small bowel CD is similar, ranging from 78%-93% and 85%-94% respectively. Intestinal ultrasound has recently been introduced as an tool for detecting small bowel CD. In a study by Wang et al, intestinal ultrasound was 80%-90% sensitive and 93%-98% specific for CD.[26]

While advantageous for evaluation beyond the bowel lumen, imaging is inferior to endoscopy for mild disease.[27] It can be difficult to perform endoscopic surveillance for jejunal and proximal ileal Crohn's disease for confirmation of mucosal healing. VCE serves as a non-invasive method for visualization of the entire small bowel in surveillance of CD. VCE is superior to barium studies and CTE in detecting small bowel disease activity in CD. MRE is comparable to VCE in monitoring small bowel CD but may miss subtle or proximal disease.[25,28] VCE allows for detailed visualization of the small bowel which can in turn influence advanced therapy. In one study, medical treatment was intensified following VCE in 48% of patients with a Lewis score 135-790 and 87% of patients with Lewis Score >790.[25] Mucosal healing is predictor for long term clinical remission based on a meta-analysis[29] (**Figure 2 a,b**). Currently, both the STRIDE II initiative and European Society of Endoscopy (ESGE) guidelines recommend using capsule endoscopy with current validated scores (Lewis or CECDAI score) to not only evaluate the response to medical treatment but also for long-term monitoring of Crohn's disease activity.[2,10]

Postoperative Recurrence

Despite the advancement in medical therapies for Crohn's disease, up to 80% of patients will need surgical intervention at some point in their lifetime.[30,31] Following surgery, biomarkers such as CRP fail to correlate adequately with postoperative recurrence.[32,33] Ileocolonoscopy is standard in detecting post operative recurrence but cannot examine the deep small bowel. VCE can detect lesions in the proximal small bowel and identify subtle inflammatory changes.[34] When comparing capsule endoscopy to ileocolonoscopy, there is moderate to good agreement in detecting lesions in the neo-terminal ileum.

Conclusions

With a growing armamentarium of medical therapies available and emphasis on sustained mucosal healing, endoscopic staging and monitoring are essential in the management of Crohn's disease.[35] In patients with small bowel CD activity, symptoms correlate poorly with disease activity while biomarkers, such as CRP and FCP, may be inaccurate. VCE allows for a non-invasive method for determining the extent and severity of small bowel involvement in CD. This information is crucial to guide treatment decisions and predict disease course.[36]

References

1. Torres J, Mehandru S, Colombel JF, Peyrin-Biroulet L. Crohn's disease. Lancet. 2017;389(10080):1741-1755.
2. Turner D, Ricciuto A, Lewis A, et al. STRIDE-II: An update on the Selecting Therapeutic Targets in Inflammatory Bowel Disease (STRIDE) initiative of the International Organization for the Study of IBD (IOIBD): Determining therapeutic goals for treat-to-target strategies in IBD. Gastroenterology. 2021;160(5):1570-1583.
3. Laterza L, Piscaglia AC, Minordi LM, et al. Multiparametric evaluation predicts different mid-term outcomes in Crohn's disease. Dig Dis. 2018;36(3):184-193.
4. Gaidos JKJ, Hashash JG. Monitoring Inflammatory Bowel Disease Activity: When, How, and Why. Am J Gastroenterol. 2025;120(8):1732-1741.
5. Solem CA, Loftus EV, Jr., Fletcher JG, et al. Small-bowel imaging in Crohn's disease: A prospective, blinded, 4-way comparison trial. Gastrointest Endosc. 2008;68(2):255-66.
6. Dubenco E, Jeejeebhoy KN, Petroniene R, et al. Capsule endoscopy findings in patients with established and suspected small bowel Crohn's disease:correlation with radiologic, endoscopic, and histologic findings. Gastrointest Endosc. 2005;62(4):538-44.
7. Annese V, Daperno M, Rutter MD, et al. European evidence-based consensus for endoscopy in inflammatory bowel disease. J Crohns Colitis. 2013;7(12):982-1018.
8. Tukey M, Pleskow D, Legnani P, Cheifetz AS, Moss AC. The utility of capsule endoscopy in patients with suspected Crohn's disease. Am J Gastroenterol. 2009;104(11):2734-2739.
9. Rosa B, Pinho R, de Ferro SM, et al. Endoscopic scores for evaluation of Crohn's disease activity at small bowel capsule endoscopy: General principles and current applications. GE Port J Gastroenterol. 2015;23(1):36-41.
10. Pennazio M, Rondonotti E, Despott EJ, et al. Small-bowel capsule endoscopy and device-assisted enteroscopy for diagnosis and treatment of small-bowel disorders: European Society of Gastrointestinal Endoscopy (ESGE) Guideline - Update 2022. Endoscopy. 2023 Jan;55(1):58-95.
11. Cotter, J, Dias de Castro F, Magalhaes J, Moreira MJ, Rosa B. Validation of the Lewis score for evaluation of small bowel Crohn's disease activity. Endoscopy. 2015; 47:330-5.
12. Rosa B, Moreira MJ, Rebelo A, Cotter J. Lewis Score: A useful clinical tool for patients with suspected Crohn's disease submitted to capsule endoscopy. J Crohns Colitis. 2012;6:692-7.
13. Monteiro S, Carvalho PB, Dias de Castro F, et al. Capsule endoscopy: Diagnostic accuracy of Lewis score in patients with suspected Crohn's disease. Inflamm Bowel Dis. 2015;21:2241-6.
14. Koulaouzidis A, Douglas S, Plevris JN. Lewis score correlates more closely with fecal calprotectin than Capsule Endoscopy Crohn's Disease Activity Index (CECDAI or Niv score): A multicenter prospective

study. Endoscopy. 2012;44:21-6.
15. Ben-Horin S, Lahat A, Amitai MM, et al. Assessment of small bowel mucosal healing by video capsule endoscopy for the prediction of short-term risk of Crohn's disease flare: A prospective cohort study. Lancet Gastroenterol Hepatol. 2019;4(7):519-28
16. Omori T, Matsumoto T, Hara T, et al. A novel capsule endoscopic score for Crohn's disease. Crohns Colitis 360. 2020;2(2):otaa040.
17. Lewis JD, Rutgeerts P, Feagan BG, et al. Correlation of stool frequency and abdominal pain measures with simple endoscopic score for Crohn's disease. Inflamm Bowel Dis. 2020;26(2):304-313.
18. Colombel JF, Panaccione R, Bossuyt P, et al. Effect of tight control management on Crohn's disease (CALM): A multicentre, randomised, controlled phase 3 trial. Lancet. 2017;390(10114):2779-2789.
19. Mosli MH, Zou G, Garg SK, et al. C-Reactive protein, fecal calprotectin, and stool lactoferrin for detection of endoscopic activity in symptomatic inflammatory bowel disease patients: A systematic review and meta-analysis. Am J Gastroenterol. 2015;110(6):802-820.
20. Shine B, Berghouse L, Jones JEL, et al. C-reactive protein as an aid in the differentiation of functional and inflammatory bowel disorders. Clin Chim Acta 1985; 148: 105–109.
21. Ponte A, Pinho R, Rodrigues A, et al. Evaluation and comparison of capsule endoscopy scores for assessment of inflammatory activity of small bowel in Crohn's disease. Gastroenterol Hepatol. 2018;41(4):245-250.
22. Yang DH, Yang SK, Park SH, et al. Usefulness of C-reactive protein as a disease activity marker in Crohn's disease according to the location of disease. Gut Liver. 2015;9(1):80-86.
23. Bar-Gil Shitrit A, Koslowsky B, Livovsky DM, et al. A prospective study of fecal calprotectin and lactoferrin as predictors of small bowel Crohn's disease in patients undergoing capsule endoscopy. Scand J Gastroenterol. 2017;52(3):328-333.
24. Kopylov U, Yung DE, Engel T, et al. Fecal calprotectin for the prediction of small-bowel Crohn's disease by capsule endoscopy: A systematic review and meta-analysis. Eur J Gastroenterol Hepatol. 2016;28:1137–1144.
25. Kopylov U, Nemeth A, Koulaouzidis A, et al. Small bowel capsule endoscopy in the management of established Crohn's disease: Clinical impact, safety, and correlation with inflammatory biomarkers. Inflamm Bowel Dis. 2015;21(1):93-100.
26. Wang YD, Zhang RN, Mao R, Li XH. Inflammatory bowel disease cross-sectional imaging: What's new? United European Gastroenterol J. 2022;10(10):1179-1193.
27. Panés J, Bouzas R, Chaparro M, et al. Systematic review: The use of ultrasonography, computed tomography and magnetic resonance imaging for the diagnosis, assessment of activity and abdominal complications of Crohn's disease. Aliment Pharmacol Ther. 2011;34(2):125-145.
28. Koulaouzidis A, Rondonotti E, Karargyris A. Small-bowel capsule endoscopy: A ten-point contemporary review. World J Gastroenterol. 2013;19(24):3726-3746.
29. Niv Y. Small-bowel mucosal healing assessment by capsule endoscopy as a predictor of long-term clinical remission in patients with Crohn's disease: A systematic review and meta-analysis. Eur. J. Gastroenterol. Hepatol. 2017;29:844–848.
30. Bernstein CN, Loftus EV Jr, Ng SC, Lakatos PL, Moum B; Epidemiology and Natural History Task Force of the International Organization for the Study of Inflammatory Bowel Disease (IOIBD). Hospitalisations and surgery in Crohn's disease. Gut. 2012;61(4):622-9.
31. Khoudari G, Mansoor E, Click B, et al. Rates of intestinal resection and colectomy in inflammatory bowel disease patients after initiation of biologics: A cohort study. Clin Gastroenterol Hepatol. 2022;20(5).
32. Yamamoto T, Shimoyama T. Monitoring and detection of disease recurrence after resection for Crohn's disease: The role of non-invasive fecal biomarkers. Expert Rev Gastroenterol Hepatol. 2017;11:899–909.
33. Nguyen GC, Loftus EV, Hirano I, et al. American Gastroenterological Association Institute guideline on the management of Crohn's disease after surgical resection. Gastroenterology. 2017;152:271–275.
34. Bourreille A, Jarry M, D'Halluin PN, et al. Wireless capsule endoscopy versus ileocolonoscopy for the diagnosis of postoperative recurrence of Crohn's disease: A prospective study. Gut. 2006;55(7):978-983.
35. Gracie DJ, Williams CJ, Sood R, et al. Poor correlation between clinical disease activity and mucosal inflammation, and the role of psychological comorbidity, in inflammatory bowel disease. Am J Gastroenterol. 2016;111(4):541-551.
36. Elosua A, Rullan M, Rubio S, et al. Does capsule endoscopy impact clinical management in established Crohn's disease? Dig Liver Dis. 2022;54(1):118-124.

Case Study Number 18

Presented by Essam Quraishi, MD

Pre-capsule Findings (included in capsule study)

A 22-year-old female college student with a history of major depression and anxiety presents for re-evaluation of chronic symptoms of abdominal bloating, decreased appetite, and intermittent diarrhea. She passes 3–4 loose bowel movements on most days and occasionally at night, waking her from sleep. She denies hematochezia or melena. Her family history was notable for a sister with moderate-to-severe Crohn's disease complicated by perianal fistula. On physical examination, the patient appears somewhat cachectic, with a thin frame and loose-fitting clothing. No abdominal tenderness or masses are appreciated, and there are no extraintestinal manifestations of inflammatory bowel disease, such as rash, sacroiliitis, or uveitis.

Laboratory evaluation reveals a mild iron deficiency anemia (hemoglobin = 11.2 g/dl). Fecal calprotectin is mildly elevated to 180 μg/mL (50–120 μg/mL). Stool testing for *Clostridioides difficile* and *Giardia lamblia* infection are negative. An endoscopic evaluation, including upper endoscopy with duodenal mucosal biopsies and colonoscopy with inspection of the terminal ileum, fails to identify a cause of the patient's symptoms.

A capsule endoscopy study is performed to evaluate for a diagnosis of Crohn's Disease. Review the capsule endoscopy study and report your findings, including: gastric passage time, small bowel passage time, and observed abnormalities. Be prepared to discuss your findings and management plan with your staff prior to reviewing the diagnosis and case discussion.

Capsule Endoscopy Findings
First Gastric Image = 0h 0min 29sec
First Duodenal Image = 0h 44min 21sec
Gastric passage time = 0h 44min
First Cecal Image = 3h 1min 55sec
Small bowel passage time = 2hr 17min

Examination of the stomach and duodenum demonstrates healthy-appearing mucosa without evidence of inflammation or ulceration. Soon after entry into the deep small bowel, a striking abnormality is identified within the lumen (**Figure 1:** 0hr 45min 0sec; **Figure 2:** 0hr 46min 30sec). The luminal finding consists of multiple square and rectangular segments arranged in a linear chain, extending continuously through the jejunum and into the ileum. In the distal ileum and cecum, individual detached segments are observed freely floating within the lumen (**Figure 3**: 3hr 1min 34sec).

Follow-up

The patient was treated with praziquantel for a diagnosis of tapeworm infection. Following therapy, she passed a large volume of tapeworm segments. Within 2 weeks, her appetite improved while her gastrointestinal complaints, previously attributed to "IBS," resolved completely. Her physical health and mental well-being improved progressively over time. She described herself as well, healthy, and happy during her 3-month follow-up visit.

Figure 1

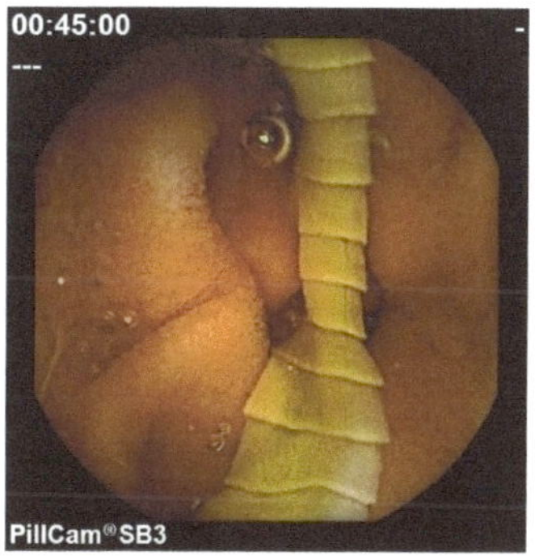

Figure 2

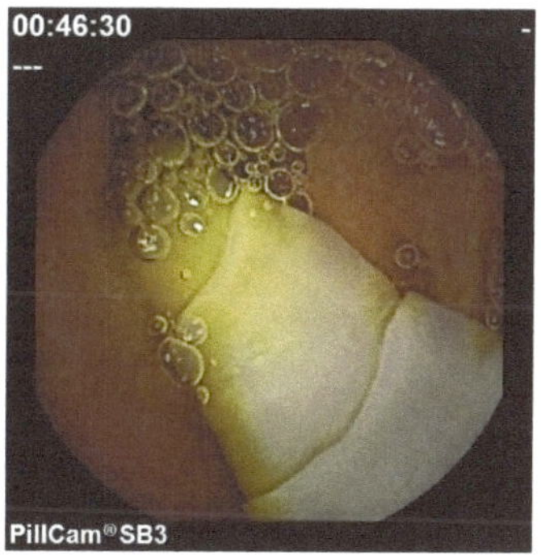

Figure 3

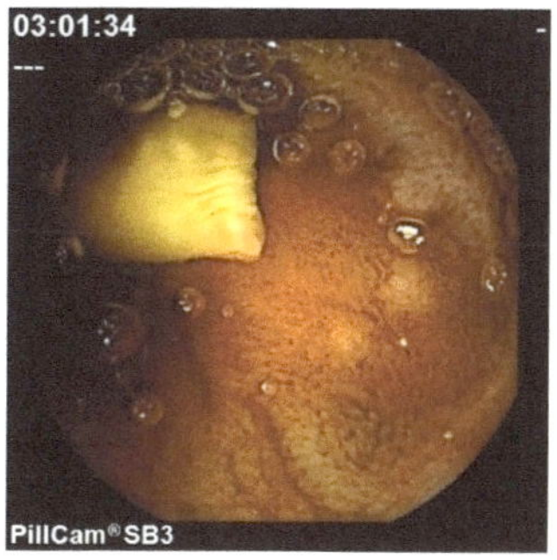

CASE STUDY DISCUSSIONS — CASE NUMBER 18

Chapter 18: Intestinal Helminths

Stephen Landreneau, MD, FACG

Introduction

Infection with intestinal helminths (parasitic worms) are prevalent in areas of poor sanitation and low socioeconomic status. An estimated 1.5 billion people are infected worldwide, primarily in Tropical and Subtropical regions.[1] While many helminth infections are asymptomatic, the impact on health and childhood development in endemic areas is substantial. In industrialized nations, helminth infections may be seen in travelers returning from endemic regions, migrants, and occasionally in local residents. Intestinal helminths are divided into nematodes (roundworms), cestodes (tapeworms) and trematodes (flukes). Nematodes and cestodes are large enough to be visualized on video capsule endoscopy (VCE) during the adult portion of their life cycles, and may be found during the evaluation for obscure gastrointestinal bleeding or diarrheal illness.[2] Clues to the diagnosis include worm morphology and location (**Table 1**).

Nematodes

Intestinal nematodes, or roundworms, are found in areas where poor sanitation and indiscriminate defecation occur. Nematodes are prevalent worldwide, with children often at the highest risk for infection.[3] Roundworms that infect humans range from 2 mm (*Strongyloides stecoralis*) to 35 cm (*Ascaris lumbricoides*) in length. Variability exists in the life cycles of individual nematodes, but they can be divided into 3 patterns.[2] *Trichuris* and *Enterobius* ova are ingested, followed by excystation and development of larvae in the gastrointestinal tract, and maturation occurs without leaving the confines of the intestine.[3] *Ascaris* ova are also ingested followed by excystation in the gastrointestinal tract. The larvae then invade the gastrointestinal mucosa and migrate via the venous circulation to the lungs. They exit the alveoli and ascend the bronchial tree to be swallowed then mature in the intestine.[4] *Acylostoma*, *Necator*, and *Strongyloides* larvae enter through the skin, often the feet, and migrate through the venous circulation to the lungs. Then, like *Ascaris*, they ascend the bronchial tree, are swallowed, and mature in the intestine.[2] Roundworms that may be identified in the intestinal lumen by capsule endoscopy include *Ascaris lumbricoides*, *Trichuris trichiura*, *Enterobius vermicularis*, *Acylostoma duodenale*, *Necator americanus*, and *Strongyloides stercoralis*.

Ascaris lumbricoides

Ascaris is found throughout the world in tropical and subtropical climates where it is transmitted through contaminated food and water. Adult worms have a lifespan of 10 months to 2 years and may grow to 35 cm in length. Clinical manifestations may relate either to the migration of the larvae through the lungs, or the presence of the adult worms in the intestine. Bronchospasm, increased secretions and urticaria can be present during the pulmonary phase. Abdominal symptoms may include pain, nausea, anorexia, and diarrhea, all of which are nonspecific, and often

Nematodes	Adult Size	Adult Location	Mechanism of Entry
Ascaris lumbricoides	35 cm	Proximal small bowel	Ingestion of ova
Trichuris trichiura "Whipworm"	3-5 cm	Cecum, colon	Ingestion of ova
Enterobius vermicularis "Pinworm"	8-13 mm	Ileum, cecum	Ingestion of ova
Ancylostoma & *Necator* "Hookworms"	5-13 mm	Distal small bowel	Skin penetration by larvae
Strongyloides stercoralis	2 mm	Proximal small bowel	Skin penetration by larvae
Cestodes	**Adult Size**	**Adult location**	**Mechanism of Entry**
Taenia saginata	4-10 m	Proximal small bowel	Ingestion of cysts
Taenia solium	2-4 m	Proximal small bowel	Ingestion of cysts

Table 1. Diagnosing parasitic worms.

difficult to ascribe to *Ascaris*, as those infected may be coinfected with other helminths. Intestinal obstruction has also been reported due to large worm burden[2] (**Figure 1**). Laboratory abnormalities include iron deficiency anemia, elevated serum IgE levels, and eosinophilia. Adult worms usually inhabit the jejunum or ileum and appear as large white or pink worms.[4,5] Diagnosis is by direct visualization of worms or stool examination for ova. First line medical therapy is albendazole in a single dose. Second line is mebendazole either single dose, twice daily for 3 days.[6]

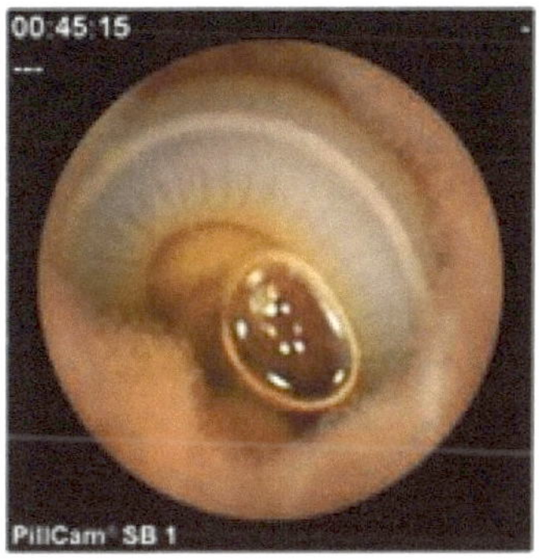

Figure 1. Ascaris lumbricoides observed in the small bowel by video capsule endoscopy.

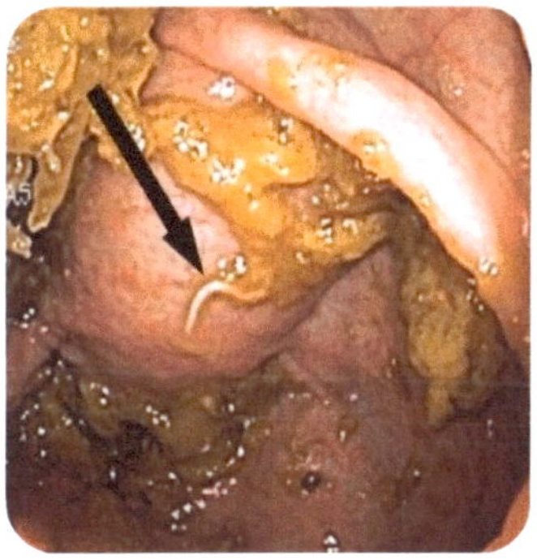
Figure 2. Whipworm observed in the lumen of the right colon in a patient undergoing screening colonoscopy.

Trichuris trichiura

Also known as "whipworm", *Trichuris* is found in the same geographic distribution as Ascaris. An estimated 500 million people are infected worldwide. In the United States, *Trichuris* is found in warm, moist climates of the southeastern region.[4] Infection results from ingesting embryonated ova. Larvae mature in the small intestine then reattach as adults in the cecum and colon. Adult worms live 4-6 years and are 30-50 mm in length. Most infections are asymptomatic, but those with heavy worm burden, especially young children, may demonstrate diarrhea, bloody mucoid stools, anemia, and growth retardation.[7] Eosinophilia may also be present. Adult worms may be seen throughout the colon, and appear as thin, thread like worms with a whip-like anterior section and more robust posterior section (**Figure 2**). Diagnosis is made by direct visualization of the adult worms in the colon or ova in the stool. First line treatment is albendazole single dose. The anti-helminth agent emodepside may be a future option as it has shown promise as a treatment in phase 2 trials.[8]

Enterobius vermicularis

Also known as the "pinworm", *Enterobius* is found in both tropical and temperate climates, and often infects children through ingestion of the ova. The adult worms populate the cecum, and adjacent ileum. Adult worms are 8-13 mm in length and live for 2-3 months.[4] Mature females migrate to the anus to lay eggs on the perineum, causing pruritus and concomitant scratching, leading to spread of the ova. Abdominal pain may occur with colonization of the appendix by adult worms mimicking appendicitis.[9] Pinworm infection has also been associated with eosinophilic enteritis.[2] Diagnosis is made by direct visualization of small white worms in the distal small bowel or cecum on endoscopy and/or by visualization of ova on low power microscopy by applying transparent tape to the perineum and then affixing the tape to a slide. Treatment options are pyrantel pamoate, mebendazole, or albendazole. A second dose of the treatment is given 2 weeks later. It is important to treat family members and meticulously sanitize linens, floors, and laundry to prevent transmission/reinfection.[10,11]

Ancylostoma duodenale & *Necator americanus*

Also known as "hookworms", *Ancylostoma* and *Necator* infections are common in humans, occurring in up to 740 million people worldwide. The highest prevalence is in sub-Saharan Africa and the Indian subcontinent. Hookworms infect humans by penetrating the skin of the feet of those who walk on contaminated soil.[12] They travel through the lymphatic system to the vasculature and then to the lungs, where they ascend the bronchial tree to be swallowed. They then attach and mature in the small intestine.[4] Infections are largely asymptomatic, but heavy infection burdens can result in nausea, fatigue, and abdominal pain. Eosinophilia and iron deficiency anemia are common. Overt gastrointestinal bleeding manifested by melena has also been reported to result from hookworm infection.[12] Treatment of human hookworm infection is with a single dose of albendazole or mebendazole.[13]

Strongyloides stercoralis

Strongyloides infects 50-100 million people worldwide and is found throughout tropical climates including Africa, Asia, Latin America, and the Southeastern United States. It follows a similar life cycle as the hookworms; it enters through the skin, migrates through the vasculature to the lungs, ascends the trachea to be swallowed, and attaches in the small intestine to mature. Ova hatch quickly, and larvae may enter though the intestinal mucosa or skin leading to autoinfection. This may result in lifelong infection or a life-threatening hyperinfection in immunocompromised hosts. Hyperinfection may present as bilateral infiltrates on chest radiograph and eosinophilia in chemotherapy patients.[14] Adult worms grow up to 2 mm in length and inhabit the proximal small bowel. Most infections are asymptomatic, but like hookworms, pulmonary symptoms such as cough and wheezing may be present during the pulmonary migration of the worms. Abdominal symptoms may include epigastric pain, nausea, diarrhea, and malabsorption. In rare cases, *Strongyloides* infection may present with acute or subacute enteritis which is identifiable by CT imaging (**Figure 3**). Diagnosis is made by stool evaluation or small bowel biopsy for larvae as adult worms are often too small to visualize on endoscopy (**Figure 4**). Ivermectin is effective for treatment.[2-4]

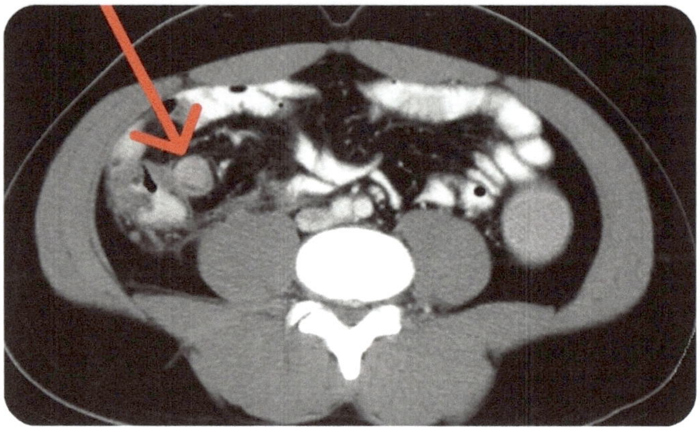

Figure 3. Ileitis with adjacent lymphadenopathy due to *Strongyloides* infection.

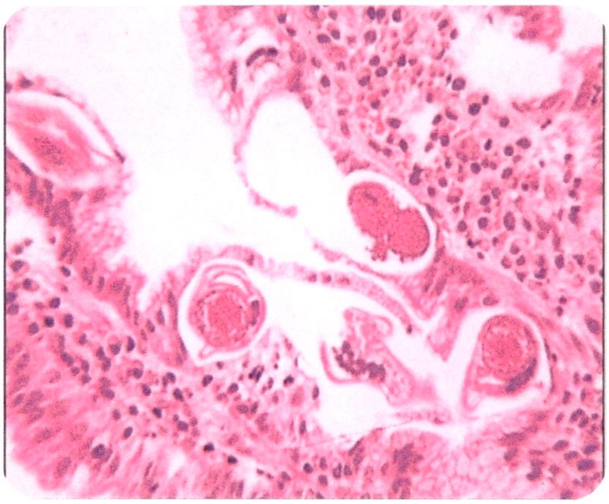

Figure 4. *Strongyloides* larva invading the submucosa of the intestine.

Cestodes

Cestodes, or tapeworms, have complex life cycles involving multiple intermediate hosts. Morphologically, tapeworms are ribbon-like worms that contain a scolex used for attachment to the host at their anterior end, followed by a strobila. The strobila consists of 3 to several thousand segments known as proglottids. Each proglottid functions as a mature individual, capable of reproduction. Tapeworms are spread through ingestion of raw or undercooked meat or flesh containing larvae. Humans are the definitive hosts for *Taenia solium* and *Taenia saginata*.[15]

Taenia saginata

Taenia saginata is known as the beef tapeworm. Approximately 50 million people are thought to be infected with *Taenia saginata*, mostly in Africa, the Middle East, and Europe. Infections are rare in the United States. Infection occurs from ingestion of raw or undercooked beef containing the larval stage of the worm. After ingestion, the scolex attaches to the jejunum and the adult worm develops. Adults may grow 4-10 meters in length and live up to 30 years. Symptoms include abdominal pain, nausea, and perineal discomfort from passage of proglottids. Diagnosis is made by stool examination for ova or proglottids. A long ribbon like worm can be seen on VCE originating in the jejunum (**Figure 5**). Treatment with praziquantel or niclosamide is effective.[2,15,16]

Taenia solium

Taenia solium is known as the pork tapeworm. Infections are common in Asia, Africa, and Latin America, in areas where hogs are raised. Humans may either serve as the definitive host, or the intermediate host. As the definitive host, infection occurs when undercooked pork meat containing cysts is ingested. Adult worms attach in the proximal jejunum and are 2-4 meters in length. Infections are typically asymptomatic but eosinophilia may occur. Diagnosis is made by stool examination. On VCE, *T. solium* is found attached in the jejunum and is visually indistinguishable from *T. saginata*. When humans serve as the intermediate host by ingesting ova from human feces, or by from internal autoinfection, cysticercosis occurs which can be life threatening. Praziquantel or niclosamide is effective for intestinal infection. Albendazole and corticosteroids are used for cysticercosis.[3,5]

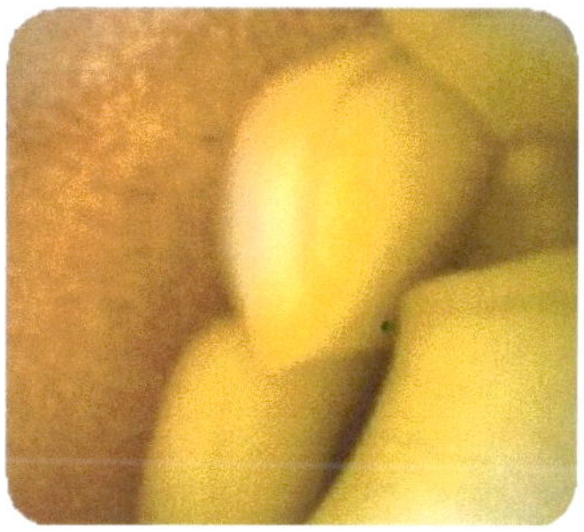

Figure 5. *Taenia saginata* observed by VCE.
Image courtesy of Dr. Michel Delvaux.

Summary

Intestinal helminths may be diagnosed in patients undergoing VCE for routine indications. In addition to worm morphology and size, location provides valuable diagnostic information. Particles of vegetable matter, hair or thread in the intestinal lumen may resemble worms but should not be confused with a true helminth infection (**Figure 6**). Strongyloides, and tapeworms may be found in the proximal small bowel while *Enterobius*, *Trichuris*, and hookworms are encountered in the distal small bowel and cecum. Effective treatment of these infections is available once a diagnosis has been made. Helminth infections can present with iron deficiency anemia and/or chronic diarrhea, potentially resulting in evaluation by video capsule endoscopy.

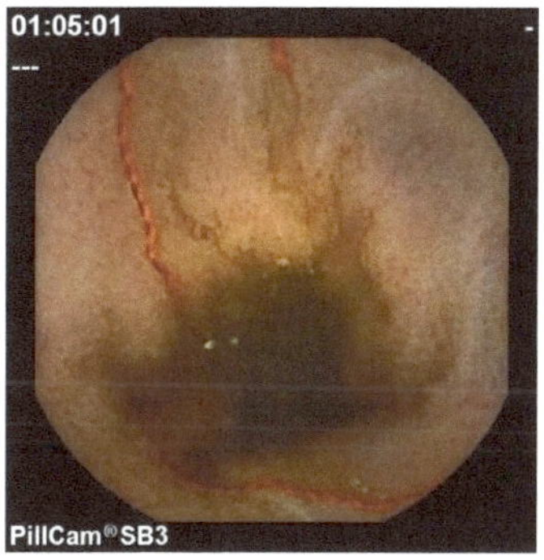

Figure 6. Braided synthetic filament, consistent with ingested thread or textile fiber. *Image courtesy of Dr. Oscar Alvarez.*

References

1. Chen J, Gong Y, Chen Q, Li S, Zhou Y. Global burden of soil-transmitted helminth infections, 1990-2021. Infect Dis Poverty. 2024;13(1):77.
2. Pearson RD: Parasitic Diseases: Helminths. In Textbook of Gastroenterology. Yamada T (ed.) Lippincott Williams and Wilkins; 1999: 2442-2459.
3. Brooker S. Estimating the global distribution and disease burden of intestinal nematode infections: Adding up the numbers--A review. Int J Parasitol. 2010;40(10):1137-44.
4. Brown HW. Basic Clinical Parasitology, 4th ed. New York: Appleton-Century-Crofts; 1975: 105-141.
5. Flierman A, Koornstra JJ, Weersma RK. An unexpected cause of iron deficiency detected by capsule endoscopy. Neth J Med. 2009;67(6):247-8.
6. Keiser J, Utzinger J. The drugs we have and the drugs we need against major helminth infections. Adv Parasitol. 2010;73:197-230
7. Grencis RK, Cooper ES. Enterobius, trichuris, capillaria, and hookworm including ancylostoma caninum. Gastroenterol Clin North Am. 1996;25(3):579-97.
8. Mrimi EC, Welsche S, Ali SM, Hattendorf J, Keiser J. Emodepside for *Trichuris trichiura* and Hookworm Infection. N Engl J Med. 2023;388(20):1863-1875.
9. Ariyarathenam AV, Nachimuthu S, Tang TY, Courtney ED, Harris SA, Harris AM. *Enterobius vermicularis* infestation of the appendix and management at the time of laparoscopic appendectomy: case series and literature review. Int J Surg. 2010;8(6):466-9.
10. Balachandran P, Prasad VG. Intestinal parasites seen on capsule endoscopy. Gastrointest Endosc. 2006;64(4):651.
11. Leung AKC, Lam JM, Barankin B, Wong AHC, Leong KF, Hon KL. Pinworm (*Enterobius vermicularis*) Infestation: An Updated Review. Curr Pediatr Rev. 2024 Jan 28.
12. Yan SL, Chu YC. Hookworm infestation of the small intestine: An unusual cause of obscure gastrointestinal bleeding. Endoscopy. 2007;39 Suppl 1:E162-3.
13. Loukas A, Hotez PJ, Diemert D, Yazdanbakhsh M, McCarthy JS, Correa-Oliveira R, Croese J, Bethony JM. Hookworm infection. Nat Rev Dis Primers. 2016;2:16088.
14. Wirk B, Wingard JR. *Strongyloides stercoralis* hyperinfection in hematopoietic stem cell transplantation. Transpl Infect Dis. 2009;11(2):143-8.
15. Howell J, Brown G. Education and imaging. Gastrointestinal: beef tapeworm (Taenia saginata). J Gastroenterol Hepatol. 2008 Nov;23(11):1769.
16. Carretero C, Borda A, Muñoz-Navas M. Face to face with teniasis. Clin Gastroenterol Hepatol. 2010;8(1):A36.

Case Study Number 19

Presented by Nisha Loganantharaj, MD

Pre-capsule Findings (included in capsule study)

A 52-year-old woman with a history of hypertension and degenerative disk disease presents for further evaluation of chronic diarrhea associated with intermittent abdominal pain. She reports 4-5 watery bowel movements per day including occasional episodes which wake her from sleep. Prior to the onset of these symptoms 2 years ago, she describes her bowel habits as "normal" with 1 soft bowel movement each morning and no abdominal pain. Her medications include lisinopril, diltiazem, Vitamin D, and acetaminophen as needed for back pain. An evaluation for diarrhea was completed prior to this visit including colonoscopy and stool tests for for *Clostridioides difficile* and *Giardia lamblia* infection. Her fecal calprotectin is mildly elevated at 169 mcg/ml (50-120 mcg/ml). Routine hematology and chemistry serologies are unremarkable except for a mild anemia (11.5 gm/dl). Testing for serum anti-TTG IgA antibodies is negative with a total IgA level within normal range.

A capsule endoscopy study is performed to evaluate for a diagnosis of Crohn's Disease. Review the capsule endoscopy study and report your findings, including: gastric passage time, small bowel passage time, and observed abnormalities. Be prepared to discuss your findings and management plan with your staff prior to reviewing the diagnosis and case discussion.

Multiple, small (3-5mm) ulcers are identified in the duodenum and proximal jejunum (**Figure 1**: 0hr 39min 49sec; **Figure 2**: 0hr 46min 16sec). An area of delayed capsule transit, or capsule hold-up, is observed beginning at 2hrs 12min. As the video capsule traverses the remaining small bowel, several areas of stenosis with deep ulceration are found (**Figure 3**: 2hr 52min 53sec; **Figure 4: 3hr 10min 28sec).**

Capsule Endoscopy Findings

First Gastric Image = 0hr 0min 25sec

First Duodenal Image = 0h 27min 48sec

Gastric passage time = 0h 27min

First Cecal Image = 3h 13min 19sec

Small bowel passage time = 2hr 44min

Figure 1

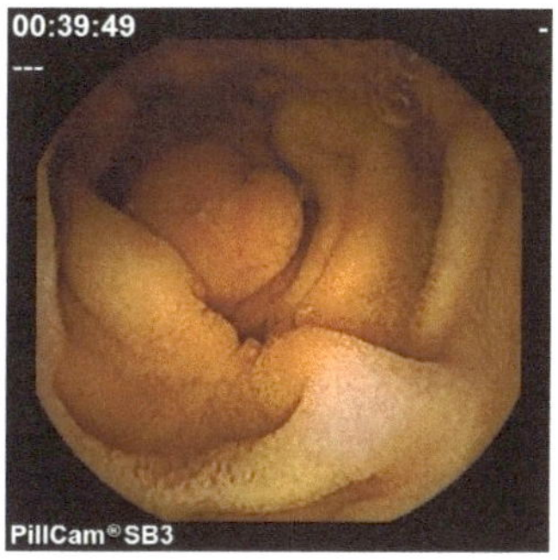

Figure 2

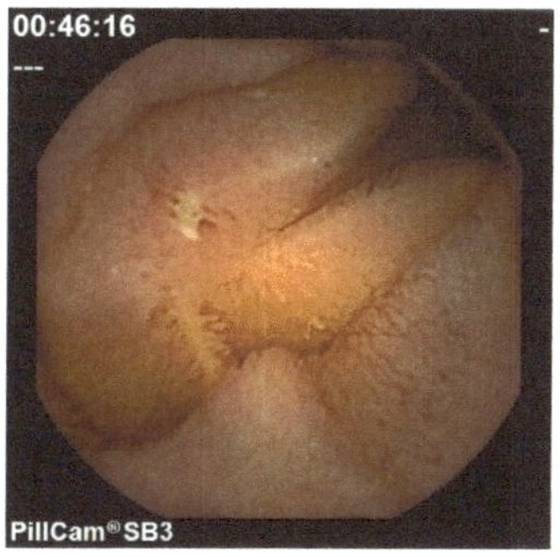

Figure 3

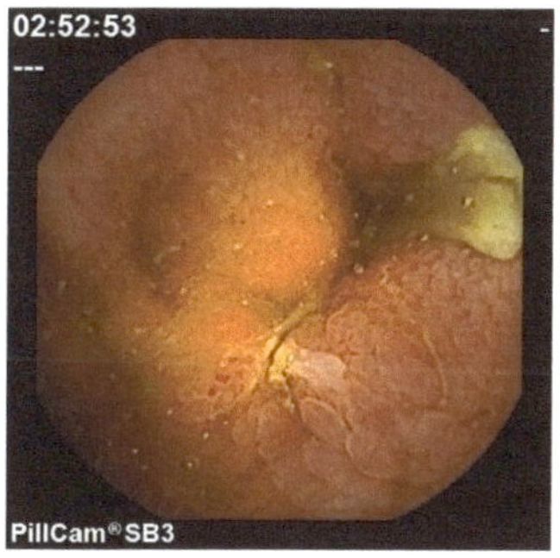

Figure 4

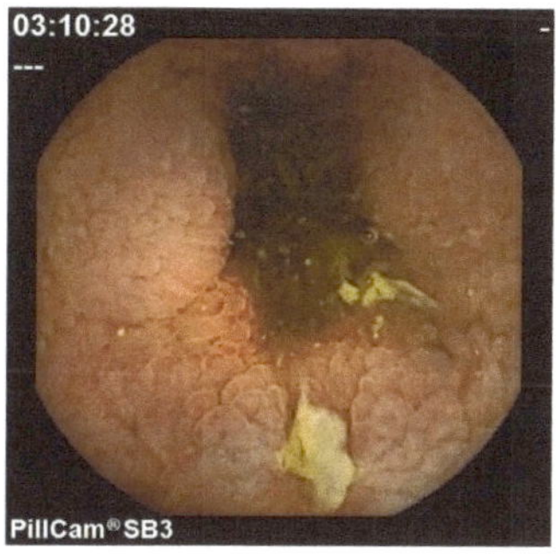

Follow-up

A retrograde double ballon enteroscopy was performed to directly visualize the distal small bowel and obtain mucosal biopsies. Serial strictures with ulceration were encountered in the distal ileum ~20 cm proximal to the ileocecal valve (**Figure 5**). Two strictures were traversed while a third stricture was too narrow to intubate. Mucosal biopsies were obtained and revealing for chronic, active inflammation most consistent with Crohn's disease and without evidence of malignant cells.

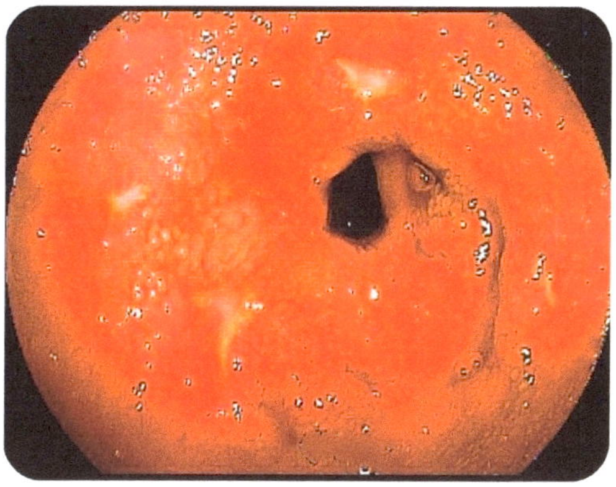

Figure 5

Chapter 19: Crohn's Disease

Nisha Loganantharaj, MD

Introduction

Crohn's disease (CD) is a chronic, progressive inflammatory condition that can affect any portion of the gastrointestinal tract from the mouth to the anus. It is characterized by patchy inflammation and transmural involvement.[1] The global incidence and prevalence of Crohn's Disease continues to rise.[2] Although the diagnosis of CD in a first degree relative is a strong risk factor for developing CD, environmental factors are also thought to play a role.[3] Smoking is a well-established environmental risk factor for the development of Crohn's and a risk factor for adverse outcomes in CD.[4,5] Other environmental factors such as antibiotic exposure and diet with ultra-processed foods have been associated with an increased risk for developing CD.[6,7] Over 1 million Americans are currently living with CD per recent estimates.[8] Crohn's is typically diagnosed between the ages of 18 and 35 years of age with a second smaller peak occurring between the ages of 50 and 60.[9] The pathophysiology of Crohn's disease is thought to stem from a combination of genetics, the host microbiome, immune dysregulation and environmental factors. The complex interaction of all these different factors result in the activation of inflammatory and pro-inflammatory cytokine cascades causing disruption of the intestinal mucosa.[10]

Clinical Features

The presenting symptoms of CD are variable and dependent on the phenotype and location of active inflammation. Due to the relapsing-remitting nature of this disease, patients may have fluctuations in their symptoms and can be often misdiagnosed with irritable bowel syndrome.[2] One study found that 70% of CD patients reported a delay in diagnosis greater than a year.[11] Symptoms can range from diarrhea, abdominal pain, bloating, nausea, vomiting, weight loss, bowel urgency, and fever or chills.[12] Fatigue is a common and underrecognized symptom in patients with CD. Extraintestinal manifestations involving the joints, skin and eyes may be present in up to 50% of patients.[13] Identification of these manifestations may result in earlier diagnosis and influence treatment choice.

Although Crohn's can affect any part of the GI tract, small bowel involvement is present in 80% of patients with approximately 30% of patients having isolated small bowel disease.[9] Approximately, one-third of patients will develop perianal fistulizing involvement of their Crohn's disease within 20 years of diagnosis. Persistent active inflammation can lead to progressive bowel damage and complications including stricture, fistula and abscesses due to the transmural involvement of the disease.[14] A recent study, PROFILE, highlighted the importance of appropriate management of CD in a top-down treatment approach as compared to a standard accelerated step up approach. Over the study period, patients treated in the top down treatment strategy had a 64 point percentage difference steroid-free and surgery-free remission in comparison to the step up treatment approach.[15] These results reinforce the importance of early diagnosis and treatment in CD in order to prevent irreversible bowel damage. Delays in diagnosis are associated with poor outcomes.[11]

Diagnosis

The diagnosis of Crohn's disease involves a careful history and physical exam, laboratory tests (including inflammatory biomarkers), imaging studies, endoscopic evaluation, and histopathological confirmation.[14] Basic laboratory testing may be revealing for anemia due to chronic blood loss, chronic inflammation, or malabsorption. Thrombocytosis may serve as marker for acute inflammation.[16] Common inflammatory markers in CD include C-reactive protein (CRP) and fecal calprotectin.[2] As a simple blood test, CRP is widely available and relatively inexpensive but is not specific for inflammation due to CD. Fecal calprotectin serves as the most sensitive screening test for inflammatory bowel disease but may be normal in some cases of isolated small bowel CD.[17]

Direct endoscopic examination with tissue biopsy remains the gold standard to confirm a diagnosis of CD. Mucosal changes characteristic of CD include patchy inflammation characterized by stricture formation and ulceration (serpiginous, linear, stellate, apthous) (**Figure 1**). Patients with isolated small bowel CD are often more difficult to diagnose due to slow progression of symptoms and limitations of

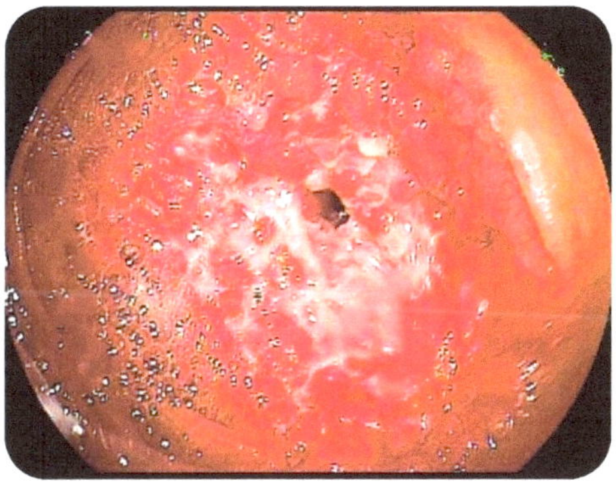

Figure 1. Ulcerated stenosis of the proximal ileum observed by anterograde DBE.

standard endoscopy in examining the small bowel. Imaging studies such as CT and MR enterography may be useful in evaluating the small bowel but do not allow for tissue confirmation and may miss disease activity in the the jejunum and proximal ileum.[16] In a cohort study of Crohn's patients, ileal CD was found to be independent risk factor for a delay in diagnosis of more than 24 months.[18]

Granulomatous inflammation on histology is pathognomonic for CD. However, granulomas are seen in only a minority of tissue specimens and are not required to diagnose CD.[19] Histology from biopsies typically has features of chronic inflammation with architectural crypt distortion.[20] Device-assisted enteroscopy is often required to confirm a diagnosis of small bowel Crohn's disease which lies out of reach standard upper endoscopy and colonoscopy.[21-28]

Role of Capsule Endoscopy

Video capsule endoscopy (VCE) allows for the visualization of the entire small bowel non-invasively. One major advantage of VCE is the ability to definitively exclude a diagnosis of CD. In patients with suspected small bowel CD, the negative predictive value of a normal VCE is 96%.[29] The diagnostic yield of VCE in patients with suspected CD has been studied and compared with other tests. Capsule endoscopy has been shown to be superior to barium studies, ileocolonoscopy, and CTE in regard to diagnostic yield. Capsule endoscopy is equivalent to MRE in detecting active inflammation. VCE is equivalent to MRE in detecting Crohn's activity in the distal small bowel and superior to MRE in detecting activity in the proximal small bowel. However, MRE can detect transmural inflammation and disease-related complications such as fistula formation.[30,31] A comparison of testing modalities currently utilized to detect small bowel CD activity is provided in **Table 1**. The Lewis score has been validated as a means to quantify the burden of inflammation based upon VCE findings of villous edema, ulceration, and strictures. A Lewis score > 135 indicates substantial inflammatory changes with a specificity of 88% for CD.[31,32] Despite this evidence, tissue biopsy is considered as the gold standard to confirm a diagnosis of CD and exclude other pathologies including nonsteroidal anti-inflammatory drug enteropathy, cryptogenic stenosing enteritis, Bechet's disease, and lymphoma.[16]

Capsule endoscopy can be used in surveillance for mucosal healing in patients with an established diagnosis of CD. Mucosal healing is a primary goal of therapy as a predictor of improved long-term outcomes with a lower risk of disease flare and hospitalizations, reduced risk of complications with a reduced need for surgery, improved quality of life and steroid-free remission.[34,35] A retrospective single center study found that capsule endoscopy was a useful tool to guide therapy, as 51% of capsule studies resulting in a change in therapy with either escalation of de-escalation of medical management.[36] The risk of capsule retention may be increased in patients with CD, ranging from 0.5% to 5.4%.[37,38] In patients with suspected or established CD, a Patency capsule may be deployed prior to VCE to evaluate for significant stenosis.[39]

Conclusions

Diagnosis of small bowel CD is commonly delayed due to lack of specific symptoms and limitations of standard EGD/colonoscopy. It is imperative to diagnose Crohn's early in the disease course to prevent progressive bowel injury and complications. Video capsule endoscopy is a non-invasive method to evaluate the small bowel for evidence of CD as well as to quantify the severity and extent of inflammation. A diagnosis of CD can be effectively excluded if VCE is negative for evidence of inflammation. Additionally, CD has a role in monitoring Crohn's disease for mucosal healing in order to make adjustments in medical therapy.

Modality	Diagnostic Yield	Tissue Acquisition	Proximal Small Bowel Detection	Radiation Exposure	Other Key Features
Video Capsule Endoscopy	Superior to SBFT, CTE, ileoscopy (incremental yield 32%, 47%, 22%)	No	Best among all modalities	No	Direct mucosal visualization; High negative predictive value (96%)
CT Enterography	Lower than VCE (yield 21%-39%)	No	Good but less sensitive than VCE	Yes	Detects mural and extramural disease
MR Enterography	Equivalent to VCE for distal disease; Lower than VCE for proximal lesions	No	Good but less sensitive for superficial inflammation	No	Detects mural and extramural disease; Preferred in young patients
Small Bowel Follow-Through	Lowest (yield: 16%-36%)	No	Poor	Yes	Limited sensitivity for early or mild disease
Ileocolonoscopy	Lower than VCE for isolated small bowel disease (yield 25-46%)	Yes	N/A	No	Gold standard for colonic/ terminal ileal disease
Device Assisted Enteroscopy	Individual case specific	Yes	Good	No	Allows for tissue biopsy to confirm CD

Table 1. Diagnostic studies used in the evaluation of small bowel Crohn's disease.

References

1. Feuerstein JD, Cheifetz AS. Crohn Disease: Epidemiology, Diagnosis, and Management. Mayo Clin Proc. 2017;92(7):1088-1103.
2. Cushing K, Higgins PDR. Management of crohn disease: A review. JAMA. 2021;325(1):69-80.
3. Moller FT, Andersen V, Wohlfahrt J, Jess T. Familial risk of inflammatory bowel disease: A population-based cohort study 1977-2011. Am J Gastroenterol. 2015;110(4):564-571.
4. Mahid SS, Minor KS, Soto RE, Hornung CA, Galandiuk S. Smoking and inflammatory bowel disease: A meta-analysis. Mayo Clin Proc. 2006;81 (11):1462–1471.
5. To N, Gracie DJ, Ford AC. Systematic review with meta-analysis: The adverse effects of tobacco smoking on the natural history of Crohn's disease. Aliment Pharmacol Ther. 2016;43(5):549–561.
6. Ungaro R, Bernstein CN, Gearry R, et al. Antibiotics associated with increased risk of new-onset Crohn's disease but not ulcerative colitis: A meta-analysis. Am J Gastroenterol. 2014;109(11):1728-1738.
7. Narula N, Wong ECL, Dehghan M, et al. Association of ultra-processed food intake with risk of inflammatory bowel disease: prospective cohort study. BMJ. 2021;374:n1554.
8. Lewis JD, Parlett LE, Jonsson Funk ML, et al. Incidence, prevalence, and racial and ethnic distribution of inflammatory bowel disease in the United States. Gastroenterology. 2023;165(5):1197-1205.e2.
9. Torres J, Mehandru S, Colombel JF, Peyrin-Biroulet L. Crohn's disease. Lancet. 2017; 389: 1741–55.
10. Petagna L, Antonelli A, Ganini C, et al. Pathophysiology of Crohn's disease inflammation and recurrence. Biol Direct. 2020;15(1):23.
11. Gallinger, Zane et al. Delayed diagnosis of Crohn's Disease is Common and associated with an increased risk disease complications. Gastroenterology. 2019; 156 (3) S21.
12. Nóbrega VG, Silva INN, Brito BS, Silva J, Silva MCMD, Santana GO. The onset of clinical manifestations in inflammatory bowel disease patients. Arq Gastroenterol. 2018;55(3):290-295.

13. Rogler G, Singh A, Kavanaugh A, Rubin DT. Extraintestinal manifestations of inflammatory bowel disease: current concepts, treatment, and implications for disease management. Gastroenterology. 2021 Oct;161(4):1118-1132.
14. Lichtenstein GR, Loftus E, Afzali A, et al. Clinical Guideline: Management of Crohn's Disease in Adults. The American Journal of Gastroenterology. 2025. 120(6):p 1225-1264.
15. Noor NM, Lee JC, Bond S, et al. A biomarker-stratified comparison of top-down versus accelerated step-up treatment strategies for patients with newly diagnosed Crohn's disease (PROFILE): A multicentre, open-label randomised controlled trial. Lancet Gastroenterol Hepatol. 2024;9(5):415-427.
16. Dolinger M, Torres J, Vermeire S. Crohn's disease. Lancet. 2024;403(10432):1177-1191.
17. Mosli MH, Zou G, Garg SK, et al. C-reactive protein, fecal calprotectin, and stool lactoferrin for detection of endoscopic activity in symptomatic inflammatory bowel disease patients: A systematic review and meta-analysis. Am J Gastroenterol. 2015;110(6):802–819.
18. Vavricka SR, Spigaglia SM, Rogler G, et al. Systematic evaluation of risk factors for diagnostic delay in inflammatory bowel disease. Inflamm Bowel Dis. 2012;18(3):496-505.
19. Molnár T, Tiszlavicz L, Gyulai C, Nagy F, Lonovics J. Clinical significance of granuloma in Crohn's disease. World J Gastroenterol. 2005;11(20):3118-3121.
20. Pasternak G, Chrzanowski G, Aebisher D, et al. Crohn's disease: Basic characteristics of the disease, diagnostic methods, the role of biomarkers, and analysis of metalloproteinases: A review. Life (Basel). 2023;13(10):2062.
21. Iacopini G, Frontespezi S, Vitale MA et al. Routine ileoscopy at colonoscopy: A prospective evaluation of learning curve and skill-keeping line. Gastrointest Endosc. 2006;63: 250-256.
22. Solitano V, Vuyyuru SK, Aruljothy A, et al. Endoscopic skipping, stricturing, and penetrating complications in crohn's disease on tandem ileo-colonoscopy and cross-sectional imaging: A retrospective cohort study. Inflamm Bowel Dis. 2025;31(6):1529-1536. Erratum in: Inflamm Bowel Dis. 2025;31(8):2325.
23. Pennazio et al. Rondonotti E, Despott EJ, Dray X, Keuchel M, Moreels T, et al. Small-bowel capsule endoscopy and device-assisted enterosocpy for diagnosis and treatment of small-bowel disorders: European Society of Gastrointestinal Endoscopy (ESGE) Guideline: Update 2022. Endoscopy. 2023;55(1):58-95.
24. Gauci J, Sammut L, Sciberras M, et al. Small bowel imaging in Crohn's disease patients. Ann Gastroenterol. 2018;31(4):395-405.
25. Mensink PB, Aktas H, Zelinkova Z, West RL, Kuipers EJ, van der Woude CJ. Impact of double-balloon enteroscopy findings on the management of Crohn's disease. Scand J Gastroenterol. 2010;45:483–489.
26. Hanscom M, Stead C, Feldman H, Marya NB, Cave D. Video capsule endoscopy and device-assisted enteroscopy. Dig Dis Sci. 2022;67(5):1539-1552.
27. Lee HH, Kim JS, Goong HJ, et al. Use of device-assisted enteroscopy in small bowel disease: an expert consensus statement by the Korean Association for the Study of Intestinal Diseases. Intest Res. 2023;21(1):3-19.
28. Rosa B, Pinho R, de Ferro SM, Almeida N, Cotter J, Saraiva MM. Endoscopic scores for evaluation of crohn's disease activity at small bowel capsule endoscopy: General principles and current applications. GE Port J Gastroenterol. 2015;23(1):36-41.
29. Hall B, Holleran G, Costigan D, McNamara D. Capsule endoscopy: High negative predictive value in the long term despite a low diagnostic yield in patients with suspected Crohn's disease. United European Gastroenterol J. 2013;1(6):461-466.
30. Mitselos IV, Fousekis FS, Lamouri C, Katsanos KH, Christodoulou DK. Current noninvasive modalities in Crohn's disease monitoring. Ann Gastroenterol. 2021;34(6):770-780.
31. Jensen MD, Nathan T, Rafaelsen SR, Kjeldsen J. Diagnostic accuracy of capsule endoscopy for small bowel Crohn's disease is superior to that of MR enterography or CT enterography. Clin Gastroenterol Hepatol. 2011;9(2):124-129.
32. Esaki M, Matsumoto T, Ohmiya N, et al. Capsule endoscopy findings for the diagnosis of Crohn's disease: a nationwide case-control study. J Gastroenterol. 2019;54(3):249-260.
33. Korman LY, Delvaux M, Gay G, Hagenmuller F, Keuchel M, Friedman S, Weinstein M, Shetzline M, Cave D, de Franchis R. Capsule endoscopy structured terminology (CEST): Proposal of a standardized and structured terminology for reporting capsule endoscopy procedures. Endoscopy. 2005;37:951–959.
34. Dave M, Loftus EV Jr. Mucosal healing in inflammatory bowel disease-a true paradigm of success? Gastroenterol Hepatol (N Y). 2012;8(1):29-38.
35. Turner D, Ricciuto A, Lewis A, et al. STRIDE-II: An update on the Selecting Therapeutic Targets in Inflammatory Bowel Disease (STRIDE) initiative of the International Organization for the Study of IBD (IOIBD): Determining therapeutic goals for treat-to-target strategies in IBD. Gastroenterology. 2021;160(5):1570-1583.
36. Elosua A, Rullan M, Rubio S, Oquiñena S, Rodríguez C, Macías E, Borda A, Fernández-Urién I, Nantes Ó. Does capsule endoscopy impact clinical management in established Crohn's disease? Dig Liver Dis. 2022 Jan;54(1):118-124.
37. Rondonotti E. Capsule retention: prevention, diagnosis

and management. Ann Transl Med. 2017;5(9):198.
38. Annese V, Daperno M, Rutter MD, et al. European Crohn's and Colitis Organisation European evidence based consensus for endoscopy in inflammatory bowel disease. J Crohns Colitis. 2013;7:982–1018.
39. Yadav A, Heigh RI, Hara AK, et al. Performance of the patency capsule compared with nonenteroclysis radiologic examinations in patients with known or suspected intestinal strictures. Gastrointest Endosc 2011;74:834-9.

Case Study Number 20

Presented by Charles Woodall, DO and David Cave, MD, PhD, FACG

Pre-capsule Findings (included in capsule study)

An 18-year-old woman with a history of trisomy 21, intellectual disability, seizure disorder, and congenital heart disease presents for transition of care to an adult gastroenterologist for continued management of Crohn's disease. She was initially diagnosed with isolated small bowel Crohn's disease at age 16 during evaluation for iron deficiency anemia. This evaluation included upper endoscopy, colonoscopy, and video capsule endoscopy (VCE). VCE was positive for an ulcerated stricture within the distal small bowel. She has been treated with adalimumab 80 mg administered subcutaneous every 2 weeks over the past 18 months.

The patient cannot provide her own history but her mother reports that her iron deficiency anemia has not improved with treatment for Crohn's disease. She denies observing her daughter experiencing abdominal pain or diarrhea. The patient's medication list includes adalimumab, cetirizine, ferrous sulfate, and vitamin D. She denies any non-steroidal anti-inflammatory drug (NSAID) use. Physical exam is unremarkable. You order an upper endoscopy, colonoscopy, and MRE for re-evaluation of disease activity but these studies are normal.

A capsule endoscopy study is performed for re-evaluation of a suspected diagnosis of small bowel Crohn's disease. Review the capsule endoscopy study and report your findings, including: gastric passage time, small bowel passage time, and observed abnormalities. Be prepared to discuss your findings and management plan with your staff prior to reviewing the diagnosis and case discussion.

The video capsule is placed endoscopically in the duodenum. Small amounts of red blood are observed in the duodenum, likely due to mucosal trauma during endoscopy. The small bowel mucosa appears to be normal until a ring-like stenosis is encountered (**Figure 1:** 4hrs 41min 18sec). The capsule traverses this stenosis only to encounter 2 additional stenoses which are characterized by thick (10 mm-20 mm) concentric ulceration (**Figure 2:** 5hrs 51min 34sec; **Figure 3**: 6hrs 9min 14sec). The video capsule is retained by a fourth stenosis until the end of battery life (**Figure 4:** 7hrs 35min 15 sec).

Figure 1

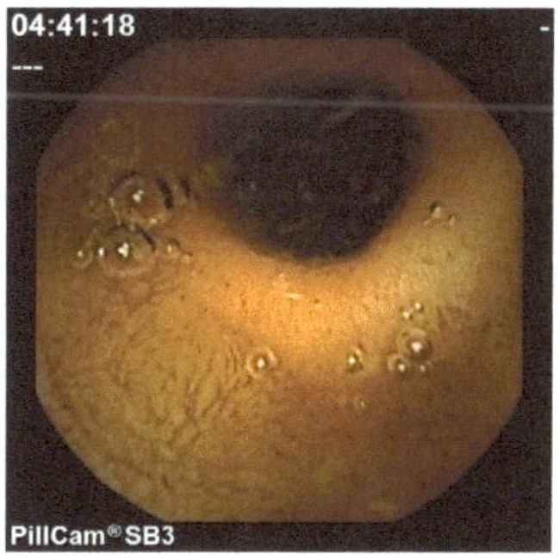

Figure 2

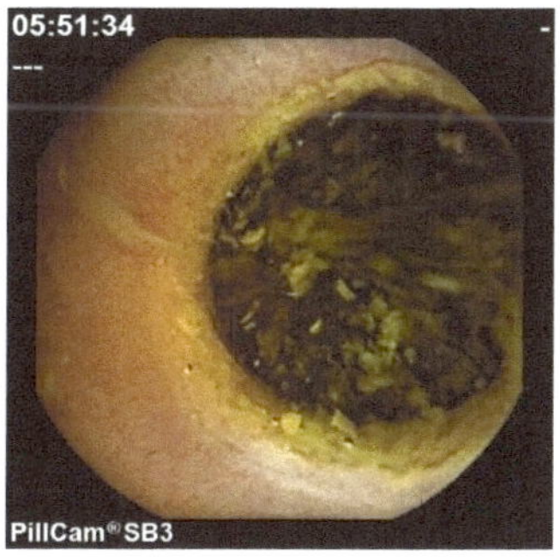

Figure 3

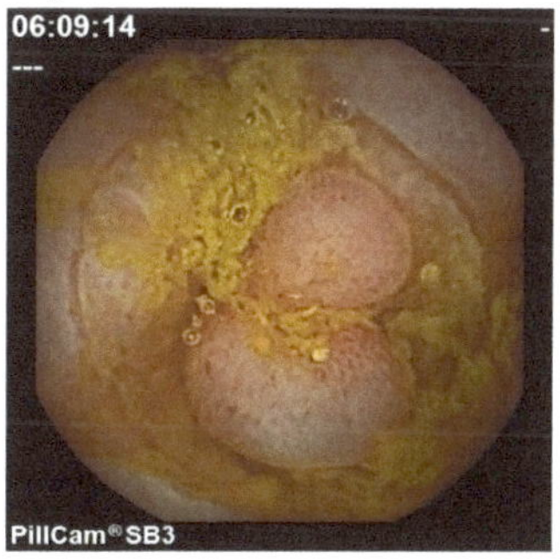

Figure 4

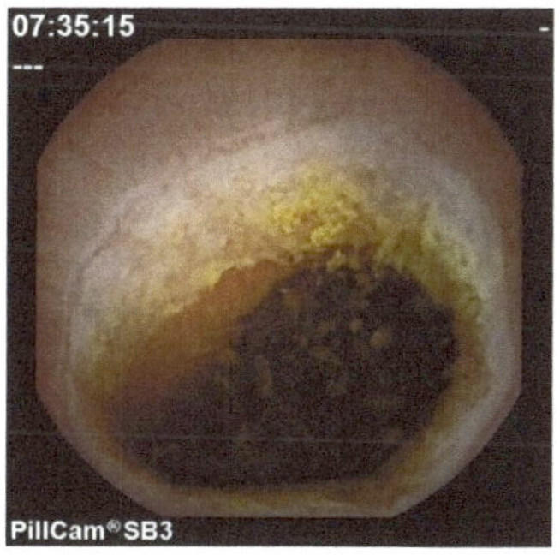

Follow-up

An abdominal x-ray performed 1 week later confirms spontaneous passage of the video capsule. An anterograde double balloon enteroscopy (DBE) exam is performed to further evaluate the ulcerated stenoses within the mid-small bowel. This exam confirms the findings observed on VCE (**Figure 5a,b**). Biopsies obtained from the ulcerated areas demonstrate an inflammatory infiltrate within lamina propria made up of plasma cells, lymphocytes, and polymorphonuclear cells. Biopsy specimens of the mucosa adjacent to ulcers show normal villous architecture without inflammation or edema.

Figure 5a

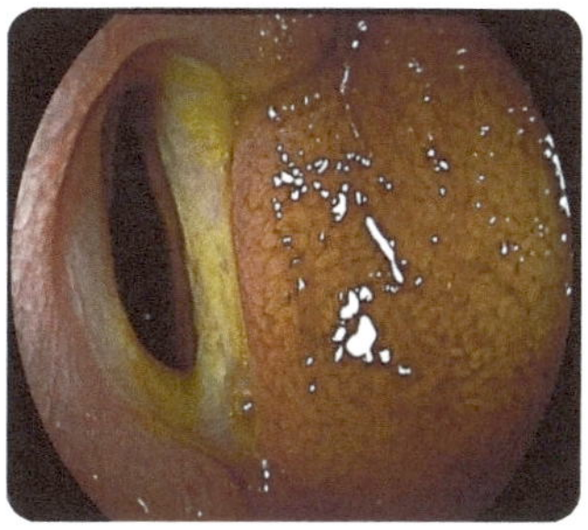

Figure 5b

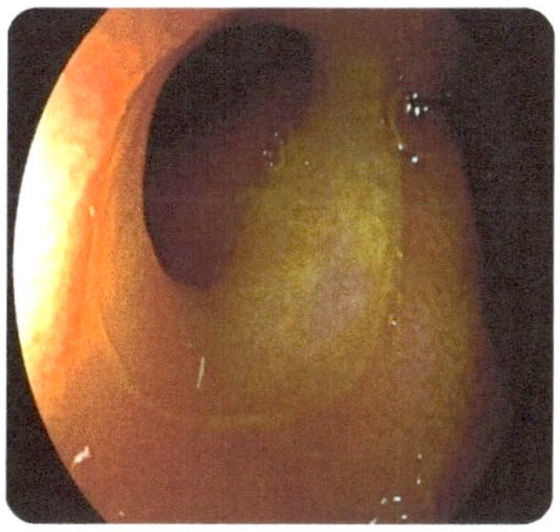

Chapter 20: Chronic Stenosing Enteritis

Charles Woodall, DO and David Cave, MD, PhD, FACG

Introduction

Chronic stenosing enteritis (CSE) is a rare condition with a chronic and relapsing course that causes multifocal ulceration and concentric stenoses/strictures of the mid small intestine.[1] Patients with CSE typically present with symptoms of abdominal pain, iron deficiency anemia, and/or small bowel obstruction.[1] Some patients have mistakenly been diagnosed with Crohn's disease (CD), which has been treated medically and/or surgically without lasting improvement in their symptoms.[1,2] CSE appears to exist as part of a spectrum of prostaglandin-associated enteropathies, which also includes cryptogenic multifocal ulcerative stenosing enteritis (CMUSE) and chronic non-specific stenosing ulcers (CNSU), with the latter of these having been renamed chronic enteropathy associated with *SLCO2A1* gene (CEAS).[1] Disease activity within this group of disorders is isolated to the small bowel, unlike CD, which can involve any segment of the gastrointestinal tract.

Epidemiology

CSE has largely only been described in the United States and India whereas CMUSE is predominantly seen in Europe and Korea and CNSU/CEAS is seen almost exclusively in Japan.[1,2] Epidemiological data for CSE are currently lacking due to its rarity. However, CSE appears to have an approximate 1.2:1 female-to-male prevalence ratio and occurs primarily in Whites based upon data from a published case study.[1] Initial presentations of CSE tend to occur during the fifth decade of life but can start in the second decade of life.[1,2] CSE likely remains under- or misdiagnosed, but is still thought to be an exceedingly rare condition.

Pathophysiology

The pathophysiology of CSE is under investigation but thought to be associated with defects in prostaglandin metabolism. Genetic mutations in *PLA2G4A*, a gene responsible for release of arachidonic acid via hydrolysis of membrane phospholipids, have been associated with multiple cases of CNSU.[1,2,3] Similarly, genetic mutations in *SLCO2A1* resulting in loss of function of a transport protein responsible for prostaglandin reuptake have been associated with CNSU/CEAS.[1,2,3] A recent study of patients with CSE by Cave et al. identified normal expression of *cPLA2A* and anti-PGT (anti-*SLCO2A1*) within 100% of small bowel tissue samples.[1] These findings suggest an undiscovered defect in the prostaglandin pathway is present in cases of CSE. Other disease variants, such as genotypes that are heterozygous for these underlying mutations, could predispose patients to NSAID-induced enteropathy. Such a relationship would link CSE, CMUSE, CNSU/CEAS, and NSAID-induced enteropathy into a spectrum of prostaglandin-associated enteropathy, as is currently theorized.[1]

Diagnosis

Chronic stenosing enteritis and other diseases of this spectrum overlap significantly in regard to their clinical presentations and endoscopic findings but can ultimately be discerned from one another, as well as from other small bowel diseases such CD and NSAID enteropathy. Abdominal pain is the most common presenting symptom shared between CSE and other small bowel disorders.[1,2] Small bowel obstruction is also a common presenting feature across the disease spectrum similar to NSAID-induced enteropathy.[1,2] Patients with CSE do not generally present with weight loss and diarrhea like those with CMUSE, CNSU/CEAS, and CD.[1,2] However iron deficiency often occurs with profound and persistent anemia. Hypoalbuminemia is often seen in patients with CMUSE but is not present in cases of CSE.[1] Extraintestinal manifestations are not seen in CSE, CMUSE, or CNSU/CEAS as may occur in CD. However, some of the Japanese patients with appropriate genetic mutations have primary hypertrophic osteoarthropathy or mild versions of it.[5]

Diagnosis of CSE relies on obtaining a thorough history, endoscopic examination of the small bowel via video capsule endoscopy (VCE), preferably preceded by a patency capsule and/or device-assisted enteroscopy (DAE), and pathologic review of tissue samples. The differential diagnosis of CSE is listed in **Table 1**. Imaging of the small intestine is often unhelpful, because the disease is not transmural and the strictures are short, mimicking valvulae conniventes.

Inflammatory	Drug-induced	Neoplastic	Infectious
Crohn's disease Radiation enteritis Behçet's disease Jejuno-ileitis of celiac disease Eosinophilic gastroenteritis Intestinal ischemia	NSAID-induced enteropathy	Lymphoma (Burkitt, MALT, marginal zone) Adenocarcinoma	Tuberculosis Cytomegalovirus

Table 1. Differential diagnosis for inflammatory or ulcerated small bowel stenosis.

The advent of VCE and DAE, specifically DBE, has allowed for improved accuracy in the diagnosis of prostaglandin-associated enteropathies including CSE. VCE is particularly useful in centers lacking availability of balloon-assisted enteroscopy, but caution must be taken to avoid its use in patients with suspected small bowel stenoses. Ulcerations in CSE are large, superficial, and sometimes circumferential with well-demarcated margins that are free of adjacent villous edema reflecting the lack of transmural involvement.[1,2,4] CSE ulcers are notably not cratered, serpiginous, or longitudinal in appearance like those characteristic of CD and are found distributed among normal mucosa.[1] Multiple ulcers are may be present and limited to an area of the small bowel encompassing the mid-jejunum to the mid-ileum with noted sparing of the terminal ileum in contrast to ulcers and diaphragms in NSAID-induced enteropathy. CMUSE can be found throughout the small intestine while CNSU/CEAS is more commonly found in the distal ileum.[1,4] Concentric stenoses or "diaphragm lesions", similar to cases of NSAID-induced enteropathy, are commonly but not always present. The ulcers present on the stenoses found in CSE are most often active in contrast to the scarred or partially healed ulcers found in NSAID-induced enteropathy.[4] The endoscopic appearance of small bowel strictures in CSE, NSAID enteroscopy, and Crohn's disease differ by pattern of ulceration (**Figures 1-3**).

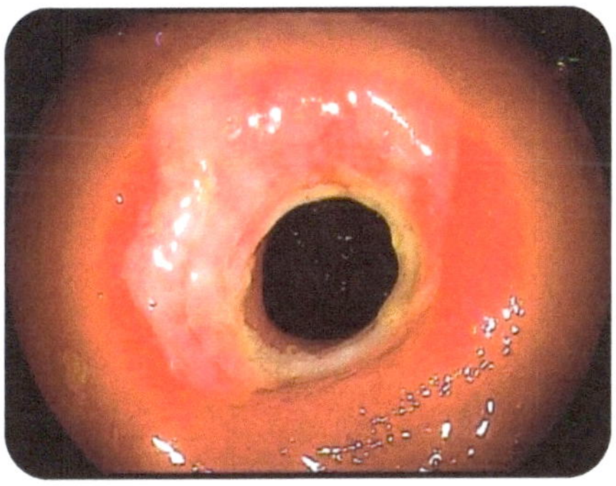

Figure 1. Stenosis of proximal ileum with broad (~3-5mm) concentric ulceration in CSE.

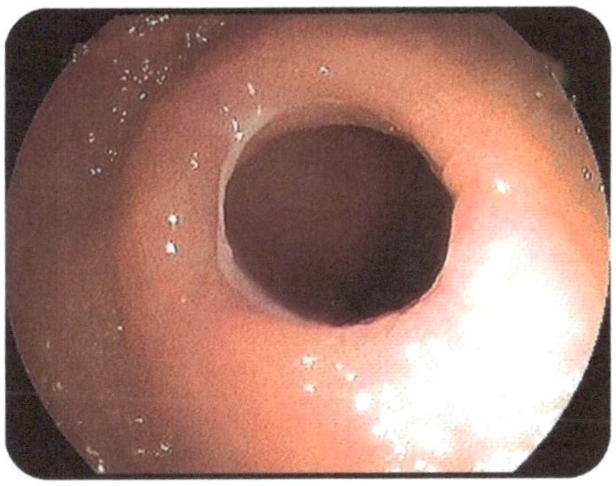

Figure 2. Thin, diaphragm stenosis of the mid ileum observed in NSAID enteropathy

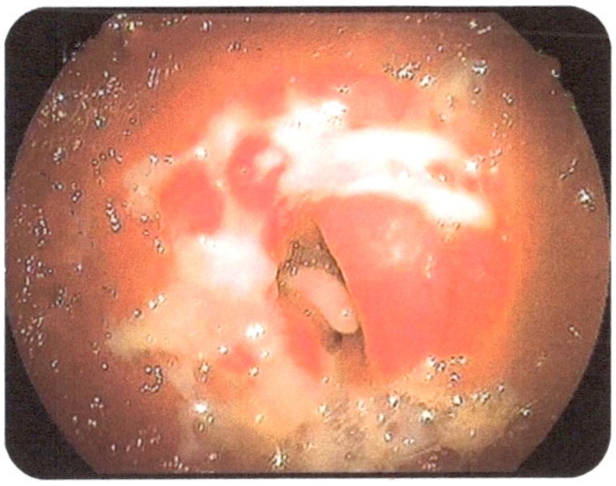

Figure 3. Ulcerated stenosis of the distal ileum in Crohn's disease.

Histopathology plays a central role in confirming the diagnosis of CSE. Characteristic findings include ulcers with clearly delineated margins which are confined to the mucosa and submucosa. Ulceration in CSE is associated with a nonspecific inflammatory infiltrate composed of plasma cells, lymphocytes, and polymorphonuclear cells.[1] Importantly, healthy mucosa is found adjacent to the ulceration.[1,4] Features characteristic of Crohn's disease, such as granuloma formation, fistulization, or transmural involvement, are absent in CSE.[1]

No specific serum or fecal testing currently exists to confirm the diagnosis of CSE, and no inflammatory markers appear to correlate with disease activity.[1] Whole-exome sequencing has been used in previous studies to identify mutations in *SLCO2A1* associated with CNSU/CEAS.[5] Genome-wide single-nucleotide polymorphism homozygosity mapping in combination with whole-exome sequencing has also been used to identify mutations in *PLA2G4A*.[6] Similar studies utilizing whole-exome sequencing are currently in progress to investigate the existence of genetic mutations associated with CSE.

Treatment

Treatment of chronic stenosing enteritis is largely anecdotal and dependent upon severity. DAE may be considered as an intervention in the acute setting to dilate stenoses/strictures.[7] Surgical resection is reserved for those patients with persistent small bowel obstruction or uncontrolled blood loss. Parenteral iron supplementation, as well as blood transfusion, may be required in patients with iron deficiency related to chronic gastrointestinal blood loss from CSE. Biologics have been used in a few cases without benefit, and no significant evidence exists to support corticosteroid therapy in CSE.[7] Misoprostol has demonstrated efficacy in treating NSAID-induced enteropathy in clinical trials but has not been investigated in CEAS.[8,9]

Conclusion

Chronic stenosing enteritis is a rare disease with a relapsing-remitting course. It belongs to a spectrum of ulcerative/stenosing small bowel diseases which can be clinically and pathologically differentiated from small bowel Crohn's disease and NSAID-induced enteropathy. Some patients with CSE have previously been misdiagnosed with CD and treated with small bowel resection. A genetic association for CSE has not yet been discovered, but whole-exome sequencing is currently being used to identify a specific genetic mutation. VCE and DAE are essential tools required to examine the deep small bowel for diagnosis and monitoring of CSE

References

1. Cave DR, Hanscom M, Bledsoe J, et al. Chronic stenosing enteritis: A variant of chronic non-specific stenosing ulceration (CNSU) that is distinct from crohn's disease. Dig Dis Sci. 2025;70(4):1449-1456.
2. Woodall CB, Raines D. S4842 CMUSE in the United States: A case series. Am J Gastroenterol. 2024;119(10S):p S3054-S3055.
3. Modi R, Storozuk T, Setia N. Genetic mutations and small bowel ulcerating disease: Role in diagnosis? Curr Gastroenterol Rep. 2025;27(1):33.
4. Matsumoto T, Nakamura S, Esaki M, et al. Endoscopic features of chronic nonspecific multiple ulcers of the small intestine: Comparison with nonsteroidal anti-inflammatory drug-induced enteropathy. Dig Dis Sci. 2006;51(8):1357-1363.
5. Umeno J, Hisamatsu T, Esaki M, et al. A hereditary enteropathy caused by mutations in the SLCO2A1 gene, encoding a prostaglandin transporter. PLoS Genet. 2015;11(11):e1005581.
6. Brooke MA, Longhurst HJ, Plagnol V, et al. Cryptogenic multifocal ulcerating stenosing enteritis associated with homozygous deletion mutations in cytosolic phospholipase A2-α. Gut. 2014;63(1):96-104.
7. Chung SH, Jo Y, Ryu SR, et al. Diaphragm disease compared with cryptogenic multifocal ulcerous stenosing enteritis. World J Gastroenterol. 2011;17(23):2873-2876.
8. Taha AS, McCloskey C, McSkimming P, McConnachie A. Misoprostol for small bowel ulcers in patients with obscure bleeding taking aspirin and non-steroidal anti-inflammatory drugs (MASTERS): A randomized, double-blind, placebo-controlled, phase 3 trial. Lancet Gastroenterol Hepatol. 2018;3(7):469-476.
9. Raskin JB, White RH, Jackson JE, et al. Misoprostol dosage in the prevention of nonsteroidal anti-inflammatory drug-induced gastric and duodenal ulcers: A comparison of three regimens. Ann Intern Med. 1995;123(5):344-350.

Case Study Number 21

Presented by Suzanne K. Lewis, MD and Peter H.R. Green, MD

Pre-capsule Findings (included in capsule study)

A 17-year-old man with a history of hemophilia presents to clinic with his parents for evaluation of a new diagnosis of anemia (serum hemoglobin = 11 g/dl) associated with a ferritin of 8 ng/ml (normal = 30-330 ng/ml). During interview, the patient admits to symptoms of watery diarrhea up to 4 episodes per day over the past few years. He denies associated rectal bleeding, vomiting, or weight loss. Medications include lisdexamfetamine (Vyvanse) for attention-deficit/hyperactivity disorder and ibuprofen 400 mg for occasional headache or muscle pain once per month, on average. His parents deny any family history of celiac disease or inflammatory bowel disease. Physical exam is unremarkable. Initial serologic studies include an elevated anti-TTG IgA antibody level of 86 U/ml (normal <20 U/ml). Following discussion of the results with the patient and his family, a video capsule endoscopy is ordered as an alternative to upper endoscopy with small bowel biopsy, given concerns about excessive bleeding in the setting of hemophilia.

A capsule endoscopy study is performed during evaluation for celiac disease. Review the capsule endoscopy study and report your findings, including: gastric passage time, small bowel passage time, and observed abnormalities. Be prepared to discuss your findings and management plan with your staff prior to reviewing the diagnosis and case discussion.

Capsule Endoscopy Findings
First Gastric Image = 0h 1min 3sec
First Duodenal Image = 0h 29min 38sec
Gastric passage time = 0h 28min
First Cecal Image = 2h 47min 21sec
Small bowel passage time = 2hr 28min

The capsule transiently enters the duodenal bulb then refluxes into the stomach prior to a second entry into the duodenum. The mucosa of the duodenum and proximal jejunum are grossly abnormal. Mucosal changes consistent with celiac disease are observed, including mosaic mucosal pattern (**Figure 1:** 0hr 36min 37sec), mucosal fissuring (**Figure 2:** 0hr 50min 29sec), and scalloped folds (**Figure 3:** 0hr 51min 15sec). The changes improve as the capsule passes into the mid-distal jejunum around 1hr 12min.

Follow Up

A diagnosis of celiac disease was confirmed by the results of this capsule study combined with positive celiac antibody testing. A gluten free diet was initiated in consultation with a dietitian experienced in celiac disease. The patient's diarrhea improves over the following 12 months with normalization of serum hemoglobin (14 g/dl) and decrease in anti-TTG IgA antibody levels to less than 20 U/ml.

Figure 1

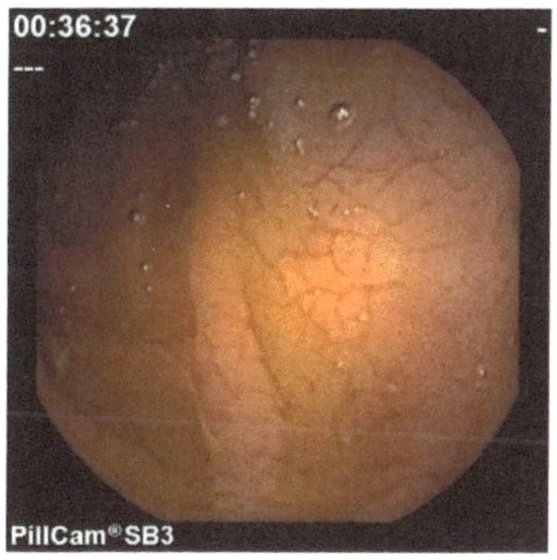

Figure 2

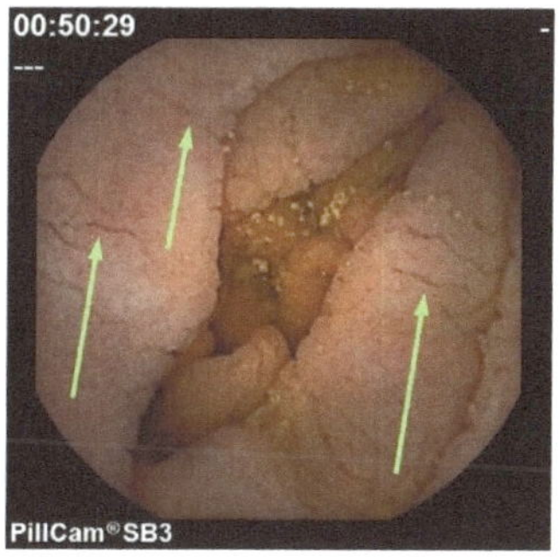

Figure 3

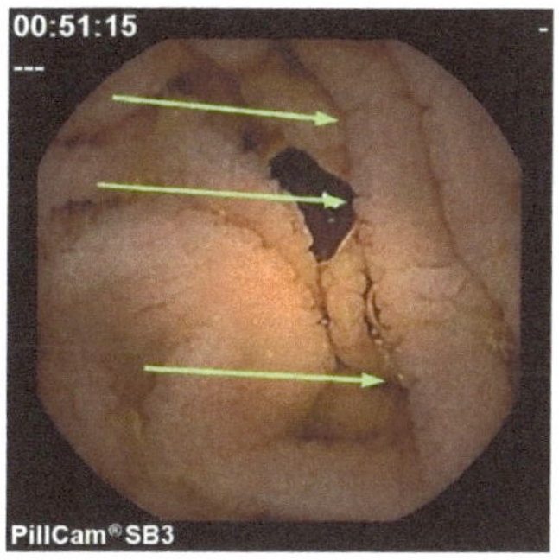

Chapter 21: Celiac Disease

Suzanne K. Lewis, MD and Peter H.R. Green, MD

Introduction

Celiac disease is a common autoimmune disease triggered in genetically predisposed individuals by the reaction to gluten, a protein component of wheat, rye, and barley.[1] Celiac disease was once considered a rare malabsorptive disorder of children, but is now recognized to be a common disease affecting approximately 1% of the population.[2] The incidence of celiac disease appears to be increasing over the past 50 years and may be associated with increased mortality when untreated.[3,4]

Pathophysiology

Celiac disease results from an abnormal T-cell mediated immune response to indigestible peptides in wheat gluten proteins (gliadins and glutenins), as well as gluten-like proteins in barley (hordeins) and rye (secalins).[5] The 33-amino-acid fragment of α2-gliadin is the best-characterized and most immunogenic peptide in celiac disease. Gliadin is deamidated by the enzyme tissue transglutaminase (TTG) in both the intestinal lumen and the intestinal lamina propria.[6] Deamidated gliadin interacts with gluten-sensitive T cells in the lamina propria expressing DQ2 or DQ8 molecules.[7,8] Activation of these cells results in T cell proliferation and production of inflammatory cytokines leading to inflammation and subsequent intestinal damage.

Clinical Presentation

Patients with celiac disease may present with classical (diarrhea-predominant) symptoms, atypical symptoms or may be asymptomatic and detected via screening.[9 10] Increased clinical suspicion of this diagnosis is appropriate for individuals with a first degree relative with celiac disease, as the incidence is increased to approximately 10%.[11] The incidence of celiac disease is approximately 4 times higher in patients diagnosed with irritable bowel syndrome.[12] Therefore, recent guidelines by the American College of Gastroenterology suggest all patients with irritable bowel syndrome (diarrhea or mixed) be screened for celiac disease.[13]

Diagnosis

Screening for celiac disease may be performed via serological testing. Individuals should be considered for screening if they have a family history of celiac disease or if they have unexplained symptoms as listed in **Table 1**. Screening should also be considered in individuals with Down Syndrome, Turner's Syndrome, and Type 1 Diabetes as celiac disease is more common in these populations.[14] Serology for the antibodies directed against tissue transglutaminase (TTG IgA) is the best screening test for celiac disease.[15] A serum IgA level should also be obtained to exclude IgA deficiency as IgA deficiency is more common in celiac patients and may result in a false negative screening result.[16] In patients with IgA deficiency, IgG antibodies to tissue transglutaminase should be obtained.[17] Testing for anti-endomysial antibody (EMA) is accurate with a high specificity for celiac disease but is expensive and labor intensive.[18] An assay to detect IgA and IgG antibodies specific for the deamidated gliadin peptide has high diagnostic accuracy.[19] but the sensitivity appears slightly decreased compared to TTG antibodies in a recent meta-analysis.[20] Antibodies usually become negative within 6-12 months of starting a gluten-free diet thus serology is not reliable in patients who are already on a gluten-free diet.

Diarrhea	Vomiting
Abdominal bloating	Abdominal Pain
Constipation	Gastroesophageal Reflux
Aphthous stomatitis	Dental Enamel Defects
Fatigue	Infertility
Anemia	Elevated Liver Enzymes
Rash (dermatitis herpetiformis)	Neurological (ataxia, neuropathy)
Hypocalcemia	Osteoporosis
Delayed puberty	Iron, folate, or other vitamin deficiency

Table 1. Manifestations of Celiac Disease

Genetic testing is available for the HLA DQ2 and DQ8 alleles associated with celiac disease. The HLA DQ2 and DQ8 alleles associated with celiac disease are present in almost all patients with celiac disease but are also found in individuals without celiac disease.[21] Genetic testing is helpful in excluding celiac disease with a negative predictive value of approximately 97%.[22] Genetic testing is useful when the diagnosis of celiac disease is uncertain, a patient has been on a gluten-free diet for an extended period of time, or to determine if family members have the potential to develop the disease. A positive genetic test does not diagnose celiac disease since the alleles are present in a significant percentage of the population. Genetic testing is available via commercial labs in the United States using samples of blood, buccal cells, or saliva.

The current gold standard for diagnosing celiac disease is upper endoscopy with small bowel biopsy. Patients with positive serology should have an upper endoscopy performed with 4-6 biopsies of the small intestine.[23] If the suspicion for celiac disease is high, an endoscopy with biopsy should be performed regardless of serology results. To maximize diagnostic yield, biopsies should be obtained in both the bulb and the second portion of the duodenum. The term ultra short celiac disease has been coined for celiac disease that is confined to the duodenal bulb.[24] It is therefore important to separate bulb from the second part of the duodenum during endoscopy. Endoscopic findings of celiac disease include villous atrophy, scalloping of folds, loss of folds, a mosaic pattern, and fissuring.[25,26] Biopsies should be obtained even if the duodenum appears endoscopically normal as findings may only be present on histology. A grading system to classify the various histological changes associated with celiac disease was originally proposed by Marsh[27] and later refined by Oberhuber[28] (**Table 2**).

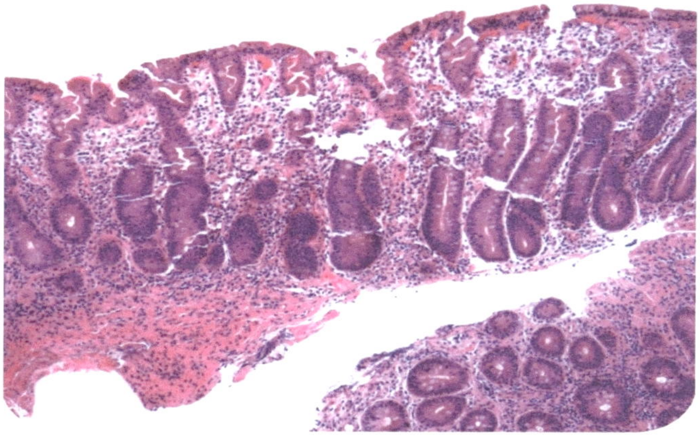

Figure 1. Histology from duodenal biopsy demonstrating increased intraepithelial lymphocytes, crypt hyperplasia, and total villous atrpny. *Image courtesy of Govind Bhagat, MD.*

Histologic changes include increased intraepithelial lymphocytosis, crypt hyperplasia, and villous atrophy (**Figure 1**). Endoscopic biopsies of the proximal duodenum are imperfect for the diagnosis of celiac disease due to several factors. Patchy disease involvement may result in sampling error. Histologic evaluation may be complicated by poor specimen orientation, lack of observer experience or presence of another condition resulting in histologic changes suggestive of celiac. Intraepithelial lymphocytosis can be caused by other conditions including infection with *Helicobacter pylori* and medications, such as aspirin and non-steroidal anti-inflammatory drugs.[29] Villous atrophy can also be caused by autoimmune enteropathy, bacterial overgrowth, common variable immunodeficiency, Crohn's disease, gastroenteritis, giardiasis, graft versus host disease, HIV enteropathy,

Marsh 0	Normal mucosa
Marsh 1	Increased intraepithelial lymphocytosis * - Normal crypt - Normal villi
Marsh 2	Increased intraepithelial lymphocytosis * - Crypt hyperplasia - Normal villi
Marsh 3a	Increased intraepithelial lymphocytosis * - Crypt hyperplasia - Partial (mild) villous atrophy
Marsh 3b	Increased intraepithelial lymphocytosis * - Crypt hyperplasia - Subtotal (marked) villous atrophy
Marsh 3c	Increased intraepithelial lymphocytosis * - Crypt hyperplasia - Total villous atrophy (villi absent)

Table 2. Modified Marsh criteria to describe the histologic changes in celiac disease. *Adapted from Oberhuber et al.*[48]

Mycobacterium tuberculosis, peptic duodenitis, radiation enteritis, eosinophilic gastroenteritis, tropical sprue and Whipple's disease. Medications causing villous atrophy include non-steroidal anti-inflammatory drugs,[3] azathioprine methotrexate, mycophenolate mofetil, angiotensin-2-receptor-blockers (A2RBs), such as olmesartan, and more recently immune checkpoint inhibitors.[30,31]

Video capsule endoscopy is a useful, non-invasive study for both the initial assessment and subsequent monitoring of celiac disease in select cases. Capsule endoscopy visualizes the entire small intestine, but symptom severity does not correlate with the extent of small bowel involvement.[32] Extent of villous atrophy on capsule endoscopy was greater in those with refractory celiac disease and correlated with malabsorption of vitamin B12 and folate.[33]

Capsule endoscopy can assist in the initial evaluation of suspected celiac disease in those unable or unwilling to undergo upper endoscopy and in those with positive celiac serology (TTG, EMA) and normal duodenal biopsies.[34] Features of celiac disease observed on capsule endoscopy include scalloping of folds, fissures, flat mucosa, layering of folds, and a mosaic pattern (**Figures 2a-d**).[35] Capsule endoscopy has a reported sensitivity of 87.5% and specificity of 90.9% in assessing for features of celiac disease as compared to the gold standard of small bowel biopsy.[36] Capsule endoscopy can also be performed when there is suspicion of complicated or refractory disease to exclude malignancy or ulcerative jejunitis. Capsule endoscopy does have some important limitations in the evaluation of celiac disease. It cannot be used to obtain biopsies or perform therapy. Partial villous atrophy may not be appreciated. Capsule interpretation is subjective and interobserver agreement may be poor among capsule readers with limited exposure to capsule endoscopy.[36] There is much potential for the use of artificial intelligence in increasing diagnostic accuracy in celiac disease. Quantitative image analysis using standardized, computer-based software provide a non subjective assessment of villous height.[37] CNN based deep learning methods are being developed and have shown good sensitivity and specificity in small studies.[37,38,39]

Figure 2a-d. Findings on capsule endoscpy in celiac disease.

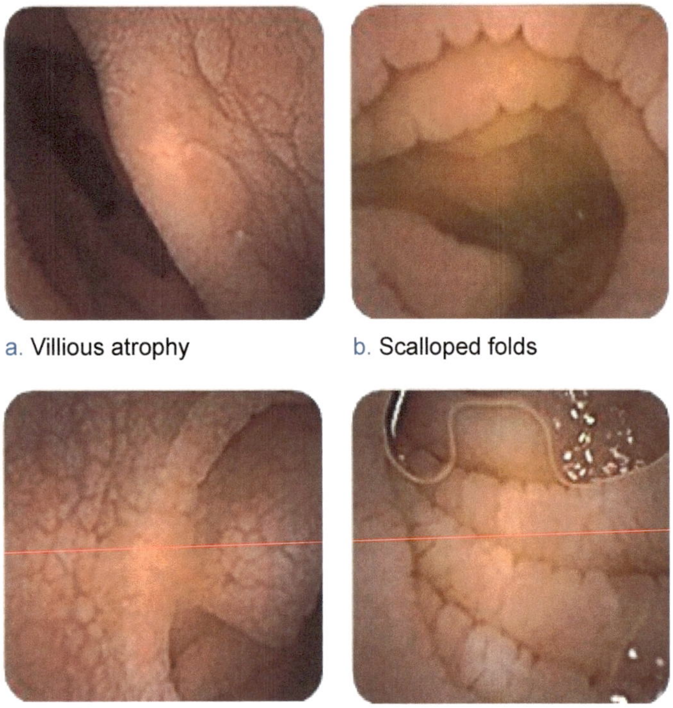

a. Villious atrophy
b. Scalloped folds
c. Mosaic pattern
d. Stacking of folds

Treatment

The only treatment for celiac disease is currently a strict gluten-free diet. Adherence to the diet improves symptoms in the majority of patients, but adherence is variable. Approximately 30% of patients experience continued symptoms on a gluten-free diet, most often due to continued gluten ingestion.[40,41] The gluten-free diet is expensive, socially restrictive, and may be lacking in certain nutritional components, such as fiber.[40,41,42] Patients with celiac disease should meet with a dietician with expertise in the gluten-free diet, however, the availability of expert dietary counseling appears to be limited.[43,44]

Nondietary therapies for celiac disease are in active development targeting points in the pathogenesis of celiac disease. These future drugs could complement or potentially replace a gluten free diet, however, none are as yet approved for use. Glutenases, such as latiglutenase, degrade immunogenic gluten peptides in the gut lumen and have been shown to improve mucosal morphology and symptoms during gluten challenge.[45] Intestinal barrier modulators are being studied to help tighten epithelial tight junctions to block intestinal permeability to gluten peptides.[46] Other therapies under studied include inhibitors of tissue transglutaminase (TTG2 inhibitors), immunotherapies to induce immune tolerance; and immunomodulators that target inflammatory cytokines (anti IL-15).[47]

Conclusion

Celiac disease is an immune-mediated enteropathy precipitated by dietary gluten in genetically predisposed individuals. Upper endoscopy with biopsy of the duodenal mucosa remains the standard for diagnosis. However, video capsule endoscopy has demonstrated utility in the initial evaluation of suspected celiac disease in patients who are unable or unwilling to undergo upper endoscopy, or in those with positive serologic markers (TTG, EMA) but normal duodenal biopsies. Capsule endoscopy may also be used to detect complications such as ulcerative jejunitis or lymphoma, and to monitor for mucosal healing in select cases. Novel therapeutic approaches targeting key checkpoints in the immune response are under active investigation and may, in the future, allow patients with celiac disease to tolerate dietary gluten.

References

1. Lebwohl B, Sanders DS, Green PHR. Coeliac disease. Lancet. 2018;391(10115):70-81.
2. Fasano A, Berti I, Gerarduzzi T, et al. Prevalence of celiac disease in at-risk and not-at-risk groups in the United States: a large multicenter study. Arch Intern Med. 2003;163(3):286-92.
3. Rubio-Tapia A, Kyle RA, Kaplan Elet al. Increased prevalence and mortality in undiagnosed celiac disease. Gastroenterology. 2009;137(1):88-93.
4. Ludvigsson JF, Montgomery SM, Ekbom A, Brandt L, Granath F. Small-intestinal histopathology and mortality risk in celiac disease. JAMA. 2009;302(11):1171-8.
5. Shan L, Molberg Ø, Parrot I, et al. Structural basis for gluten intolerance in celiac sprue. Science. 2002;297(5590):2275-9.
6. Meling MT, Kleppa L, Besser HA, Khosla C, du Pré MF, Sollid LM. Enterocyte-derived and catalytically active transglutaminase 2 in the gut lumen of mice: Implications for celiac disease. Gastroenterology. 2024;167(5):1026-1028.e4.
7. Molberg O, Mcadam SN, Körner R, et al. Tissue transglutaminase selectively modifies gliadin peptides that are recognized by gut-derived T cells in celiac disease. Nat Med. 1998;4(6):713-7.
8. Qiao SW, Bergseng E, Molberg Ø, Xia J, Fleckenstein B, Khosla C, Sollid LM. Antigen presentation to celiac lesion-derived T cells of a 33-mer gliadin peptide naturally formed by gastrointestinal digestion. J Immunol. 2004;173(3):1757-62.
9. Lo W, Sano K, Lebwohl B, Diamond B, Green PH. Changing presentation of adult celiac disease. Dig Dis Sci. 2003;48(2):395-8.
10. Green PH. The many faces of celiac disease: clinical presentation of celiac disease in the adult population. Gastroenterology. 2005;128(4 Suppl 1):S74-8.
11. Ford AC, Chey WD, Talley NJ, Malhotra A, Spiegel BM, Moayyedi P. Yield of diagnostic tests for celiac disease in individuals with symptoms suggestive of irritable bowel syndrome: systematic review and meta-analysis. Arch Intern Med. 2009;169(7):651-8.
12. Dubé C, Rostom A, Sy R, et al. The prevalence of celiac disease in average-risk and at-risk Western European populations: a systematic review. Gastroenterology. 2005;128(4 Suppl 1):S57-67.
13. Rubio-Tapia A, Hill ID, Semrad C, Kelly CP, Greer KB, Limketkai BN, Lebwohl B. American College of Gastroenterology Guidelines Update: Diagnosis and Management of Celiac Disease. Am J Gastroenterol. 2023;118(1):59-76. Erratum in: Am J Gastroenterol. 2024 Jul 1;119(7):1441.
14. Crowe SE. In the clinic. Celiac disease. Ann Intern Med. 2011;154(9):ITC5-1-ITC5-15.
15. Rostom A, Dubé C, Cranney A, et al. The diagnostic accuracy of serologic tests for celiac disease: a systematic review. Gastroenterology. 2005;128(4 Suppl 1):S38-46.
16. Cataldo F, Marino V, Ventura A, Bottaro G, Corazza GR. Prevalence and clinical features of selective immunoglobulin A deficiency in celiac disease. Gut. 1998; 42: 362-365.
17. Korponay-Szab6 IR, Dahlbom I, Laurila K, et al. Elevation of IgG antibodies against tissue transglutaminase as a diagnostic tool for coeliac disease in selective IgA deficiency. Gut. 2003; 52: 1567-1571.
18. Lewis NR, Scott BB. Systemic review: The use of serology to exclude or diagnose coeliac disease (a comparison of the endomysial and tissue transglutaminase antibody tests). Aliment Pharmacol Ther. 2006; 24:47-54.
19. Kaukinen K, Collin P, Laurila K, Kaartinen T, Partanen J, Maki M. Resurrection of gliadin antibodies in coeliac disease. Deamidated gliadin peptide antibody test provides additional diagnostic benefit. Scand J Gastroenterol. 2007; 42:1428-1433.
20. Lewis NR, Scott BB. Meta-analysis: deamidated gliadin peptide antibody and tissue transglutaminase antibody compared as screening tests for coeliac disease. Aliment Pharmacol Ther. 2010;31(1):73-81.
21. Sollid LM, Markussen G, Ek J, et al. Evidence for a primary association of celiac disease to a particular HLA-DQ alpha/beta heterodimer. J Exp Med. 1989;

169: 345-350.
22. Hadithi M, von Blomberg BM, Crusius JB, et al. Accuracy of serologic tests and HLA-DQ typing for diagnosing celiac disease. Ann Intern Med. 2007;147(5):294-302.
23. Rostom A, Murray JA, Kagnoff MF. American Gastroenterological Association (AGA) Institute technical review on the diagnosis and management of celiac disease. Gastroenterology. 2006;131(6):1981-2002.
24. Raju SA, Greenaway EA, Schiepatti A, et al. New entity of adult ultra-short coeliac disease: the first international cohort and case-control study. Gut. 2024;73(7):1124-1130.
25. Magazzu G, Bottari M, Tuccari G, et al. Upper gastrointestinal endoscopy can be a reliable screening tool for celiac sprue in adults. J Clin Gastro 1994; 19:255-257.
26. Mauriño E, Capizzano H, Niveloni S, Kogan Z, Valero J, Boerr L, Bai JC. Value of endoscopic markers in celiac disease. Dig Dis Sci. 1993;38(11):2028-33.
27. Marsh MN. Gluten, major histocompatibility complex, and the small intestine. A molecular and immunobiologic approach to the spectrum of gluten sensitivity ('celiac sprue'). Gastroenterology. 1992;102(1):330-54.
28. Oberhuber G, Granditsch, Vogelsang H. The histopathology of coeliac disease: a time for a standardized report scheme for pathologists. Eur Journal of Gastro Hepatol 1999, 11:1185-1194.
29. Aziz I, Evans KE, Hopper AD, Smillie DM, Sanders DS. A prospective study into the aetiology of lymphocytic duodenosis. Alimen Pharma Ther 2010; 32: 1392-1397.
30. Mi K, Cao S, Adams D. Non-celiac Enteropathies. Curr Gastroenterol Rep. 2025;27(1):27.
31. Schiepatti A, Premoli A, Maimaris S, et al. Small bowel villous atrophy due to immune-checkpoint inhibitors: report of two cases and literature review. Drugs Context. 2022;11:2022-6-3.
32. Cellier C, Green PH, Collin P, Murray J; ICCE. ICCE consensus for celiac disease. Endoscopy. 2005;37(10):1055-9.
33. Chetcuti Zammit S, Kurien M, Sanders DS, Sidhu R. What is the role of small bowel capsule endoscopy in established coeliac disease? Clin Res Hepatol Gastroenterol. 2020;44(5):753-761.
34. Rondonotti E, Spada C, Cave D, et al. Video capsule enteroscopy in the diagnosis of celiac disease: A multicenter study. Am J Gastroenterol. 2007; 102:1624-1631.
35. Ciaccio EJ, Tennyson CA, Lewis SK, Krishnareddy S, Bhagat G, Green PH. Distinguishing patients with celiac disease by quantitative analysis of videocapsule endoscopy images. Comput Methods Programs Biomed. 2010;100(1):39-48.
36. Petroniene R, Dubcenco E, Baker JP, et al. Given capsule endoscopy in celiac disease: evaluation of diagnostic accuracy and interobserver agreement. Am J Gastroenterol. 2005;100(3):685-94.
37. Zhou T, Han G, Li BN, et al. Quantitative analysis of patients with celiac disease by video capsule endoscopy: A deep learning method. Comput Biol Med. 2017 1;85:1-6.
38. Wang X, Qian H, Ciaccio EJ, et al. Celiac disease diagnosis from videocapsule endoscopy images with residual learning and deep feature extraction. Comput Methods Programs Biomed. 2020;187:105236.
39. Ciaccio EJ, Lewis SK, Bhagat G, Green PH. Color masking improves classification of celiac disease in videocapsule endoscopy images. Comput Biol Med. 2019;106:150-156.
40. O'Mahony S, Howdle PD, Losowsky MS et al. Review article: management of patients with non-responsive coeliac disease. Aliment Pharmacol Ther. 1996;10: 671-680.
41. Abdulkarim AS, Burgart LJ, See J, Murray JA. Etiology of nonresponsive celiac disease: results of a systematic approach. Am J Gastroenterol. 2002;97(8):2016-21.
42. Lee AR, Ng DL, Zivin J, Green PH. Economic burden of a gluten-free diet. J Hum Nutr Diet. 2007;20(5):423-30.
43. Thompson T, Dennis M, Higgins LA, Lee AR, Sharrett MK. Gluten-free diet survey: are Americans with coeliac disease consuming recommended amounts of fibre, iron, calcium and grain foods? J Hum Nutr Diet. 2005;18(3):163-9.
44. Nelson M, Mendoza N, McGough N. A survey of provision of dietetic services for coeliac disease in the UK. J Hum Nutr Diet. 2007;20(5):403-11.
45. Murray JA, Syage JA, Wu TT, et al. Latiglutenase Protects the Mucosa and Attenuates Symptom Severity in Patients With Celiac Disease Exposed to a Gluten Challenge. Gastroenterology. 2022;163(6):1510-1521.e6.
46. Kelly CP, Green PH, Murray JA, et al. Larazotide acetate in patients with coeliac disease undergoing a gluten challenge: a randomised placebo-controlled study. Aliment Pharmacol Ther. 2013;37(2):252-62.
47. Discepolo V, Kelly CP, Koning F, Schuppan D. How Future Pharmacologic Therapies for Celiac Disease Will Complement the Gluten-Free Diet. Gastroenterology. 2024;167(1):90-103.
48. Oberhuber G, Granditsch G, Vogelsang H. The histopathology of coeliac disease: time for a standardized report scheme for pathologists. Eur J Gastroenterol Hepatol. 1999;11(10):1185-94.

Case Study Number 22

Presented by David Hass, MD, FACG and Daniel Raines, MD, FACG

Pre-capsule Findings (included in capsule study)

A 59-year-old man with a past medical history significant for hypertension, coronary artery disease, and prostate cancer presents for further evaluation of complicated celiac disease. He was initially diagnosed with celiac disease 18 months ago during an evaluation for chronic diarrhea. Duodenal biopsies at that time showed typical histologic features of celiac disease including increased intra-epithelial lymphocytes, crypt hyperplasia, and total villous atrophy (Marsh 3c). The patient's diarrhea has failed to improve despite adherence to a strict gluten free diet (GFD) and counseling by an experienced dietitian. He has lost 40 lbs over the past year following transition to a GFD. Serologic testing for anti-TTG IgA is negative on a GFD. Repeat duodenal biopsies obtained by upper endoscopy 8 weeks ago demonstrate persistent, severe villous atrophy. The patient currently denies any recent travel or change in medications. He has no family history of celiac disease, inflammatory bowel disease or colorectal cancer. Physical exam is remarkable for an underweight male wearing loose fitting clothes.

A capsule endoscopy study is performed for evaluation of a case of complicated celiac disease.. Review the capsule endoscopy study and report your findings, including: gastric passage time, small bowel passage time, and observed abnormalities. Be prepared to discuss your findings and management plan with your staff prior to reviewing the diagnosis and case discussion.

The capsule is placed endoscopically into the duodenal bulb. Within the duodenum, a small (6 mm) ulcer is observed in the duodenal bulb followed by small amounts of red blood associated with sites of recent endoscopic biopsy. Areas of mucosal scalloping are observed early in the study (**Figure 1:** 0hr 30min 4sec). Multiple frames of the jejunum capture a pattern of mucosal folds which are adherent to each other or "stacked" close together. (**Figure 2:** 0hr 47min 4sec; **Figure 3:** 0hr 56min 1sec) The mucosa of the deep small bowel is grossly atrophic along its entire length. (**Figure 4:** 2hr 30min 7sec) Capsule transit is slow through the small bowel to reach the cecum in 10 hours. The study is negative for evidence of mass lesions or areas of ulceration to suggest lymphoma.

Figure 1

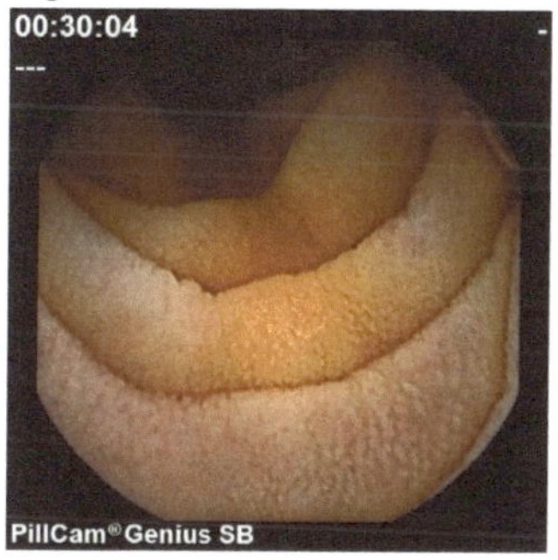

Figure 2

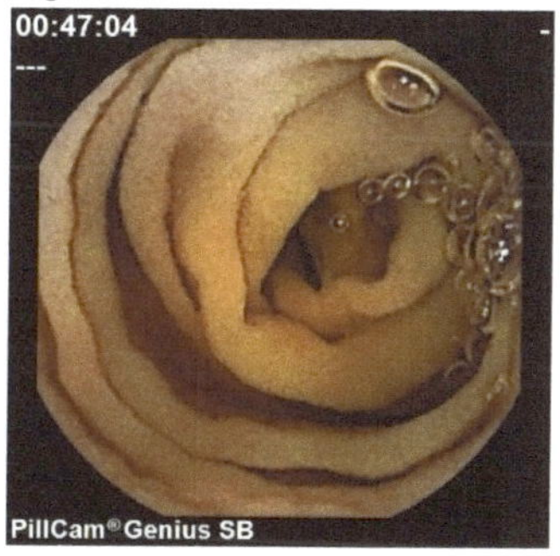

Figure 3

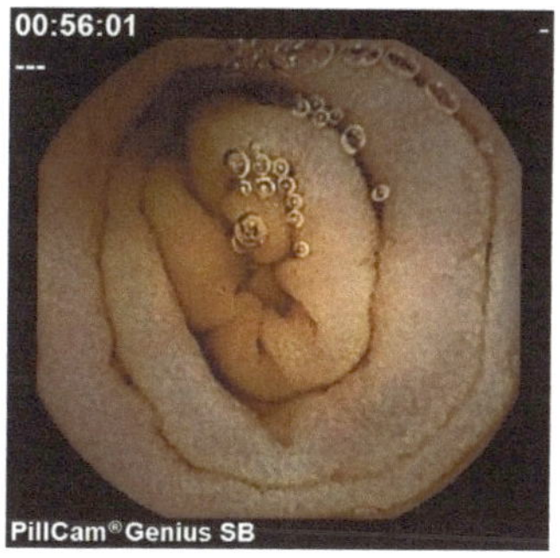

Figure 4

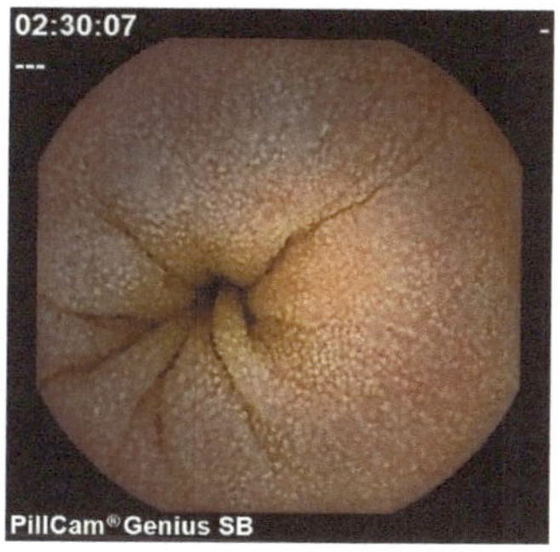

Capsule Endoscopy Findings
First Duodenal Image = 0h 3min 21sec
Gastric passage time = *Endoscopic capsule placement*
First Cecal Image = 10h 22min 50sec
Small bowel passage time = 10hr 19min

Follow-up

A survey of the patient's prior treatment for prostate cancer was negative for radiation therapy. His medications were reviewed, including prescription and non-prescription drugs. Olmesartan was identified as a potential cause of villous atrophy, diarrhea, and weight loss. This medication was withdrawn due to concern for drug-induced enteropathy and lack of indication with a reduced blood pressure (108/60 mmHg). Genetic testing was ordered for the presence of human leukocyte antigens (HLA) alleles DQ2 or DQ8. At clinic follow-up 1 month later, the patient reported that his diarrhea improved dramatically, and his weight had stabilized. Testing was negative for HLA DQ2 and HLA DQ8 alleles.

Chapter 22: Seronegative Villous Atrophy (SNVA)

David Hass, MD, FACG and Daniel Raines, MD, FACG

Introduction

The small intestine is a vast repository of absorptive surface area consisting of circular folds, villi, and microvilli. It serves as the primary site of absorption of organic nutrients (carbohydrates, proteins, fats, vitamins) and inorganic nutrients (minerals). Disease of the small intestine, or "enteropathy," may impact nutrient absorption. Video capsule endoscopy can detect gross features of small bowel mucosal damage, such as scalloping, fissuring, and mosaic appearance. Histologically, this corresponds to villous atrophy. Cases of small bowel villous atrophy with negative testing for celiac antibodies are classified as seronegative villous atrophy (SNVA). This chapter will review etiologies of villous atrophy which cannot be readily attributed to celiac disease.

Etiologies of Non-Celiac Villous Atrophy

Medication-Induced Villous Atrophy

Medications may lead to damage of the intestinal mucosa. The most well-known association of this phenomenon is that of angiotensin II receptor blockers (ARBs). Olmesartan is an angiotensin II receptor antagonist which has been prescribed for the treatment of hypertension since 2002.[1] The association of olmesartan therapy with symptoms of diarrhea and weight loss was formally described by Tapia-Rubio et al. in 2012, in which 22 cases of SNVA associated with olmesartan use were reported[1] (**Figure 1**). This cohort of patients developed symptoms of chronic diarrhea and weight loss. Although onset of symptoms correlated poorly with initiation of olmesartan therapy (range of 6 months to 7 years), resolution of diarrhea following suspension of olmesartan was observed in all cases. Several clinical features listed in this study now serve as criteria for defining enteropathy associated with olmesartan including chronic diarrhea, weight loss, histologic evidence of villous atrophy, and negative testing for anti-tissue transglutaminase (anti-TTG) IgA antibodies in the absence of IgA deficiency. A publication by the same Mayo clinic group in 2014 provided additional pertaining to enteropathy associated with the ARB drug class.[2] Further, additional retrospective case series and case reports have added to the clinical evidence of ARB medications as a cause of enteropathy.[1,3,4,6,7,8]

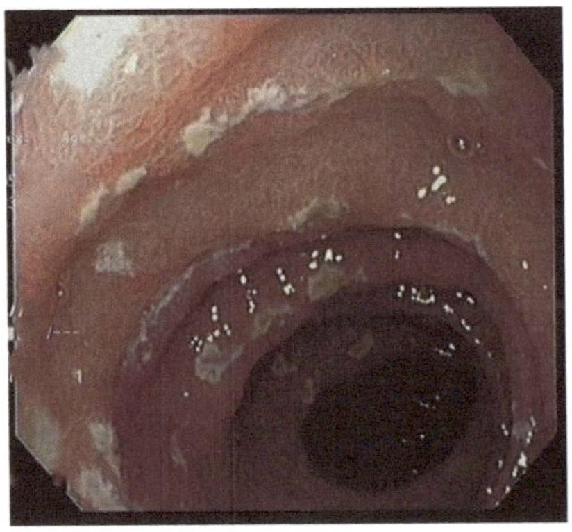

Figure 1. Olmesartan associated villous atrophy observed by enteroscopy.

Medication-induced SNVA has been reported with other drug classes. Azathioprine has been reported as a cause of chronic diarrhea associated with villous atrophy which develops and resolves within several weeks of drug initiation and withdrawal, respectively.[9] Chronic diarrhea associated with duodenal villous atrophy has also been reported to be associated with mycophenolate mofetil, methotrexate, and oxcarbazepine.[10,11] Recently, immune checkpoint inhibitor therapies have been identified as a cause of SNVA.[12]

The frequency of medication-related enteropathy diagnoses varies significantly between 2 large studies of SNVA. In a retrospective study of 72 patients with SNVA, 19 patients (26%) were diagnosed with medication-related villous atrophy including 16 patients with unclassified sprue whom the researchers "reclassified" as olmesartan associated enteropathy, presumably due to discovery of olmesartan on a medication list. A larger, prospective study of 200 patients with SNVA encountered between 2000 to 2015 classified only 13 patients (6.5%) with medication-related villous atrophy.[13]

Autoimmune Enteropathy

Autoimmune enteropathy (AIE) is rare disease observed in both children and adults which manifests as intractable diarrhea coupled with small bowel villous atrophy, lack of improvement with a GFD and positive testing for anti-enterocyte antibodies and/or anti-goblet cell antibodies.[14] The presence of anti-enterocyte antibodies are also observed in patients with celiac disease, inflammatory bowel disease, and HIV enteropathy. The pathophysiology of AIE appears to involve hyperactive cell-mediated immunity with activation of CD4+ and CD8+ lymphocytes. Patients with AIE respond to respond to immunosuppressive therapy to achieve and maintain remission.[15,16] Budesonide is recommended as initial therapy with specific dose administration to allow for adequate distribution to the entire small intestine mucosal surface area.

Collagenous Sprue

Collagenous sprue (CS) is characterized by symptoms of diarrhea associated with a peculiar histologic finding of subepithelial collagen combined with villous atrophy and increased intra-epithelial lymphocytes. The pathophysiology of collagenous sprue is unknown but has been associated with celiac disease, as well as multiple medications, including non-steroidal anti-inflammatory agents (NSAIDs), proton pump inhibitors, angiotensin receptor inhibitors, and ARBs.[17] The treatment of collagenous sprue is based upon the associated condition. For example, patients with CS associated with celiac disease can be successfully treated with a gluten free diet with or without steroids. Patients with CS associated with a specific medication exposure may improve with suspension of the offending medication and/or immunosuppression.[17] If immunosuppressive therapy is initiated in combination with medication withdrawal, the underlying cause of illness may remain undefined.[3,7,8]

Tropical Sprue

Tropical sprue (TS) is an acquired chronic diarrheal illness often complicated by folic acid and/or B12 deficiency. It is observed in residents of or travelers to tropical areas in the Caribbean, Central America, India, and Southeast Asia.[18,19] In the Western Hemisphere, TS is prevalent in the countries of Haiti, Dominican Republic, Puerto Rico, and Cuba. Tropical sprue is seldom seen in travelers who visit an endemic area for less than 2 weeks. This disorder histologically characterized by villous atrophy, crypt hyperplasia and increased intra-epithelial lymphocytes (IEL's) as observed in celiac disease. Subtle histologic features have been reported as useful in differentiating tropical and celiac sprue.[20,21,22] In celiac disease, the intraepithelial lymphocytosis occurs in a "crescendo pattern" (mostly in the upper third of villous mucosa) in contrast with tropical sprue, where intraepithelial lymphocytosis occurs in a decrescendo pattern (basal one third of the villi or mucosal crypts).[23] Eosinophilic infiltration of the lamina propria is more commonly observed in TS than in CD.

Despite its prevalence worldwide, the cause of TS is still unknown. An infectious pathogen may be culprit, acting as either a persistent infection or through a "post-infectious" immune-mediated inflammatory response.[20] Treatment with doxycycline and folic acid supplementation are the primary therapies for tropical sprue. Clinical improvement in response to antibiotic therapy, typically occurring within 2-6 weeks, supports the diagnosis.[21]

Whipple's Disease

Whipple's Disease (WD) is an infectious cause of SNVA related to *T. whipplei*, a gram-positive bacillus. Patients with WD typically present with diarrhea, weight loss, and abdominal pain coincidental with joint pain. Histologic features of small bowel injury due to WD include villous atrophy and accumulation of "foamy" macrophages in the lamina propria with intensely periodic acid-Schiff (PAS)-positive intracellular material (**Figure 2**). Treatment for this condition includes doxycycline and hydroxychloroquine. Patients with evidence of systemic infection, such as endocarditis, may require additional therapy.[24,25]

Common Variable Immunodeficiency

Common variable immunodeficiency (CVID) is associated with SNVA (**Figure 3**). This condition

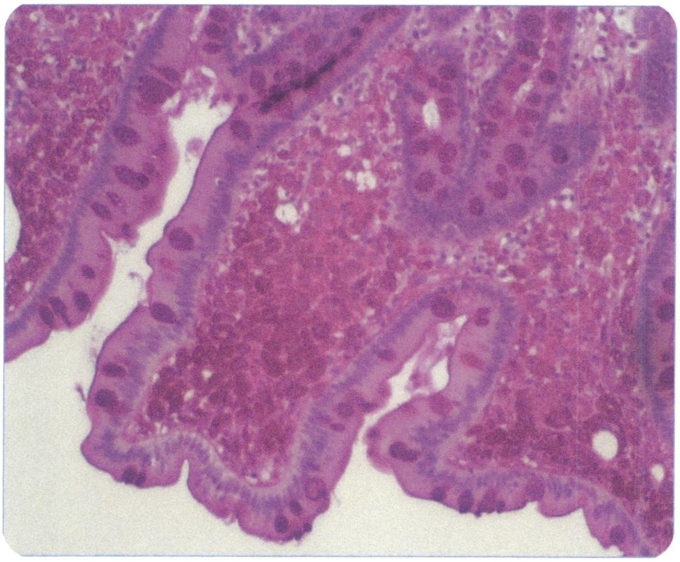

Figure 2. Positive PAS staining of submucosal macrophages in Whipple's Disease.

results in recurrent upper airway and/or sinus infections and persistent diarrhea/steatorrhea due to enteropathy. The conspicuous absence of plasma cells in the lamina propria is a key histologic finding on small bowel biopsy. CVID is confirmed by low titer of 2 or more immunoglobulin classes (IgG, IgA, or IgM).[26] Treatment for enteropathy in CVID consists of IVIG supplementation with or without oral budesonide.

Other Disorders Associated with SNVA

- *Peptic duodenitis* accounted for 11.5% of cases of SNVA in one prospective analysis.[13] Villous atrophy attributed to peptic injury should improve with acid suppressive therapy. In severe peptic injury, a diagnosis of Zollinger Ellison Syndrome should be suspected (**Figure 4**).
- *Small intestinal bacterial overgrowth (SIBO)* may result in villous atrophy and has been reported as a complication of celiac disease. SIBO is diagnosed by positive hydrogen breath testing and/or quantitation of small bowel bacterial content, although these tests are not always accurate. Patients who demonstrate a true diagnosis of SIBO should respond clinically and/or histologically to treatment with antibiotics.
- *Helicobacter pylori* infection is a common infection that can affect up to 25% of the U.S. population. This has been associated with villous atrophy in some cases. Aziz et al. reported that 10% of their cases of SNVA were attributed to *H. pylori*. *H. pylori* is responsive to antibiotic therapy and eradication must be documented following therapy by objective testing given its known association with gastric neoplasia.[13]
- *Giardiasis* is known to cause SNVA. This infection is characterized by diarrhea, abdominal pain, and weight loss. A diagnosis of giardiasis may be made through observation of trophozoites in villi and/or positive PCR from duodenal aspirate or stool sample.
- *HIV Enteropathy* is associated with villous atrophy and should be excluded through antibody testing for HIV infection.[27]

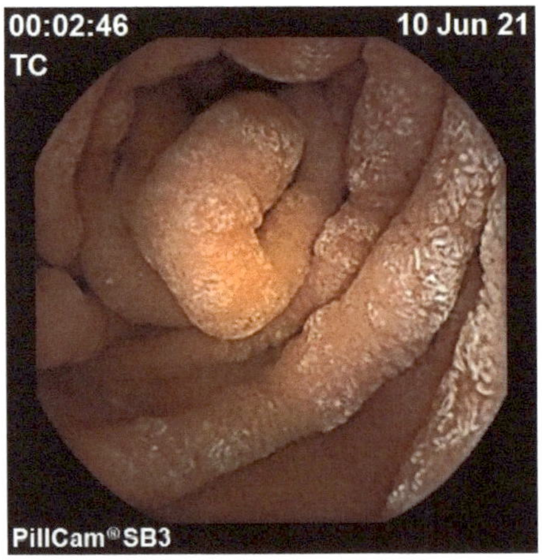

Figure 3. Mucosal fissuring observed by video capsule study in CVID

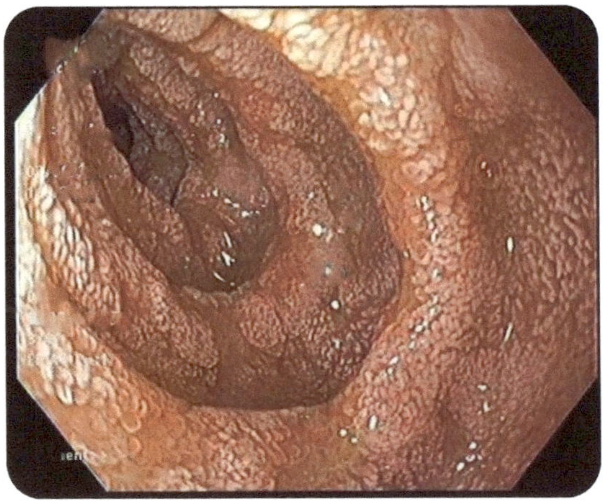

Figure 4. Enteropathy due to Zollinger-Ellison Syndrome.

Diagnostic Evaluation

The evaluation of cases of SNVA may follow the algorithm described by Aziz et al (**Figure 5**).[13] Patients should continue a gluten-containing diet until a diagnosis is established. Premature initiation of a GFD may complicate the evaluation of SNVA due to subjective improvement in patients with non-celiac villous atrophy or a delayed improvement in symptoms and/or histology in sero-negative celiac disease.[28] The introduction of a GFD may also limit the utility of additional celiac antibody serologies such as anti-deminated gliadin (DGGL) antibodies and anti-endomysial (EMA) antibodies.

Screening for selective IgA deficiency is the first step in evaluation of patients with villous atrophy and negative testing for anti-TTG IgA. Patients diagnosed with selective IgA deficiency should be testing for TTTG IgG and DGGL IgG antibodies. If testing for IgA deficiency is negative, a medication review should be performed followed by testing of 1 or more HLA alleles required for CD (HLA DQ2 or DQ8). As approximately 30% of the general population possesses 1 or more HLA-DQ2/DQ8 alleles, the presence of these alleles

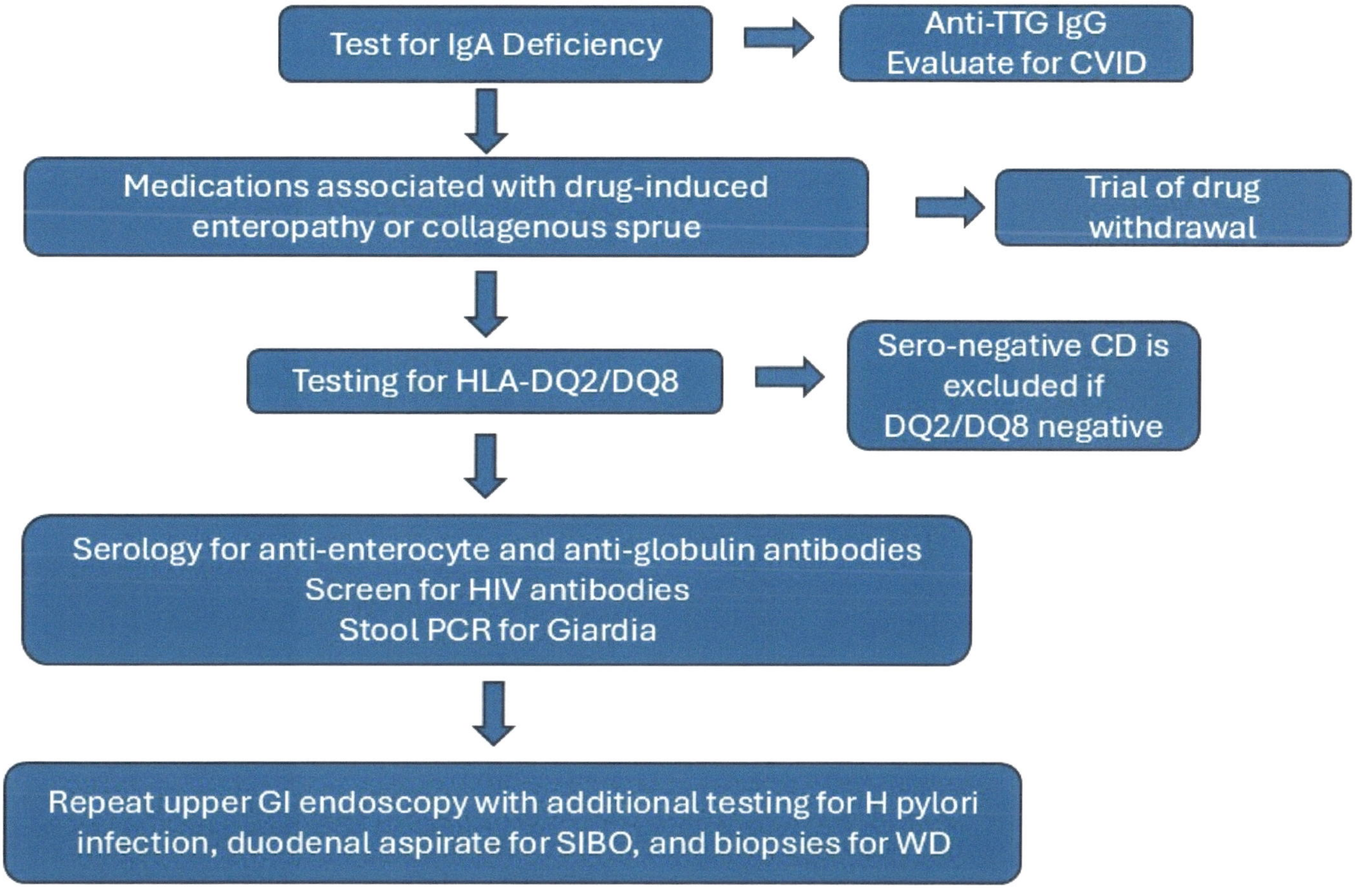

Figure 5. Diagnostic evaluation of SNVA. Adapted from Aziz et al[13].

is non-diagnostic for CD but the absence of these alleles excludes a diagnosis of CD.[29] Patients who possess at least 1 allele should be evaluated for specific pathologies associated with SNVA including antibody testing of AIE, screening for HIV, stool Giardia PCR, and repeat EGD with additional testing for *H. pylori*, SIBO, and duodenal biopsies. This sequence of testing should be successful in categorizing most cases of SNVA as sero-negative celiac disease or non-celiac villous atrophy.

Conclusion

Villous atrophy observed by video capsule endoscopy is a marker of small bowel disease which may indicate additional testing. In patients with known or suspected enteropathy, VCE may be considered as an additional study to support a final diagnosis as well as evaluate for complications of enteropathy such as stricture formation or malignancy. Small bowel mucosal atrophy is a feature of multiple enteropathies in addition to celiac disease. In patients diagnosed with villous atrophy which fails to correlate with elevations in antibodies observed in celiac disease, a diagnostic evaluation will allow for physicians to determine an etiology and exclude treatable causes.

References

1. Tapia-Rubio A, Herman ML, Ludvigsson JF, et al. Severe Spruelike Enteropathy Associated with Olmesartan. Mayo Clin Proc. 2012 87(8):732-738.
2. Cartee AK, Murray JA. Sprue-like Enteropathy associated with olmesartan. Curr Cadiovasc Risk Rep 2014; 8:420:1-8.
3. DeGaetani M, Tennyson CA, Lebwohl B, et al. Villous atrophy and negative celiac serology: a diagnostic and therapeutic dilemma. Am J Gastroenterol 2013;108:647-53.
4. Theophile H, David XR, Miremont-Salame G, Haramburu F. Five cases of sprue-like enteropathy

in patients treated by olmesartan. Dig Liver Dis 2014;46:465-9.
5. Bhat N, Anupama N, Yelsangikar A, Vizhi K. Olmesartan related sprue-like enteropathy. Indian J Gastroenterol 2014;33: 564-7.
6. Ianiro G, Bibbo S, Montalto M, Ricci R, Gasbarrini A, Cammarota G. Systematic review: sprue-like enteropathy associated with olmesartan. Aliment Pharmacol Ther 2014;40:16-23.
7. Marthey L, Cadiot G, Seksik P, et al. Olmesartan-associated enteropathy: results of a national survey. Aliment Pharmacol Ther 2014;40:1103-9.
8. Scialom S, Malamut G, Meresse B, et al. Gastrointestinal disorder associated with olmesartan mimics autoimmune enteropathy. PLoS One 2015;10:e0125024.
9. Ziegler TR, Estivariz-Fernandez C, Gu LH, et al. Severe Villus Atrophy and Chronic Malabsorption Induced by Azathioprine. Gastroenterology 2003; 124:1950-1957.
10. Ducloux D, Ottignon Y, Semhoun-Ducloux S et al. Mycophenolate mofetil-induced villous atrophy. Transplantation 1998; 66:1115-1116.
11. Bosca MM, Anon R, Mayordomo E, et al. Methotrexate induced sprue-like syndrome. World J Gastroenterol 2008;14:7009-11.
12. Alsaadi D, Shah NJ, Charabaty A, Atkins MB. A case of checkpoint inhibitor-induced celiac disease. J Immunother Cancer. 2019;7(1):203.
13. Aziz I, Peerally MF, Barnes JH, et al. The clinical and phenotypical assessment of seronegative villous atrophy; a prospective UK centre experience evaluating 200 adult cases over a 15-year period (2000-2015). Gut. 2017;66(9):1563-1572.
14. Gentile NM, Murray JA, Pardi DS. Autoimmune enteropathy: a review and update of clinical management. Curr Gastroenterol Rep. 2012:14(5):380-385.
15. Montalto M, D'Onofrio F, Santoro L, et al. Autoimmune enteropathy in children and adults. Scand J Gastroenterol 2009;44(9):1029-1036.
16. Ruemmele FM, Brousse N, Goulet I. Autoimmune enteropathy: molecular concepts. Curr Opin Gastroenterol. Nov; 2004: 20(6):587-591.
17. Lan N, Shen B, Yuan L, Liu X. Comparison of Clinical Features, Treatment and Outcomes of Collagenous Sprue, Celiac Disease and Collagenous Colitis. J Gastroenterol Hepatol. 2017;32(1):120-127.
18. Nath SK. Tropical sprue. Curr Gastroenterol Rep. 2005;7:343-349.
19. Batheja MJ, Leighton J, Azueta A, Heigh R. The face of tropical sprue in 2010. Case Rep Gastroenterol 2010;4:168-172.
20. Brown IS, Bettington A, Bettington M, Rosty C. Tropical sprue: revisiting an underrecognized disease. Am J Surg Pathol. 2014; 38(5): 666-672.
21. Green PH, Cellier C. Celiac disease. N Engl J Med 2007, 357: 1731-1743.
22. Lo W, Sano K, Lebwohl B, Diamond B, Green PH. Changing presentation of adult celiac disease. Dig Dis Sci 2003, 48:395-398.
23. Sharma P, Baloda V, Gahlot GP, et al. Clinical, endoscopic, and histological differentiation between celiac disease and tropical sprue: A systematic review. J Gastroenterol Hepatol. 2019;34(1):74.
24. Swartz MN. Whipple's disease--past, present, and future. N Engl J Med 2000; 342:648.
25. Bai JC, Mazure RM, Vazquez H, et al. Whipple's disease. Clin Gastroenterol Hepatol 2004;2:849-860.
26. Malamut G, Verkarre V, Suarez F, et al. The enteropathy associated with common variable immunodeficiency. Am J Gastroenterol 2010; 105:2262-2275.
27. Batman PA, Kapembwa MS, Griffin GE. Enteropathy associated with HIV. Gut 1990;31:960.
28. Wahab PJ, Meijer JW, Mulder CJ. Histologic follow-up of people with celiac disease on a gluten-free diet: slow and incomplete recovery. Am J Clin Pathol 2002;118:459–63.
29. Brown NK, Guandalini S, Semrad C, Kupfer SS. A clinician's guide to celiac disease HLA genetics. Am J Gastroenterol. 2019;114(10):1587-1592.

Case Study Number 23

Presented by Yichun Fu, MD and Carol E. Semrad, MD, FACG

Pre-capsule Findings (included in capsule study)

A 62-year-old woman with a history of celiac disease (CD) and osteoporosis is referred for an 18-month history of ongoing diarrhea, abdominal bloating, and weight loss of 20 pounds. Celiac disease was diagnosed more than 2 decades ago based upon positive antibody testing (anti-tissue transglutaminase [TTG] IgA) and duodenal biopsy with villous atrophy. Following transition to a strict gluten-free diet (GFD), her anti-TTG IgA antibody remained weakly positive for 2 years then converted to negative. Outside duodenal biopsies performed 9 months prior to this clinic visit showed moderate to severe villous atrophy with increased intraepithelial lymphocytes (IELs) and crypt loss, normal goblet cells, and no increase in apoptosis to suggest autoimmune enteropathy. Family history is positive for celiac disease and inflammatory bowel disease. Repeat upper endoscopy is performed to obtain duodenal biopsies for histology, immunohistochemistry, and flow cytometry. A video capsule is deployed during endoscopy to evaluate the deep small bowel.

A capsule endoscopy study is performed for further evaluation of refractory celiac disease. Review the capsule endoscopy study and report your findings, including: gastric passage time, small bowel passage time, and observed abnormalities. Be prepared to discuss your findings and management plan with your staff prior to reviewing the diagnosis and case discussion.

Capsule Endoscopy Findings
First Gastric Image = endoscopically placed*
First Duodenal Image = 0h 2min 30sec
First Cecal Image = 3h 11min 59sec
*Small bowel passage time = 3h 9min

The mucosa of the entire duodenum and jejunum appears fissured and scalloped as observed in **Figure 1** (0hrs 4min 2 sec) and **Figure 2** (0hrs 4min 23sec). Scalloping is milder in the distal jejunum (**Figure 3**: 0hrs 19min 42 sec) and within the ileum (**Figure 4**: 2hrs 42min 37sec). No mass lesions or deep ulcers are observed on this study.

Figure 1

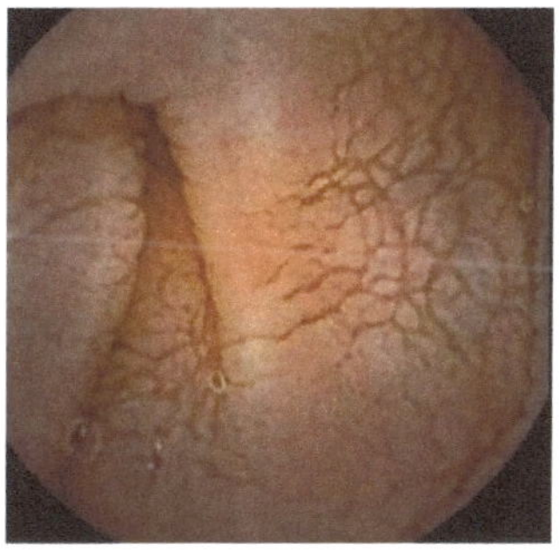

Figure 2

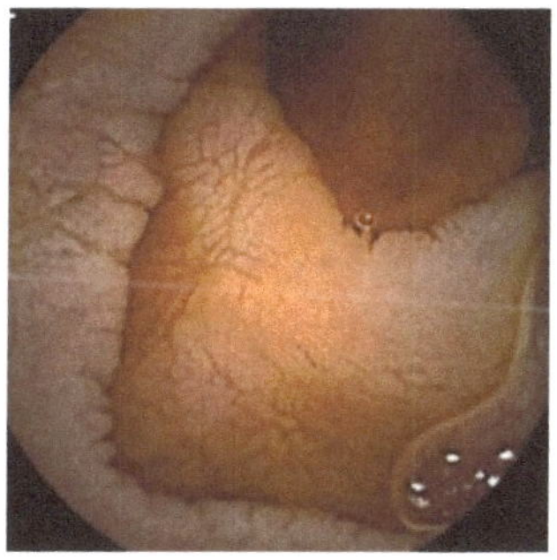

Figure 3

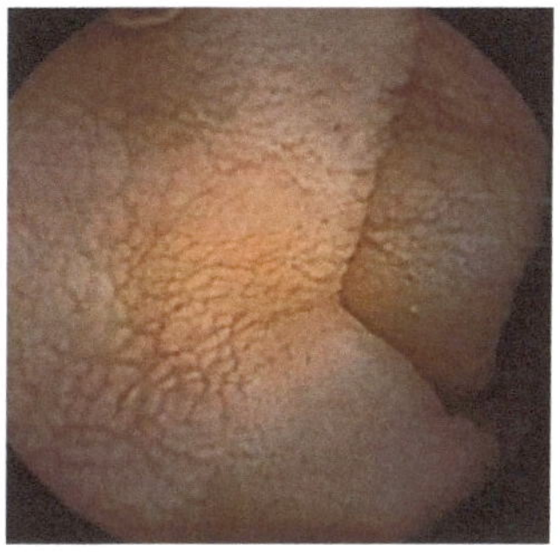

Figure 4

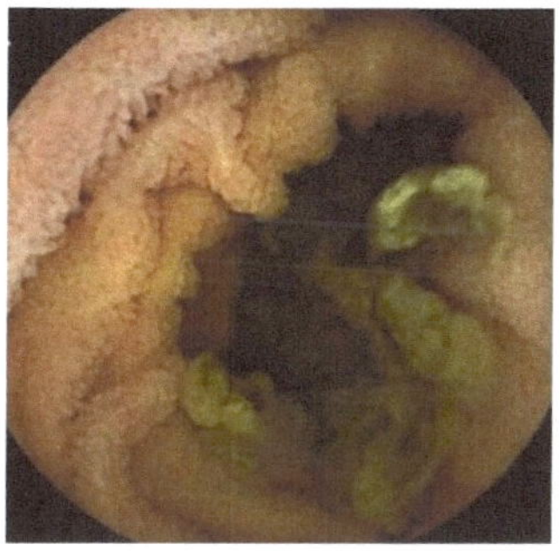

Follow-up

Pathologic review of duodenal biopsies was notable for villous blunting, increased IELs, and marked plasmacytosis (Marsh 3b). Flow cytometry showed 13% of events were atypical CD8+ T cells with loss of CD5 but no loss of CD3+ surface cells. After a joint conference with pathology and hematology, the patient was diagnosed with RCD type 1. Preservation of CD3+ expression excluded a diagnosis of RCD type II but close clinical monitoring was recommended as aberrant IELs are a risk factor for T cell lymphoma.[1]

This patient was treated with oral budesonide 3 mg 3 times a day (2 capsules opened and 1 capsule closed). Her symptoms of diarrhea and bloating improved progressively with this therapy. Repeat upper endoscopy was performed annually to assess for possible lymphocyte transformation to RCD II or enteropathy-associated T cell lymphoma (EATL). Budesonide was slowly tapered to 6 mg and then 3 mg as the patient gained weight. Follow-up duodenal biopsies showed improvement in duodenal villous blunting and a stable lymphocyte pattern by flow cytometry.

Chapter 23: Refractory Celiac Disease

Yichun Fu, MD and Carol E. Semrad, MD, FACG

Introduction

Celiac disease (CD) is an immune-mediated disorder triggered by ingestion of dietary gluten in individuals with HLA-DQ2/-DQ8 haplotype.[2,3] The pathogenesis of celiac disease upon exposure of gluten involves changes in intestinal permeability, innate and adaptive immune responses which leads to creation of serum autoantibodies, and eventually enteropathy of predominantly the proximal small bowel.[4] The disease affects approximately 1% of the population worldwide, with wide regional differences.[5,6] Clinical manifestations are systemic. The gastrointestinal symptoms include diarrhea, gas/bloating, abdominal distension, and weight loss, which occurs in 40%-50% of patients.[3] Malabsorption from intestinal inflammation leads to iron deficiency with or without anemia, vitamin deficiencies (particularly folate), decreased bone mineral density, peripheral neuropathy and chronic fatigue. Other clinical features include dermatitis herpetiformis, nephrolithiasis and infertility.[3,6] The only available treatment at present is a strict GFD.

Most patients with CD have symptom improvement within the first 2 weeks of a GFD along with return of duodenal biopsy to normal and conversion of serum antibodies to negative.[2] Approximately 7%-30% of adults with celiac disease experience persistent symptoms despite at least 6 months on a GFD. These patients are referred to as non-responsive or "slow-response" celiac disease.[7,8] The most common cause is persistent villous atrophy due to gluten contamination. Other causes for persistent symptoms include constipation, microscopic colitis, lactose or fructose intolerance and small intestinal bacterial overgrowth.[7] A rare but important cause is refractory celiac disease (RCD). This is distinct from nonresponsive disease due to accidental gluten exposure. RCD is characterized by diarrhea, malabsorption, and weight loss with persistent villous atrophy after more than 1 year on a strict gluten free diet.[2] Although most patients with RCD show initial response to a GFD, up to 65% of these patients experience a recurrence of symptoms.[2] RCD affects less than 1% of patients with celiac disease.[7] These patients are clinically sicker than those with non-responsive CD. Although rare, a missed diagnosis can lead to detrimental complications.

Diagnosis and Evaluation

There are 2 types of RCD based on the immunophenotype and clonality of small bowel intraepithelial lymphocytes (IELs).[9,10] RCD I is characterized by normal, polyclonal cells on flow cytometry, similar to active CD, and is associated with a favorable prognosis. RCD II is characterized by aberrant clonal cells with high risk of conversion to enteropathy-associated T cell lymphoma (EATL).[2,7] RCD usually presents 5-10 years after CD diagnosis.[11,12] Both subtypes of RCD present as persistent diarrhea and villous atrophy. Patients with RCD often suffer from debilitating diarrhea and nutrient malabsorption.

The clinical and endoscopic features of RCD I are similar to active uncomplicated celiac disease.[12,13] (**Figure 1a, b**) Gluten contamination must be excluded by a knowledgeable dietitian and testing for gluten immunogenic peptides in the urine or stool that are now commercially available.[2,14] One must also exclude alternative diagnoses such as drug-induced enteropathy (e.g., olmesartan, mycophenolate), tropical sprue, common variable immunodeficiency, and autoimmune enteropathy. On histopathology, the typical findings of RCD I include villous atrophy, crypt hyperplasia, increased IELs with normal cytologic appearance, a predominant CD3+CD8+ immunophenotype and a polyclonal T-cell receptor repertoire.[2]

Patients with RCD II typically present at an older age with diarrhea, weight loss and hypoalbuminemia. Fifty percent of patients exhibit resistance to a GFD.[12] Besides villous atrophy, 60%-70% of patients develop ulcerative jejunoileitis with large ulcers which may be

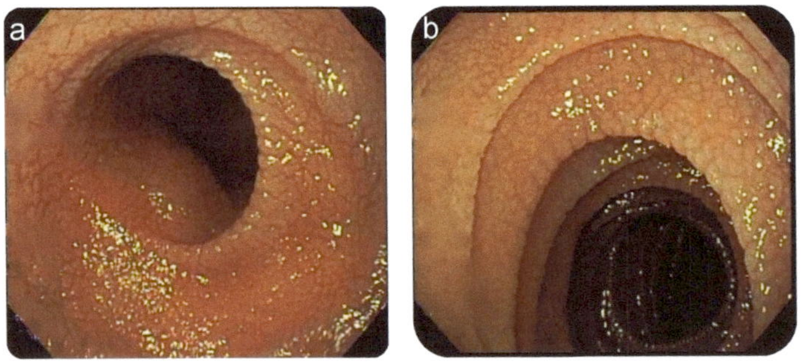

Figure 1: Endoscopic features of refractory celiac disease are similar to active uncomplicated celiac disease.

associated with strictures.[12] Such ulcers in patients with known celiac disease are highly correlated with RCD II. However, use of nonsteroidal anti-inflammatory drugs also causes ulcers and may confound these findings. On flow cytometry, aberrant IELs are surface CD3 negative, cytoplasmic CD3 positive, CD4 negative, and CD8 negative in more than 20% of the total IEL population.[2]

The clinical features of RCD I and RCD II correlate with complications and mortality. Patients with RCD II had a higher frequency of moderate to severe villous atrophy (Marsh 3b-3c) than RCD I patients, as well as high frequency of strictures, all localized beyond the ligament of Treitz.[11] Patients with RCD I still have a small risk of transformation to RCD II and development of EATL.[2] A study of 83 patients reported that the 5-year risk of developing EATL was 14.3% in RCD I and 32.6% in RCD II.[12] These observations highlight the importance of diligent follow-up. When alarming symptoms arise, the small bowel requires full examination with radiologic imaging, video capsule endoscopy (VCE) and deep enteroscopy. A computed tomorgraphy (CT) or magnetic resonance (MR) enterography is needed to assess for asplenism, mesenteric adenopathy, and small bowel wall thickening, strictures, or mass suggestive of RCD II. VCE is a non-invasive way to examine the entire small bowel mucosa, particularly for distal lesions more common in RCD II, provided the patient does not have obstructive symptoms. The diagnostic accuracy of VCE in celiac disease has been examined in prior studies. Identifying villous atrophy of Marsh 3 histology was 90.9%-100% specific in multiple studies while the sensitivity ranged from 70% to 92% compared to upper endoscopy (60%).[15–17] A retrospective study of 163 patients found that capsule endoscopy identified villous atrophy in more than 50% of the patients with positive serology and negative atrophy in duodenal biopsy.[18]

Several studies have examined the features of RCD on VCE, thus emphasizing its utility in diagnosis, risk stratification and management. A retrospective study of 48 adult patients found no difference in gastric and small bowel transit time in uncomplicated celiac disease, RCD and EATL. In the multivariable analysis, the presence of proximal erythema and absence of progression of the capsule to the distal intestine were independently associated with a risk of poor prognosis. The highest mortality was observed in patients with both features on capsule endoscopy (80% for both features vs none for neither).[19] In one study, the small bowel transit time of the capsule was significantly longer in RCD II than in RCD I and uncomplicated celiac disease ($P = 0.03$).[20] A systemic review and metanalysis comprising 22 studies and over 1,500 patients examined the yield of capsule endoscopy regarding celiac disease. Sixteen of the studies included a total of 393 patients with RCD. Mucosal atrophy ($P < 0.0001$), scalloping ($P = 0.015$) and ulcers ($P < 0.0001$) were significantly higher in RCD versus uncomplicated celiac disease.[21] However, a high level of heterogeneity was found among the study populations.

There are several limitations of capsule endoscopy: lack of tissue sampling, lower sensitivity and specificity among inexperienced capsule readers, and risk of retention with obstructive symptoms.[22] There is no data for retention rate specific to celiac disease. Overall, it is estimated to be similar to the retention rate of 2.1% in the general population.[23,24] VCE is indicated in celiac disease in patients with persistent or unexplained anemia, weight loss, gastrointestinal bleeding, and refractory celiac disease.[9,22] When combined with deep enteroscopy, it is useful to diagnose complicated celiac disease and to identify those who warrant tissue sampling.[22]

Treatment

For both subtypes of RCD, corticosteroids are the first line of treatment combined with dietary counseling to assure a strict GFD.[9,11] Despite their best efforts, many patients still ingest measurable amounts of gluten.[25] Certified processed gluten-free foods generally contain less then 20 parts per million of gluten, tolerable for most but not all patients. A stricter GFD that limits processed and restaurant food may be needed. Oral budesonide capsules (3 mg open in applesauce, 3 mg open in water, and 3 mg closed every day) is preferred over the more systemically bioavailable prednisone to avoid a myriad of side effects.[2,9] In an open-label study, budesonide led to clinical and histologic response in 90% of patients with RCD I.[26] Patients responsive to steroids experienced weight gain, fewer bowel movements and improvement in abdominal pain. The evidence for second-line treatment in RCD I is lacking. Previously trialed therapies included thiopurines with clinical response rate of 71%.[2,9] In case reports and small trials, second-line therapies for RCD II included anti-tumor necrosis factor alpha, cladribine, pentostatin and fludarabine. These improved symptoms but aberrant IELs persisted, and some progressed to EATL. A trial of an anti-interleukin 15 monoclonal antibody AMG 714 improved symptoms but failed the primary endpoint to eliminate aberrant IELs.[27] Cyclosporine did not have any therapeutic effect in a retrospective study.[11] Azathioprine, although effective, should be avoided due to the risk of EATL.[2] Autologous stem cell transplant is a promising therapeutic option in younger patients with RCD II resistant to budesonide therapy.[28] When severe malnutrition is present, parenteral nutrition should be initiated. The prognosis for RCD II remains poor and the overall 5-year survival rate is estimated 20%-25%.[11] In one study, the causes of death included progression of EATL, severe malnutrition, septic shock and hemorrhagic shock from ulcerative jejunitis.[11] It is imperative to survey these patients on long-term therapy for both subtypes of RCD with flow cytometry on small bowel biopsies, although there is no current guideline for specific intervals.

References

1. Verbeek WHM, Goerres MS, Von Blomberg BME, et al. Flow cytometric determination of aberrant intra-epithelial lymphocytes predicts T-cell lymphoma development more accurately than T-cell clonality analysis in Refractory Celiac Disease. Clin Immunol. 2008;126(1):48-56.
2. Malamut G, Soderquist CR, Bhagat G, Cerf-Bensussan N. Advances in Nonresponsive and Refractory Celiac Disease. Gastroenterology. 2024;167(1):132-147.
3. Fasano A, Catassi C. Clinical practice. Celiac disease. N Engl J Med. 2012;367(25):2419-26.
4. Green PH, Cellier C. Celiac disease. N Engl J Med. 2007;357(17):1731-43.
5. Singh P, Arora A, Strand TA, et al. Global prevalence of celiac disease: Systematic review and meta-analysis. Clin Gastroenterol Hepatol. 2018;16(6):823-836.e2.
6. Zingone F, Bai JC, Cellier C, Ludvigsson JF. Celiac Disease-Related Conditions: Who to Test? Gastroenterology. 2024;167(1):64-78.
7. Tye-Din JA. Review article: Follow-up of coeliac disease. Aliment Pharmacol Ther. 2022;56 Suppl 1(Suppl 1):S49-S63.
8. Leffler DA, Dennis M, Hyett B, Kelly E, Schuppan D, Kelly CP. Etiologies and predictors of diagnosis in nonresponsive celiac disease. Clin Gastroenterol Hepatol. 2007;5(4):445-50.
9. Green PHR, Paski S, Ko CW, Rubio-Tapia A. AGA clinical practice update on management of refractory celiac disease: Expert review. Gastroenterology. 2022;163(5):1461-1469.
10. Soderquist CR, Bhagat G. Cellular and molecular bases of refractory celiac disease. Int Rev Cell Mol Biol. 2021;358:207-240.
11. Elli L, Soru P, Roncoroni L, et al. Clinical features of type 1 and 2 refractory celiac disease: Results from a large cohort over a decade. Dig Liver Dis. 2023 Feb;55(2):235-242.
12. Malamut G, Afchain P, Verkarre V, et al. Presentation and long-term follow-up of refractory celiac disease: comparison of type I with type II. Gastroenterology. 2009;136(1):81-90.
13. Rubio–Tapia A, Kelly DG, Lahr BD, Dogan A, Wu T, Murray JA. Clinical staging and survival in refractory celiac disease: A single center experience. Gastroenterology. 2009;136(1):99-107.
14. Elli L, Leffler D, Cellier C, et al. Guidelines for best practices in monitoring established coeliac disease in adult patients. Nat Rev Gastroenterol Hepatol. 2024;21(3):198-215.
15. Murray JA, Rubio-Tapia A, Van Dyke CT, et al. Mucosal atrophy in celiac disease: Extent of involvement, correlation with clinical presentation, and response to treatment. Clin Gastroenterol Hepatol. 2008;6(2):186-193.
16. Petroniene R, Dubcenco E, Baker JP, et al. Given capsule endoscopy in celiac disease: evaluation of diagnostic accuracy and interobserver agreement. Am J Gastroenterol. 2005 Mar;100(3):685-94.
17. Rokkas T, Niv Y. The role of video capsule endoscopy in the diagnosis of celiac disease: A meta-analysis. Eur J Gastroenterol Hepatol. 2012;24(3):303-308.
18. Luján-Sanchis M, Pérez-Cuadrado-Robles E, García-Lledó J, et al. Role of capsule endoscopy in suspected celiac disease: A European multi-centre study. World J Gastroenterol. 2017;23(4):703.
19. Van Weyenberg SJB, Smits F, Jacobs MAJM, Van Turenhout ST, Mulder CJ. Video dapsule endoscopy in patients with nonresponsive celiac disease. J Clin Gastroenterol. 2013;47(5):393-399.
20. Barret M, Malamut G, Rahmi G, et al. Diagnostic yield of capsule endoscopy in refractory celiac disease. Am J Gastroenterol. 2012;107(10):1546-1553.
21. Shapiro M, Niv Y. Diagnostic yield of video capsule endoscopy (VCE) in celiac disease (CD): A systematic review and meta-analysis. J Clin Gastroenterol. 2025; 59(7): 598-606.
22. Lewis SK, Semrad CE. Capsule endoscopy and enteroscopy in celiac disease. Gastroenterol Clin North Am. 2019;48(1):73-84.
23. Topa M, Corradi M, Elli L, et al. Navigating celiac disease with small bowel capsule endoscopy: current state and future horizons. Ther Adv Gastrointest Endosc. 2025;18:26317745251340120.
24. Cortegoso Valdivia P, Skonieczna-Żydecka K, Elosua A, et al. Indications, detection, completion and retention

rates of capsule endoscopy in two decades of use: A systematic review and meta-analysis. Diagnostics. 2022;12(5):1105.
25. Silvester JA, Comino I, Kelly CP, et al. Most patients with celiac disease on gluten-free diets consume measurable amounts of gluten. Gastroenterology. 2020;158(5):1497-1499.e1.
26. Mukewar SS, Sharma A, Rubio-Tapia A, Wu TT, Jabri B, Murray JA. Open-capsule budesonide for refractory celiac disease. Am J Gastroenterol. 2017;112(6):959-967.
27. Cellier C, Bouma G, Van Gils T, et al. Safety and efficacy of AMG 714 in patients with type 2 refractory coeliac disease: A phase 2a, randomised, double-blind, placebo-controlled, parallel-group study. Lancet Gastroenterol Hepatol. 2019;4(12):960-970.
28. Al-toma A, Visser OJ, Van Roessel HM, et al. Autologous hematopoietic stem cell transplantation in refractory celiac disease with aberrant T cells. Blood. 2007;109(5):2243-2249.

CAPSULE ENDOSCOPY BY CASE STUDY

Case Study Number 24

Presented by Pablo Machado, MD

Pre-capsule Findings (included in capsule study)

A 21-year-old woman with a history of Peutz-Jeghers Syndrome (PJS) presents for surveillance of intestinal polyposis. PJS was initially mentioned by her dermatologist who identified melanocytic macules on her lips. A diagnosis of PJS was confirmed after her younger brother was found to have PJS. Genetic testing is positive for same *STK11* gene mutation in both siblings. After diagnosis, an endoscopic evaluation was performed by standard upper endoscopy and colonoscopy. Three small (<5 mm) polyps were identified in the gastric body and removed by cold snare technique. Two additional polyps (6-8 mm) were observed in the proximal jejunum. Analysis of the removed gastric polyps confirmed hamartomas.

A capsule endoscopy study is performed to evaluate for surveillance of an intestinal polyposis syndrome. Review the capsule endoscopy study and report your findings, including: gastric passage time, small bowel passage time, and observed abnormalities. Be prepared to discuss your findings and management plan with your staff prior to reviewing the diagnosis and case discussion.

Capsule Endoscopy Findings
First Gastric Image = 0h 0min 15sec
First Duodenal Image = 1h 6min 4sec
Gastric passage time = 1h 6min
First Cecal Image = 3h 29min 20sec
Small bowel passage time = 2hr 23min

Examination of the proximal small bowel is positive for at least 4 hamartomatous polyps with an estimated size ranging from 8mm to 12mm (**Figure 1:** 1hr 13min 16sec; **Figure 3**: 1hr 22min 19sec; **Figure 3**: 1hr 35min 35sec). Within the mid small bowel, a larger (>20mm) hamartoma is observed which partially obstructs the bowel lumen (**Figure 4:** 1hr 44min 36sec). Capsule transit is delayed in this segment for approximately 25 minutes. Evaluation of the distal small bowel is remarkable only for benign lymphoid hyperplasia in the terminal ileum.

Follow-up

An anterograde double balloon enteroscopy exam was performed to remove all small bowel hamartomas >15 mm in size. The exam was successful in resection of one 15 mm hamartoma within the jejunum as well as one large (35 mm) hamartoma within the proximal ileum which partially obstructed the bowel lumen. This anterograde exam was complete to the cecum (total enteroscopy).

Figure 1

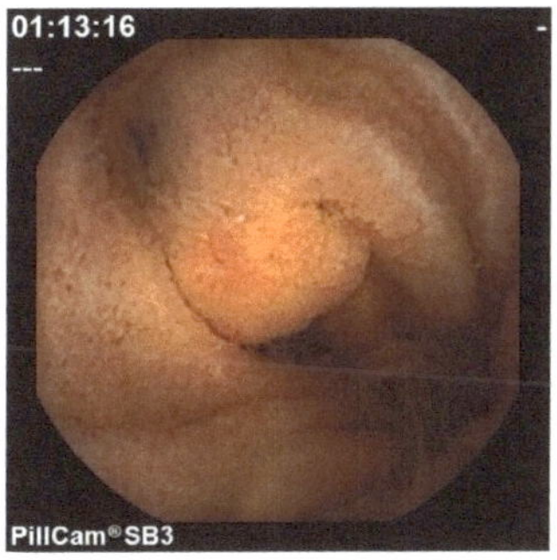

Figure 2

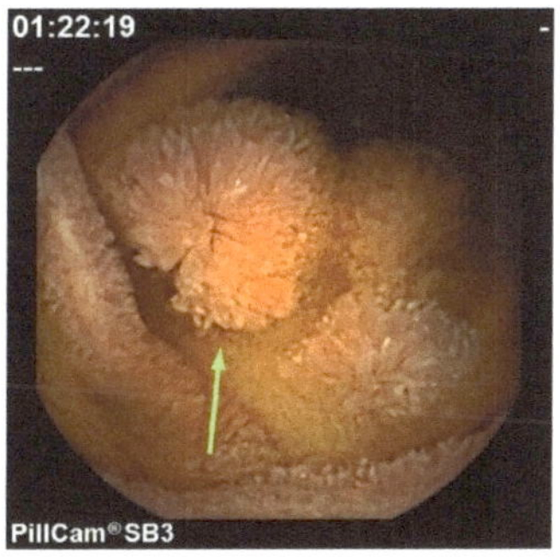

Figure 3

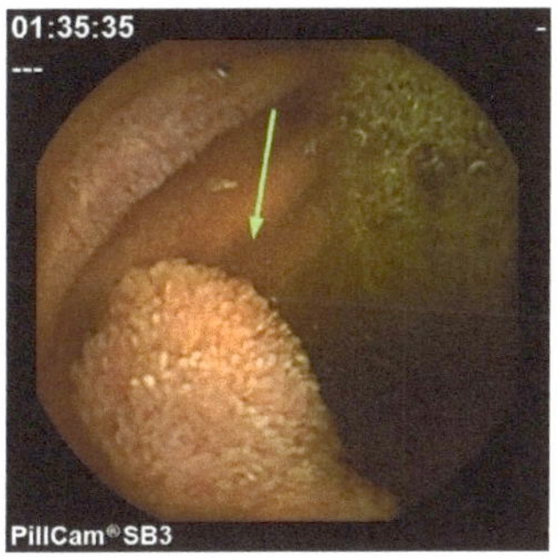

Figure 4

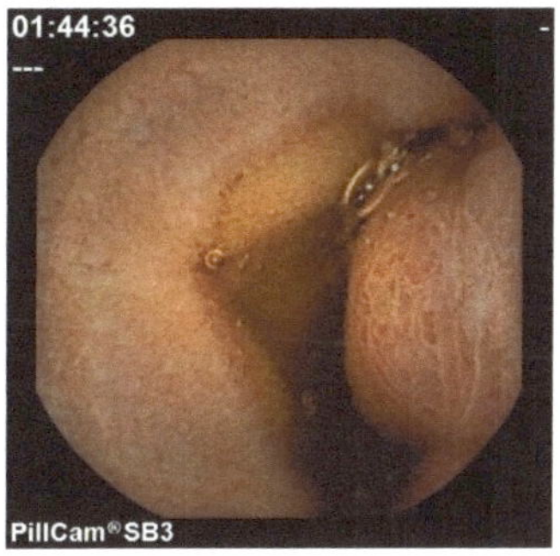

Chapter 24: Peutz-Jeghers Syndrome

Abraham Z. Cheloff, MD, MS and Seth A. Gross, MD, FACG

Introduction

Peutz-Jeghers syndrome (PJS) is a rare, autosomal dominant genetic disorder[1] characterized by gastrointestinal polyposis and mucocutaneous pigmentation.[2] Prevalence estimates range from 1:50,000 to 1:200,000 people, with an incidence of 1:8,300 to 1:200,000 births.[3] The average age of diagnosis is 23 years old in men and 26 years old in women.[4] This chapter will review the clinical features, diagnosis, management, and surveillance recommendations for patients diagnosed with PJS.

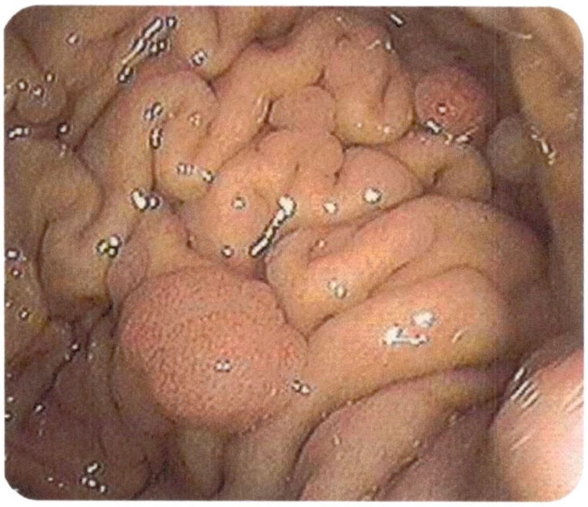

Figure 1. Gastric hamartomas observed by standard upper endoscopy.

Clinical Features

Gastrointestinal

Hamartomatous polyps of the gastrointestinal (GI) tract are a key characteristic of PJS. These polyps are smooth, lobulated growths that can appear anywhere along the GI tract,[5,6] with histopathology showing normal cells with distorted architecture.[7] The number, size, and distribution of hamartomas may vary significantly between individual patients.[8,9] Studies of large groups of PJS patients suggest that hamartomatous polyps are most prevalent in the small intestine (64%), followed by the stomach (48.6%), colon (53.2%), and rectum (32%). The esophagus is typically spared[4] (**Figure 1, 2).**

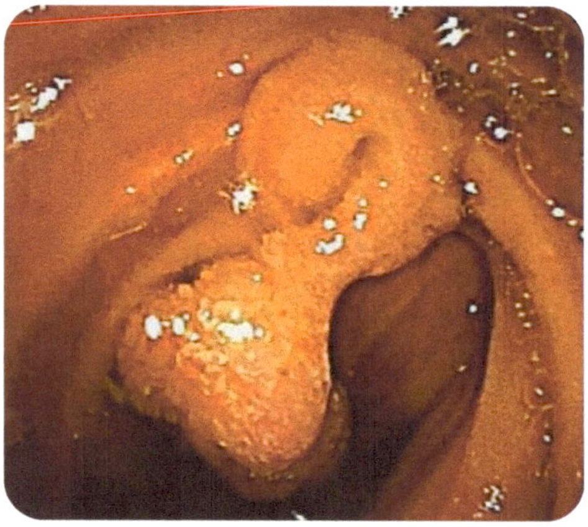

Figure 2. Pedunculated hamartoma of the jejunum observed by DAE

The majority of PJS patients initially present with complications related GI hamartomas, including small bowel intussusception with obstruction (42.8%), abdominal pain (23.4%), or rectal bleeding (13.5%). Most (69%) patients experience at least 1 episode of small bowel intussusception and multiple episodes are common. The risk of intussusception by age 20 is 50%, while a median age of first intussusception of 16 years old. As small bowel hamartomas >15 mm in size are more likely to intussuscept, endoscopic surveillance with proactive resection of larger polyps may prevent future episodes.[2]

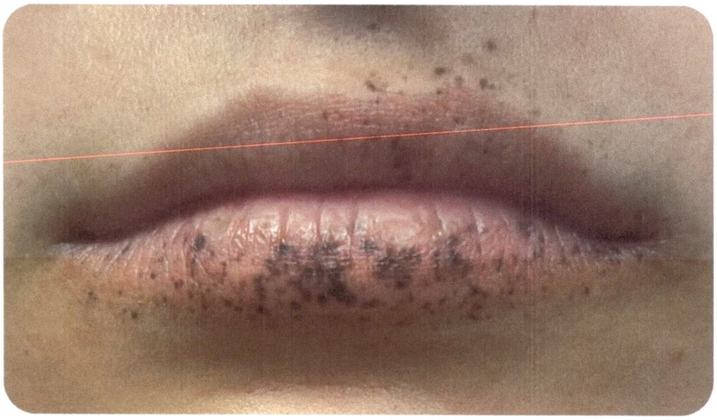

Figure 3. Pigmented lesions in Peutz-Jeghers syndrome.

Mucocutaneous Pigmentation

Another primary feature of PJS is mucocutaneous pigmentation or "melanocytic macules," which is present in 52% of patients upon diagnosis. These lesions appear as dark brown or blue macules, described as freckle-like, and can be found on skin or mucous membranes including the lips, buccal mucosa, genitalia, and fingertips[10] (**Figure 3**). Melanocytic macules usually emerge in infancy and made fade during puberty or early adulthood.[11] Although these macules are benign, recognition of their presence as associated with PJS is crucial for early diagnosis.

Diagnosis

PJS is a clinical diagnosis which requires 1 or more of the following criteria to be met. As sporadic GI hamartomas are occasionally encountered during routine endoscopy, a single hamartomatous polyp is not sufficient for a diagnosis of PJS. Patients who meet at least 1 criterion should be referred for genetic testing.

- Two or more Peutz-Jeghers-type polyps, confirmed on histology
- Mucocutaneous hyperpigmentation characteristic of PJS in an individual with a family history of PJS in close relatives
- At least 1 Peutz-Jeghers-type polyp in an individual with characteristic mucocutaneous hyperpigmentation
- At least 1 Peutz-Jeghers-type polyp in an individual with a family history of PJS in close relatives[12]

The genetic mutations associated with PJS have been mapped to chromosome 19p13.3, the location of *STK11* (*LKB1*) gene. This gene encodes for serine/threonine kinase that acts as a tumor suppressor.[13,14] Mutations in *STK11* are detected in 50%-80% of families with PJS, suggesting the presence of another gene locus[15-18] or genetic mosaicism.[19,20] Individuals with PJS associated a *STK11* mutation not found in any relatives are assumed to have *de novo* PJS.[21]

As some genetic mutations remain unidentified, a negative genetic test does not rule out a diagnosis of PJS unless a specific familial mutation has been found. Individuals and at-risk family members with clinical criteria for PJS but negative genetic testing should follow the same surveillance recommendations as other PJS patients. Only patients who test negative for a known mutation identified in other family members are excluded.[6]

Surveillance Recommendations

Malignancy is the primary cause of death in patients with PJS. The lifetime risk of cancer by age 70 is 55%-83%.[22] The lifetime risks of gastrointestinal cancers are greatest for colorectal cancer (39%) followed by pancreatic cancer (11%-36%), gastric cancer (29%), and malignancy of the small bowel (13%). Non-gastrointestinal cancers are also common, with a cumulative risk of 32%-54% for breast cancer, 21% for ovarian cancer, 7%-17% for lung cancer, 10% for cervical cancer, and 9% for uterine or testicular cancers.[22]

Surveillance recommendations for patients with PJS are designed for prevention or early detection of malignancies. The American College of Gastroenterology (ACG) publishes clinical guidelines on appropriate screening for patients with PJS, and recommend monitoring for colon, stomach, small intestine, pancreas, breast, ovary, endometrial, cervical, and testicular cancers.[23]

Gastrointestinal Surveillance

Surveillance for GI malignancy is recommended first at age 8 including esophagogastroduodenoscopy (EGD), colonoscopy, and video capsule endoscopy (VCE). If polyps are found, testing should continue every 3 years. If initial endoscopy surveillance is negative for polyps, surveillance may be deferred until age 18, then resumed at an interval of every 3 years.[23] While VCE is recommended as the primary means of examining the small bowel in PJS, other techniques have been studied, including small bowel follow-through (SBFT), fluoroscopic enteroclysis, CT enterography (CTE), and magnetic resonance enterography (MRE). VCE is recommended over imaging by fluoroscopy or CTE in pediatrics, due to concern for risk of cumulative radiation exposure. VCE has been shown to be superior to SBFT[24,25] and MRE[26] in the detection of small bowel hamartomas, particularly for polyps <5 mm in size.

Double balloon enteroscopy (DBE) is capable of examining the entire gastrointestinal tract to surveil for gastrointestinal malignancy in PJS and to proactively resect small bowel hamartomas >10-15 mm in size. Published research from high-volume DBE referral centers illustrates the utility of combined upper and lower DBE every 3 years in select PJS patients.[27,28] DBE may also be considered as an alternative to surgery in the management of small bowel obstruction due to intussusception. In these cases, the balloon-tipped enteroscope is used to reduce the intussusception then resect the polyp by hot snare technique after injection of the stalk with saline (**Figure 4a-d**). Surgery may be required to remove large hamartomas in cases in which endoscopic removal is not feasible. Laparoscopic-assisted endoscopic polypectomy may

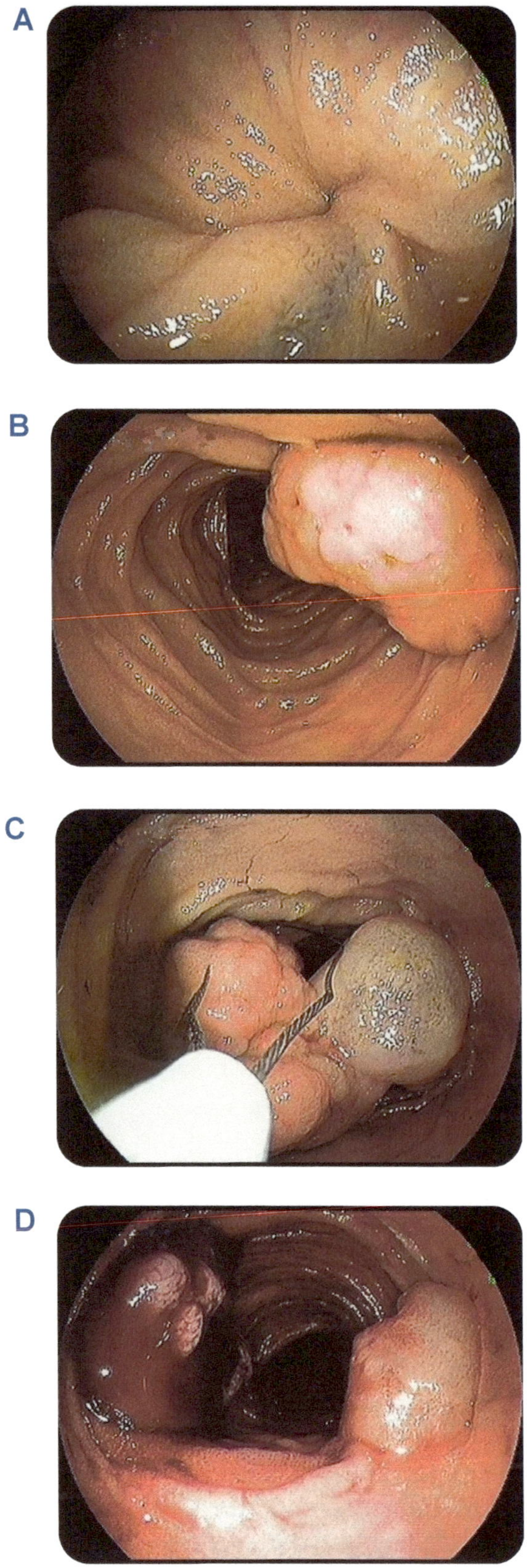

Figure 4A-D: The balloon-tipped enteroscope is used to reduce the intussusception then resect the polyp by hot snare technique after injection of the stalk with saline.

be evaluated as an alternative to standard small bowel resection, depending upon individual case specifics and local expertise.[29]

Surveillance for pancreatic cancer every 1-2 years should be considered in adults with PJS using magnetic resonance cholangiopancreatography (MRCP) or endoscopic ultrasound (EUS). However, the utility of pancreatic cancer surveillance in this patient population has been questioned due to lack of proven benefit and associated costs.[12] Current society recommendations, including the most recent ACG guidelines,[23,30] support continued surveillance for pancreatic cancer in patients with PJS.

Additional Surveillance

The ACG recommends the following additional surveillance in patients with PJS:

- Monthly self-exam of the breast starting at age 18, with a transition to annual screening via breast MRI or mammogram starting at age 25
- Yearly pelvic exams with a pelvic or transvaginal ultrasound starting at age 25 to screen for ovarian and endometrial malignancies as well as sex cord tumor with annular tubules (SCTAT). The ACG *does not* recommend the use of routine blood work such as CA-125
- Yearly pap smear starting at age 25
- Yearly testicular exam from birth through adolescence with follow up ultrasound for any abnormalities
- Education on lung cancer symptoms and smoking cessation. Annual radiography and CT *are not* recommended for PJS patients.

Conclusion

Peutz-Jeghers syndrome (PJS) is a rare but clinically significant hereditary polyposis syndrome characterized by mucocutaneous pigmentation and hamartomatous polyps of the gastrointestinal tract. Timely recognition of this diagnosis through clinical criteria, histologic confirmation, and genetic testing, is critical for initiating appropriate surveillance for malignancy and mitigating the risk of complications. Individuals with PJS carry markedly elevated lifetime risks for both gastrointestinal and extraintestinal malignancies, necessitating a comprehensive, multidisciplinary surveillance strategy beginning in early childhood. Evidence-based screening protocols, as outlined by the ACG, emphasize early endoscopic evaluation and organ-specific cancer surveillance to reduce morbidity and mortality. Continued research into the genetic heterogeneity and optimal management strategies for PJS remains essential to improving long-term outcomes in this high-risk population.

References

1. Pai RK, Wilcox R, Hart J. Chapter 23 - Molecular Gastrointestinal, Liver, and Pancreatic Pathology. In: Tubbs RR, Stoler MH, eds. Cell and Tissue Based Molecular Pathology. Philadelphia: Churchill Livingstone; 2009:269-295.
2. Wu L, di Pietro M. Screening and surveillance of hereditary upper GI cancers. Best Pract Res Clin Gastroenterol. 2025;75:102018.
3. Tacheci I, Kopacova M, Bures J. Peutz-Jeghers syndrome. Curr Opin Gastroenterol. 2021;37(3):245-254.
4. Utsunomiya J, Gocho H, Miyanaga T, Hamaguchi E, Kashimure A. Peutz-Jeghers syndrome: Its natural course and management. Johns Hopkins Med J. 1975;136(2):71-82.
5. Richter JE. Eosinophilic esophagitis dilation in the community--Try it--You will like it--But start low and go slow. Am J Gastroenterol. 2016;111(2):214-216.
6. Amru RL, Dhok A. Peutz-Jeghers syndrome: A comprehensive review of genetics, clinical features, and management approaches. Cureus. 2024;16(4):e58887.
7. Soravia C, Pocard M. Hereditary colorectal cancer associated with polyposis syndromes. Ann Chir. 1999;53(10):979-984.
8. Tanaka A, Sasaki F, Kanmura S, Ido A. Magnified endoscopic imaging of a Peutz-Jeghers-type polyp in the jejunum. Dig Liver Dis. 2021;53(7):920-921.
9. Blatter R, Tschupp B, Aretz S, et al. Disease expression in juvenile polyposis syndrome: a retrospective survey on a cohort of 221 European patients and comparison with a literature-derived cohort of 473 *SMAD4/ BMPR1A* pathogenic variant carriers. Genet Med. 2020 Sep;22(9):1524-1532.
10. McGarrity TJ, Amos CI, Baker MJ. Peutz-Jeghers Syndrome. 2001 Feb 23 [updated 2021 Sep 2]. In: Adam MP, Feldman J, Mirzaa GM, Pagon RA, Wallace SE, Amemiya A, editors. GeneReviews [Internet]. Seattle (WA): University of Washington, Seattle; 1993–2025.
11. Hearle N, Schumacher Vr, Menko FH, et al. Frequency and spectrum of cancers in the Peutz-Jeghers syndrome. Clin Cancer Res. 2006 May 15;12(10):3209-15.
12. Beggs AD, Latchford AR, Vasen HF, et al. Peutz-Jeghers syndrome: A systematic review and recommendations for management. Gut. 2010;59(7):975-986.
13. Resta N, Pierannunzio D, Lenato GM, et al. Cancer risk associated with germline mutations in Peutz-Jeghers syndrome patients: Results of an Italian multicenter study. Dig Liver Dis. 2013;45(7):606-611.
14. Mehenni H, Blouin J-L, Radhakrishna U, et al. Peutz-Jeghers syndrome: confirmation of linkage to chromosome 19p13.3 and identification of a potential second locus, on 19q13.4. Am J Hum Genet. 1997;61(6):1327-34.
15. Lim W, Hearle N, Shah B, et al. Further observations on *LKB1/STK11* status and cancer risk in Peutz-Jeghers syndrome. Br J Cancer. 2003;89(2):308-313.
16. Volikos E, Robinson J, Aittomäki K, et al. *LKB1* exonic and whole gene deletions are a common cause of Peutz-Jeghers syndrome. J Med Genet. 2006;43(5):e18.
17. Mehenni H, Gehrig C, Nezu J, et al. Loss of *LKB1* kinase activity in Peutz-Jeghers syndrome, and evidence for allelic and locus heterogeneity. Am J Hum Genet. 1998;63(6):1641-1650.
18. Wang HH, Xie NN, Li QY, Hu YQ, Ren JL, Guleng B. Exome sequencing revealed novel germline mutations in Chinese Peutz-Jeghers syndrome patients. Dig Dis Sci. 2014;59(1):64-71.
19. Jelsig AM, Bertelsen B, Forss I, Karstensen JG. Two cases of somatic STK11 mosaicism in Danish patients with Peutz-Jeghers syndrome. Fam Cancer. 2021;20(1):55-59.
20. McKay V, Cairns D, Gokhale D, Mountford R, Greenhalgh L. First report of somatic mosaicism for mutations in STK11 in four patients with Peutz-Jeghers syndrome. Fam Cancer. 2016;15(1):57-61.
21. Hernan I, Roig I, Martin B, Gamundi MJ, Martinez-Gimeno M, Carballo M. De novo germline mutation in the serine-threonine kinase STK11/LKB1 gene associated with Peutz-Jeghers syndrome. Clin Genet. 2004;66(1):58-62.
22. Yehia L, Heald B, Eng C. Clinical spectrum and science behind the hamartomatous polyposis syndromes. Gastroenterology. 2023;164(5):800-811.
23. Syngal S, Brand RE, Church JM, Giardiello FM, Hampel HL, Burt RW. ACG Clinical Guideline: Genetic testing and management of hereditary gastrointestinal cancer syndromes. Am J Gastroenterol. 2015;110(2):223-262.
24. Brown G, Fraser C, Schofield G, et al. Video capsule endoscopy in Peutz-Jeghers syndrome: A blinded comparison with barium follow-through for detection of small-bowel polyps. Endoscopy. 2006;38(4):385-390.
25. Mata A, Llach J, Castells A, et al. A prospective trial comparing wireless capsule endoscopy and barium contrast series for small-bowel surveillance in hereditary GI polyposis syndromes. Gastrointest Endosc. 2005;61(6):721-725.
26. Caspari R, von Falkenhausen M, Krautmacher C, Schild H, Heller J, Sauerbruch T. Comparison of capsule

endoscopy and magnetic resonance imaging for the detection of polyps of the small intestine in patients with familial adenomatous polyposis or with Peutz-Jeghers' syndrome. Endoscopy. 2004;36(12):1054-1059.
27. Mohamed Elfeky OW, Panjwani S, Cave D, Wild D, Raines D. Device-assisted enteroscopy in the surveillance of intestinal hamartomas in Peutz-Jeghers syndrome. Endosc Int Open. 2024;12(1):E128-e134.
28. Wang YX, Bian J, Zhu HY, et al. The role of double-balloon enteroscopy in reducing the maximum size of polyps in patients with Peutz-Jeghers syndrome: 12-year experience. J Dig Dis. 2019;20(8):415-420.
29. Goneidy A, Ross AR, Roberts R, Hyer W, Choudhry M. Laparoscopic-assisted polypectomy: A promising minimally-invasive solution for endoscopically irresectable polyps in children. J Pediatr Surg. 2025;60(7):162329.
30. van Lier MG, Wagner A, Mathus-Vliegen EM, Kuipers EJ, Steyerberg EW, van Leerdam ME. High cancer risk in Peutz-Jeghers syndrome: A systematic review and surveillance recommendations. Am J Gastroenterol. 2010;105(6):1258-1264.

Case Study Number 25

Presented by Felice Schnoll-Sussman, MD, FACG and Daniel Raines, MD FACG

Pre-capsule Findings (included in capsule study)

A 37-year-old man with a history of familial adenomatous polyposis (FAP) is referred to your office by his colorectal surgeon for a small bowel evaluation. A video capsule study is requested to "clear" the jejunum and ileum of any significant lesions prior to duodenectomy. The patient has a previous history of stage II colon cancer diagnosed at age 30 in the setting of numerous (>100) colonic adenomas. Treatment at that time included colectomy with end ileostomy without adjunctive chemotherapy or radiation. Following colectomy, his surgeon has carefully surveilled the patient's distal ileum and upper GI tract for adenomatous polyps every 1-2 years. Examination of the duodenum was recently positive for multiple polyps including 1 lesion in the third portion of the duodenum which was marked with an ink tattoo.

During interview, the patient expresses considerable anxiety about the prospect of another major operation. His previous colectomy was complicated by intra-abdominal infection resulting in a prolonged hospitalization. He currently reports intermittent abdominal pain after meals, occasionally accompanied by nausea, symptoms that have persisted since his prior surgery. Physical examination is notable for a prominent midline abdominal scar but is otherwise unremarkable.

Capsule Endoscopy Findings

First Gastric Image = 0h 0min 21sec

First Duodenal Image = 0h 59min 10sec

Gastric passage time = 0h 59min

First Cecal Image = 8h 15min 6sec

Small bowel passage time = 7hr 16min

A capsule endoscopy study is performed for evaluation of the small bowel prior to duodenectomy. Review the capsule endoscopy study and report your findings, including: gastric passage time, small bowel passage time, and observed abnormalities. Be prepared to discuss your findings and management plan with your staff prior to reviewing the diagnosis and case discussion.

Upon entry into the gastric body, multiple sub centimeter polyps are encountered in the gastric body. Examination of the duodenum is revealing for 2–3 small (5 mm) adenomas (**Figure 1:** 1hr 4min 32sec), as well as 2 larger adenomas (>1 cm) located adjacent to an ink tattoo (**Figure 2:** 1hr 0min 57sec; **Figure 3:** 1hr 5min 25 sec). Capsule transit is delayed in this segment and in multiple areas of the deep small bowel between 1.5-2.5hrs; 3-4hrs; and 6-7hrs. The small bowel lumen is irregularly contoured in these areas of capsule hold-up, likely due to adhesions external to the bowel wall. Luminal deformities and benign bulges observed in these areas may mimic pathology (**Figure 4**: 6hr 34min 45sec).

Figure 1

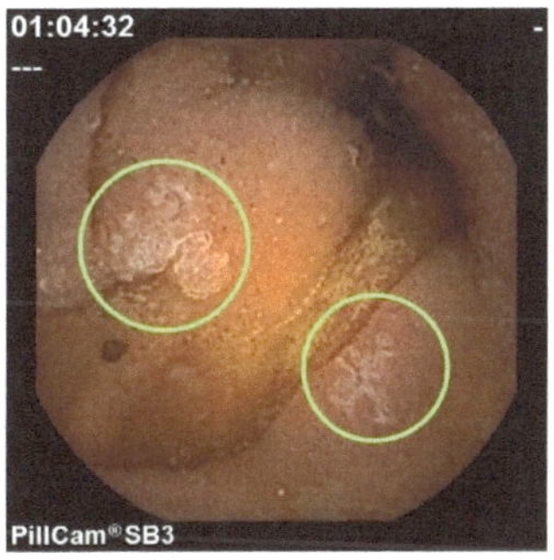

Figure 2

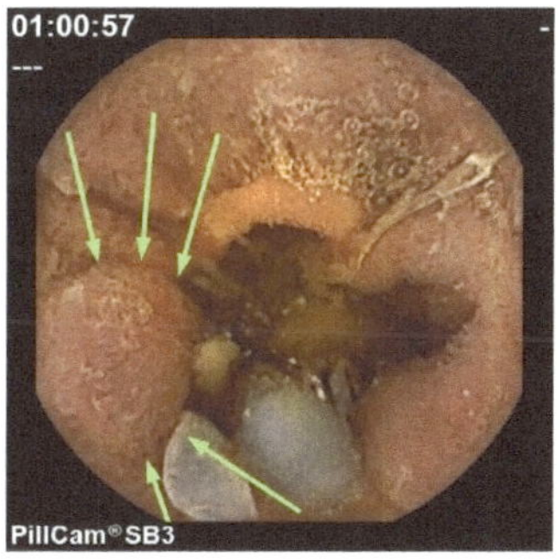

Figure 3

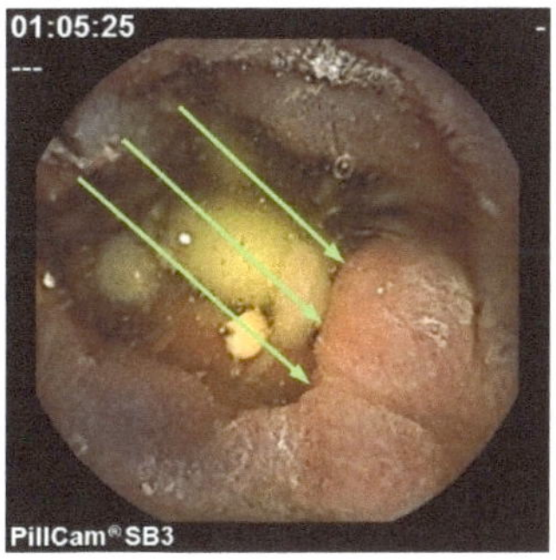

Figure 4

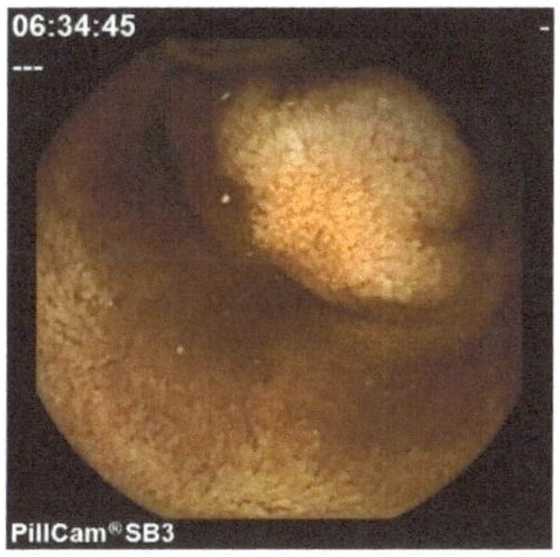

Follow-up

An anterograde double balloon enteroscopy exam was performed as next step in management. This exam was successful in removing the 2 duodenal adenomas >1 cm in size (**Figure 5**). Detailed examination of the remaining small bowel including the neoterminal ileum (total enteroscopy) was negative for additional adenomas >1 cm in size. Examination of the ampulla with a duodenoscope was normal. Following review of pathology results and endoscopy findings colorectal surgery, the patient was elected for continued endoscopic surveillance as an alternative to duodenectomy.

Figure 5

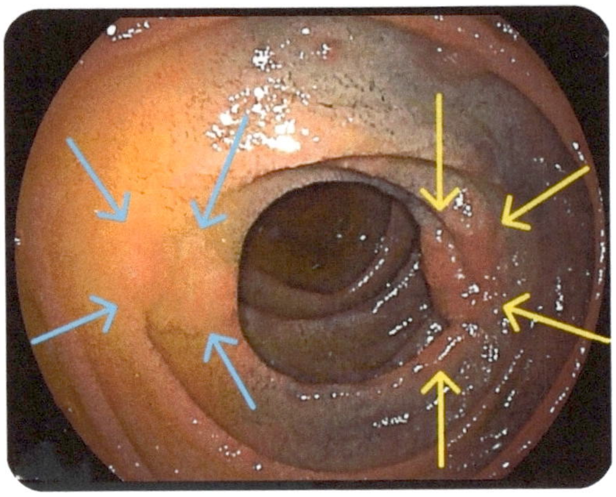

Chapter 25: Familial Adenomatous Polyposis

Felice Schnoll-Sussman, MD, FACG and Daniel Raines, MD FACG

Introduction

Familial adenomatous polyposis (FAP) is an inherited syndrome caused by mutations in the adenomatous polyposis coli (*APC*) gene located on chromosome 5 (Sq21-Sq22). This gene plays an important role in tumor suppression by regulating cell growth and adhesion, particularly in the intestinal epithelium. FAP is uncommon, with a prevalence of 1:10,000 to 1:30,000 births.[1] While most cases follow an autosomal dominant inheritance pattern, approximately 25% result from de novo mutations.[2] This chapter will review the clinical features, diagnosis, and management of FAP, with emphasis on endoscopic surveillance in FAP patients post-colectomy.

Clinical Features

Classical FAP is characterized by the development of hundreds of adenomatous polyps within the colon and rectum. Polyposis typically begins in early adolescence with eventual progression to colorectal cancer in virtually all cases if untreated. An attenuated form of FAP exists, which is characterized by a reduced number of polyps, delayed presentation (age 50-70 years), and average lifetime risk of colorectal cancer of 70%.[3]

The lifetime risk of other gastrointestinal cancers is increased in FAP, including cancer of duodenum/ampulla (4%-12%), pancreas (2%), and stomach (1%). Adenomatous lesions of the duodenum and ampulla are a major source of morbidity and mortality in patients after colectomy.[3] FAP is also associated with an increased risk of follicular or papillary thyroid cancer, childhood hepatoblastoma, and medulloblastoma of the CNS.[4]

Extraintestinal manifestations of FAP include dental abnormalities (supernumerary or unerupted teeth), congenital hypertrophy of the retinal pigment epithelium, benign cutaneous cysts or fibromas, osteomas, desmoid tumors, and adrenal adenomas.[5] These disease manifestations are increasingly recognized as major contributors to morbidity in FAP patients.[3]

Diagnosis

A diagnosis of FAP is established primarily through clinical criteria and confirmed by genetic testing. Classic FAP is defined by the presence of more than 100 colorectal adenomatous polyps, while attenuated FAP is characterized by 30 to 100 adenomas in the colon. Genetic testing should be considered in all patients with ≥10 cumulative colorectal adenomas as an *APC* gene mutation may be present but not yet fully expressed. Screening for these mutations is particularly important in patients with a family history of colorectal cancer or extracolonic manifestations of FAP. Testing typically involves sequencing of the *APC* gene as well as testing for other polyposis-related genes (e.g., *MUTYH, POLE, POLD1*). Identification of a pathogenic *APC* variant confirms the diagnosis and enables predictive testing of at-risk relatives. If genetic testing is negative but clinical suspicion remains high, the patient should be managed with a clinical diagnosis of FAP due to an unknown mutation.[5,6]

Endoscopic Surveillance After Colectomy

Endoscopic surveillance in FAP post-colectomy includes serial examination of ileal anastomosis, upper gastrointestinal tract, and deep small bowel (jejunum/ileum). Surveillance guidelines were most recently published by the American Society of Colon and Rectal Surgeons (ASCRS) in 2024 and the American Society for Gastrointestinal Endoscopy (ASGE) in 2020.[3,4] Recommendations for surveillance of the gastrointestinal (GI) tract for adenomas vary based upon anatomic location and disease severity.

Ileoscopy (with proctoscopy or pouchoscopy)

Following subtotal colectomy, patients with an ileorectal anastomosis should undergo proctoscopy with ileoscopy every 6 to 12 months. Patients with an ileal pouch-anal anastomosis or permanent end ileostomy should be examined every 1 to 2 years, including careful examination of the anal transition zone, pouch body, and afferent limb using high-definition endoscopy, often with dye-based (indigo carmine, methylene blue) or virtual chromoendoscopy to highlight subtle adenomas. Endoscopic polypectomy should be performed for all visible adenomas, and the interval may be shortened if there is a high polyp burden or advanced histology.[3,4,7]

Upper GI Endoscopy

Adenocarcinoma of the duodenum/ampulla is the most common cause of cancer death in FAP patients after colectomy. The overall risk of duodenal cancer in patients with FAP is predicted by the extent of duodenal polyposis. The Spigelman classification system incorporates polyp number, size, histology, and degree of dysplasia to assign a Spigelman stage (**Table 1**).[8] The clinical utility of this staging system was demonstrated in a prospective cohort study of 114 FAP patients followed for 10 years. In this population, Spigelman stages II, III, and IV were associated with duodenal cancer rates of 2.3%, 2.4%, and 36%, respectively.[9] A separate prospective study of FAP patients undergoing upper GI surveillance over 15 years demonstrated a reduced risk of duodenal cancer compared to non-surveilled historical controls.[10]

Upper endoscopy is recommended every 5 years for Spigelman stage 0, every 2-3 years for Spigelman Stage I, every 1-2 years for Spigelman Stage II, and every 6-12 months for Spigelman Stage III. Spigelman stage IV patients should be managed by a multidisciplinary team with individualized decision-making regarding endoscopic surveillance versus surgical resection.[3,4] Management of polyps identified by upper endoscopy varies based upon polyp location and size.

Gastric Body. Polyps are found in the gastric body in up to 88% of adults with FAP. The vast majority of these polyps are fundic gland polyps (FGP) (**Figure 1**). These polyps are generally benign but mild dysplasia may be present in up to 40%. FGPs rarely transform into adenocarcinoma. However, adenomas of the gastric body may develop into adenocarcinoma within a background of numerous FGDs (**Figure 2**). Adenomas >1 cm in size are at risk for progression while lesions >3 cm in size may be malignant. Polyps in the gastric body should be removed if greater than 1 cm in size or atypical in appearance.[3,4,11] The optimal strategy for monitoring of gastric polyposis in FAP remains under investigation as the incidence of gastric cancer is rising in Western FAP populations despite active surveillance.[12]

Gastric Antrum. Adenomas can occur anywhere within the stomach but occur more commonly in the antrum. Antral adenomas are usually sessile and poorly circumscribed. All antral polyps encountered during upper endoscopy should be removed due to the likelihood of adenoma in this location.[12]

Duodenum. Most duodenal polyps are adenomatous but the risk of progression to malignancy is low for small (<10 mm) lesions. The extent of duodenal polyposis is useful for predicting risk of duodenal cancer as well as risk of gastric adenocarcinoma and adenomas of the deep small bowel. Current guidelines recommend removal of all duodenal polyps >1 cm in size.[3,4]

Ampulla of Vater. Surveillance of the major ampulla

Criteria	1 point	2 points	3 points
Polyp number	1-4	5-20	>20
Polyp size (mm)	1-4	5-10	>10
Histology	Tubular	Tubulovillous	Villous
Dysplasia	Low grade dysplasia		High grade dysplasia

Spigelman Stage	Total Score
Stage 0	0 points
Stage 1	1-4 points
Stage 2	5-6 points
Stage 3	7-8 points
Stage 4	9-12 points

Table 1. Spigelman Stage (modified). Points are assigned based on the number, size, histology, and dysplasia of duodenal polyps. The sum of points from each of these 4 criteria determines the Spigelman Stage.

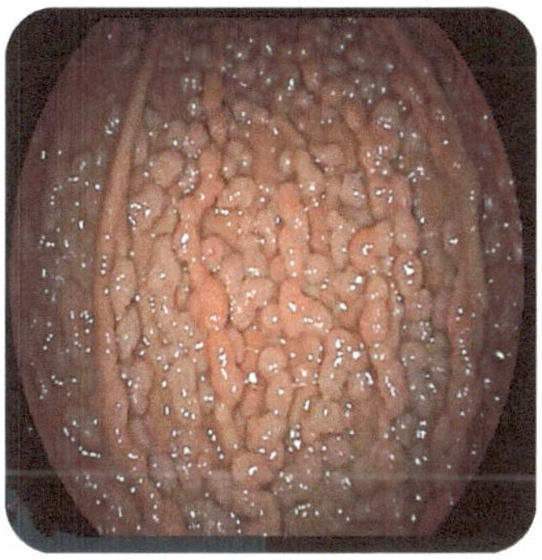

Figure 1. Multiple fundic gland polyps observed in the gastric body.

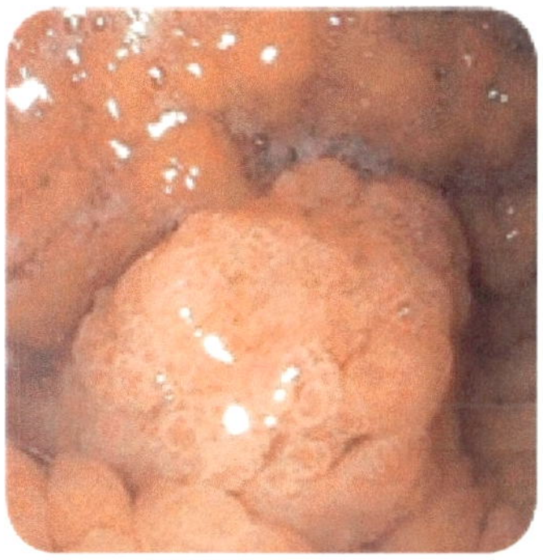

Figure 2. Large adenomatous polyp in a background of FGPs.

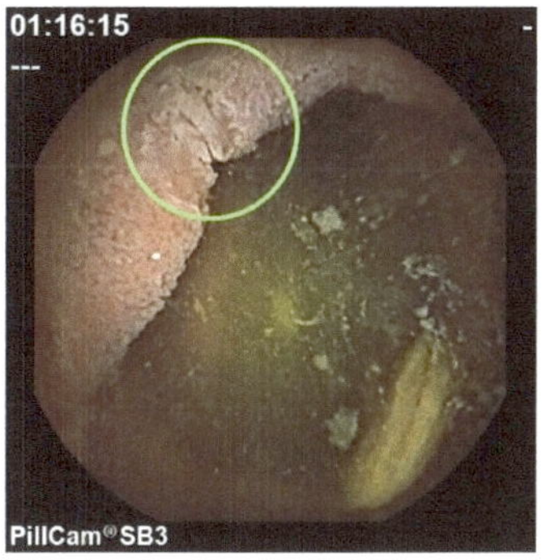

Figure 3. Subtle jejunal adenoma less than 1 cm in size.

should be performed using a side-viewing endoscope (duodenoscope) for close inspection and biopsy of any mucosal irregularities such as ulceration, friability, or firmness. Cap-assisted upper endoscopy is an acceptable alternative if a duodenoscope is unavailable, as it improves visualization by flattening duodenal folds and stabilization of the endoscope. Endoscopic ampullectomy is the treatment of choice for non-invasive ampullary adenomas. However, some research suggests that ampullary adenomas <1 cm in size might be closely observed for evidence of progression prior to ampullectomy. Surgical resection is recommended in cases of confirmed or suspected malignancy or if the lesion is not suitable for endoscopic removal. Endoscopic ultrasound can assist in evaluating the depth of invasion and suitability for endoscopic resection.[13,14,15]

Video Capsule Endoscopy (VCE)

Adenomas of the jejunum and ileum are less common than duodenal adenomas in FAP, with an estimated prevalence ranging from 45% to 75% and 10% to 20%, respectively.[16] Endoscopic evaluation of the jejunum and ileum is recommended for routine surveillance in patients with Spigelman stage III or IV disease, as well as during preoperative assessment of FAP patients prior to duodenectomy. VCE is recommended as the primary modality for surveillance of the jejunum and ileum in FAP while device-assisted enteroscopy (DAE) is often reserved for removal of polyps or evaluation of suspicious lesions observed by VCE. A small bowel surveillance algorithm described by Plum et al indicates VCE every 2 years if small bowel polyps <1 cm are identified vs 4 years if initial VCE is negative for small bowel polyps. DAE is recommended for removal of polyps >1 cm.[17]

Evidence supporting small bowel surveillance in FAP is derived from multiple sources. In a longitudinal study by Günther et al., serial VCE demonstrated progression of small bowel polyposis in FAP patients: 1 individual developed medium-sized adenomas in the proximal jejunum after previously having only small polyps, while another was found to have a large flat adenoma in the upper small intestine that had gone undetected on earlier VCE studies.[18] Reports of polyp growth and malignant transformation detected by VCE have been described in multiple cases. More recently, a pooled analysis of FAP patients undergoing upper single-balloon enteroscopy revealed that 8.8% of 319 patients harbored advanced jejunal lesions—defined as polyps >1 cm or with high-grade dysplasia.[19]

Prospective studies have demonstrated that VCE is more sensitive than magnetic resonance enterography (MRE) for detecting small bowel polyps[20] (**Figure 3**). In one study of patients with FAP and PJS, VCE identified 448 polyps, including numerous lesions <5 mm, whereas MRE detected only 24 polyps, all >5 mm.[21] A separate prospective study in patients with PJS found that VCE detected significantly more polyps ≥10 mm than MRE (47 vs 14, $P = 0.02$).[22] In a prospective, blinded study of FAP patients, Tescher et al. reported that VCE identified significantly more polyps in the jejunum and ileum compared to MRE or small bowel follow-through.[23] These findings are consistent with earlier reports by

Burke, Katsinelos, and Mata, which further highlight the high sensitivity of VCE for detecting small bowel polyps in hereditary polyposis syndromes.[24-26]

Conclusion

Endoscopic surveillance after colectomy in FAP includes serial examination of the ileal anastomosis, stomach, duodenum, and deep small bowel (**Table 2**). Monitoring for duodenal and ampullary lesions is critical to prevent or treat malignant transformation in this segment. Gastric polyps are managed based upon location, size, and endoscopic features . For polyps of the jejunum and ileum, video capsule endoscopy offers the most sensitive and least invasive assessment, with device-assisted enteroscopy reserved for therapeutic removal. Comprehensive evaluation across these sites remains essential to reducing morbidity and mortality in familial adenomatous polyposis.

Endoscopic Examination	Location	Target Lesions	Surveillance Recommendation
Ileoscopy with proctoscopy or pouchoscopy	Ileorectal (IRA)	Adenomas *any size	Ileoscopy with proctoscopy every 6 -12 months
		Adenocarcinoma	
	Ileal pouch-anal anastomosis (IPAA)		Ileoscopy with pouchoscopy every 1-2 years
	End ileostomy		Ileoscopy every 1-2 years
Upper GI Endoscopy *standard view and side-view	Gastric Body	Polyps >1cm *majority are benign (FGP)	Upper endoscopy (EGD) with interval based upon Spigelman Stage • Stage 0 = every 5 years • Stage I = every 2-3 years • Stage II = every 1-2 years • Stage III = every 6-12 months • Stage IV *individual case specific
	Gastric Antrum	All polyps *majority are adenomas	
	Ampulla of Vater	Any abnormal tissue	Inspection of the ampulla requires a side-viewing endoscope (duodenoscope) or cap-assisted gastroscope exam
	Duodenum	Polyps >1cm *majority are adenomas	
Video Capsule Endoscopy (VCE)	Jejunum & ileum	Polyps >1 cm *majority are adenomas	VCE prior to duodenectomy or every 2-4 years for surveillance with Spigelman Stage III or IV

Table 2: Summary of endoscopic surveillance in FAP after colectomy.

References

1. Karstensen JG, Burisch J, Pommergaard HC, et al. colorectal cancer in individuals with familial adenomatous polyposis, based on analysis of the Danish Polyposis Registry. Clin Gastroenterol Hepatol. 2019;17(11):2294-2300.e1.
2. Aelvoet AS, Buttitta F, Ricciardiello L, Dekker E. Management of familial adenomatous polyposis and MUTYH-associated polyposis; new insights. Best Pract Res Clin Gastroenterol. 2022;58-59:101793.
3. Poylin VY, Shaffer VO, Felder SI, et al. The American Society of Colon and Rectal Surgeons Clinical Practice Guidelines for the management of inherited adenomatous polyposis syndromes. Dis Colon Rectum. 2024;67(2):213-227.
4. Yang J, Gurudu SR, Koptiuch C, et al. American Society for Gastrointestinal Endoscopy Guideline on the Role of endoscopy in familial adenomatous polyposis syndromes. Gastrointest Endosc. 2020;91(5):963-982.e2.
5. Hampel H, Bennett RL, Buchanan A, Pearlman R, Wiesner GL; Guideline Development Group, American College of Medical Genetics and Genomics Professional Practice and Guidelines Committee and National Society of Genetic Counselors Practice Guidelines Committee. A practice guideline from the American College of Medical Genetics and Genomics and the National Society of Genetic Counselors: referral indications for cancer predisposition assessment. Genet Med. 2015;17(1):70-87.
6. Short E, Thomas LE, Davies A, et al. APC transcription studies and molecular diagnosis of familial adenomatous polyposis. Eur J Hum Genet. 2020;28(1):118-121.
7. Anele CC, Xiang J, Martin I, et al. Regular endoscopic surveillance and polypectomy is effective in managing rectal adenoma progression following colectomy and ileorectal anastomosis in patients with familial adenomatous polyposis. Colorectal Dis. 2022;24(3):277-283.
8. Spiegelman AD, Williams CB, Talbot IC, et al. Upper gastrointestinal cancer in patients with familial adenomatous polyposis. Lancet 1989, 11:783-785.
9. Groves CJ, Saunders BP, Spigelman AD, Phillips RK. Duodenal cancer in patients with familial adenomatous polyposis (FAP): Results of a 10 year prospective study. Gut. 2002;50:636–641
10. Serrano PE, Grant RC, Berk TC, et al. Progression and manage ment of duodenal neoplasia in familial adenomatous polyposis: A cohort study. Ann Surg. 2015;261:1138–1144.
11. Mankaney GN, Cruise M, Sarvepalli S, et al. Surveillance for pathology associated with cancer on endoscopy (SPACE): Criteria to identify high-risk gastric polyps in familial adenomatous polyposis. Gastrointest Endosc. 2020;92(3):755-762.
12. Wang KK, Kim K, Bancila L, et al. Novel endoscopic polypectomy surveillance technique for fundic gland polyps in familial adenomatous polyposis can improve early detection of dysplasia and gastric cancer. Am J Gastroenterol. 2022;117(8):1246-1254.
13. Chadalavada P, Shah TU. Updates in endoscopic management of ampullary and duodenal adenomas. Curr Opin Gastroenterol. 2023;39(6):496-502.
14. Angsuwatcharakon P, Ahmed O, Lynch PM, et al. Management of ampullary adenomas in familial adenomatous polyposis syndrome: 16 years of experience from a tertiary cancer center. Gastrointest Endosc. 2020;92(2):323-330.
15. Björk J, Akerbrant H, Iselius L, et al. Periampullary adenomas and adenocarcinomas in familial adenomatous polyposis: cumulative risks and APC gene mutations. Gastroenterology. 2001;121(5):1127-35.
16. Fukushi G, Tanaka K, et al. Genotype–phenotype correlation of small intestinal polyps on small bowel capsule endoscopy in familial adenomatous polyposis. Gastrointestinal Endoscopy. 2023; 97 (1):59–68.e7
17. Plum N, May A, Manner H, Ell C. Small-bowel diagnosis in patients with familial adenomatous polyposis: comparison of push enteroscopy, capsule endoscopy, ileoscopy, and enteroclysis. Z Gastroenterol. 2009;47(4):339–346.
18. Gunther U, Bojarski C, Buhr HJ, Zeitz M, Heller F. Capsule endoscopy in small-bowel surveillance of patients with hereditary polyposis syndromes. Int J Colorectal Dis. 2010 (11):1377-1382.
19. Ruys AT, Alderlieste YA, Gouma DJ, Dekker E, Mathus-Vliegen EM. Jejunal cancer in patients with familial adenomatous polyposis. Clin Gastroenterol Hepatol. 2010;8(8):731-3.
20. Alderlieste YA, Rauws EA, Mathus-Vliegen EM,

Fockens P, Dekker E. Prospective enteroscopic evaluation of jejunal polyposis in patients with familial adenomatous polyposis and advanced duodenal polyposis. Fam Cancer. 2013;12(1):51-6.

21. Crook DW, Knuesel PR, Froehlich JM, et al. Comparison of magnetic resonance enterography and video capsule endoscopy in evaluating small bowel disease. Eur J Gastroenterol Hepatol. 2009;21(1):54-65.
22. Caspari R, von Falkenhausen M, Krautmacher C, Schild H, Heller J, Sauerbruch T. Comparison of capsule endoscopy and magnetic resonance imaging for the detection of polyps of the small intestine in patients with familial adenomatous polyposis or with Peutz-Jeghers' syndrome. Endoscopy. 2004;36(12):1054-9.
23. Urquhart P, Grimpen F, Lim GJ, et al. Capsule endoscopy versus magnetic resonance enterography for the detection of small bowel polyps in Peutz-Jeghers syndrome. Fam Cancer. 2014;13(2):249-55.
24. Tescher P, Macrae FA, Speer T, et al. Surveillance of FAP: A prospective blinded comparison of capsule endoscopy and other GI imaging to detect small bowel polyps. Hered Cancer Clin Pract. 2010, 8(1):3.
25. Burke CA, Santisi J, Church J, Levinthal G. The utility of capsule endoscopy small bowel surveillance in patients with polyposis. Am J Gastroenterol. 2005;100(7):1498-1502.
26. Katsinelos P, Kountouras J, Chatzimavroudis G, et al. Wireless capsule endoscopy in detecting small-intestinal polyps in familial adenomatous polyposis. World J Gastroenterol. 2009;15(48):6075-9.
27. Mata A, Llach J, Castells A, et al. A prospective trial comparing wireless capsule endoscopy and barium contrast series for small-bowel surveillance in hereditary GI polyposis syndromes. Gastrointest Endosc. 2005;61(6):721-5.

www.ingramcontent.com/pod-product-compliance
Ingram Content Group UK Ltd.
Pitfield, Milton Keynes, MK11 3LW, UK
UKHW061014121026
15625UKWH00069B/618
* 9 7 9 8 2 1 8 7 4 7 2 9 9 *